Circadian Rhythm Sleep Disorders

Guest Editor

KENNETH P. WRIGHT, Jr., PhD

SLEEP MEDICINE CLINICS

www.sleep.theclinics.com

June 2009 • Volume 4 • Number 2

SAUNDERS an imprint of ELSEVIER, Inc.

W.B. SAUNDERS COMPANY
A Division of Elsevier Inc.

1600 John F. Kennedy Boulevard ● Suite 1800 ● Philadelphia, PA 19103-2899

http://www.sleep.theclinics.com

SLEEP MEDICINE CLINICS Volume 4, Number 2
June 2009, ISSN 1556-407X, ISBN-13: 978-1-4377-0541-6, ISBN-10: 1-4377-0541-3

Editor: Sarah E. Barth
Developmental Editor: Donald Mumford

Sleep Medicine Clinics (ISSN 1556-407X) is published quarterly by Elsevier, 360 Park Avenue South, New York, NY 10010. Months of issue are March, June, September and December. Business and Editorial Office: 1600 John F. Kennedy Blvd., Suite 1800, Philadelphia, PA 19103-2899. Accounting and Circulation Offices: 11830 Westline Industrial Drive, St. Louis, MO 63146. Periodicals postage paid at New York, NY, and additional mailing offices. Subscription prices are $150.00 per year (US individuals), $76.00 (US students), $339.00 (US institutions), $149.00 (Canadian individuals), $106.00 (Canadian students), $373.00 (Canadian institutions), $185.00 (foreign individuals), $106.00 (foreign students), and $373.00 (foreign institutions). Foreign air speed delivery is included in all *Clinics* subscription prices. All prices are subject to change without notice. **POSTMASTER:** Send change of address to *Sleep Medicine Clinics*, Elsevier, Periodicals Customer Service, 11830 Westline Industrial Drive, St. Louis, MO 63146. Customer Service (orders, claims, online, change of address): **Elsevier Periodicals Customer Service, 11830 Westline Industrial Drive, St. Louis, MO 63146. Tel: 1-800-654-2452 (U.S. and Canada); 314-453-7041 (outside U.S. and Canada). Fax: 314-453-5170. E-mail: journalscustomerservice-usa@elsevier.com (for print support); journalsonlinesupport-usa@elsevier.com (for online support).**

Reprints. For copies of 100 or more of articles in this publication, please contact the Commercial Reprints Department, Elsevier Inc., 360 Park Avenue South, New York, NY 10010-1710. Tel.: 212-633-3812; Fax: 212-462-1935; E-mail: reprints@elsevier.com.

Printed and bound by CPI Group (UK) Ltd, Croydon, CR0 4YY

Transferred to Digital Print 2011

GOAL STATEMENT

The goal of *Sleep Clinics of North America* is to keep practicing physicians up to date with current clinical practice by providing timely articles reviewing the state of the art in patient care.

ACCREDITATION

The *Sleep Clinics of North America* is planned and implemented in accordance with the Essential Areas and Policies of the Accreditation Council for Continuing Medical Education (ACCME) through the joint sponsorship of the University of Virginia School of Medicine and Elsevier. The University of Virginia School of Medicine is accredited by the ACCME to provide continuing medical education for physicians.

The University of Virginia School of Medicine designates this educational activity for a maximum of *15 AMA PRA Category 1 Credits*™ for each issue, 60 credits per year. Physicians should only claim credit commensurate with the extent of their participation in the activity.

The American Medical Association has determined that physicians not licensed in the US who participate in this CME activity are eligible for a maximum of *15 AMA PRA Category 1 Credits*™ for each issue, 60 credits per year.

Credit can be earned by reading the text material, taking the CME examination online at http://www.theclinics.com/home/cme, and completing the evaluation. After taking the test, you will be required to review any and all incorrect answers. Following completion of the test and evaluation, your credit will be awarded and you may print your certificate.

FACULTY DISCLOSURE/CONFLICT OF INTEREST

The University of Virginia School of Medicine, as an ACCME accredited provider, endorses and strives to comply with the Accreditation Council for Continuing Medical Education (ACCME) Standards of Commercial Support, Commonwealth of Virginia statutes, University of Virginia policies and procedures, and associated federal and private regulations and guidelines on the need for disclosure and monitoring of proprietary and financial interests that may affect the scientific integrity and balance of content delivered in continuing medical education activities under our auspices.

The University of Virginia School of Medicine requires that all CME activities accredited through this institution be developed independently and be scientifically rigorous, balanced and objective in the presentation/discussion of its content, theories and practices.

All authors/editors participating in an accredited CME activity are expected to disclose to the readers relevant financial relationships with commercial entities occurring within the past 12 months (such as grants or research support, employee, consultant, stock holder, member of speakers bureau, etc.). The University of Virginia School of Medicine will employ appropriate mechanisms to resolve potential conflicts of interest to maintain the standards of fair and balanced education to the reader. Questions about specific strategies can be directed to the Office of Continuing Medical Education, University of Virginia School of Medicine, Charlottesville, Virginia.

The faculty and staff of the University of Virginia Office of Continuing Medical Education have no financial affiliations to disclose.

The authors/editors listed below have identified no professional or financial affiliations for themselves or their spouse/partner: Sabra M Abbott, MD, PhD; Torbjörn Åkerstedt, PhD; Simon N. Archer, PhD; R. Robert Auger, MD; Sarah Barth (Acquisitions Editor); Vivien Bromundt, MSc; Cynthia Brown, MD (Test Author); Tina M. Burke, MS; Allie Buti, BS; Christian Cajochen, PhD; Daniel A. Cohen, MD; Jeanne F. Duffy, MBA, PhD; Charmane I. Eastman, PhD; Jonathan S. Emens, MD; Steven C. Fiala, BA; Martha U. Gillette, PhD; Leon C. Lack, PhD; Aaron D. Laposky, PhD; Amber Lynn Laurie, BA; Alfred J. Lewy, MD, PhD; Mikhail Litinski, MD; Steven W. Lockley, PhD; Frank A.J.L. Scheer, PhD; Steven A. Shea, PhD; Neelam Sims, BS; Jeannie B. Songer, BA; Fred W. Turek, PhD; Michael V. Vitiello, PhD; and Helen R. Wright, PhD.

The authors/editors listed below identified the following professional or financial affiliations for themselves or their spouse/partner:

Richard R. Bootzin, PhD is an industry funded research/investigator for Takeda Pharmaceuticals, NA, and is a consultant for Consolidated Research.

Helen J. Burgess, PhD is a consultant for American College of Physicians.

Charles A. Czeisler, PhD, MD is a consultant for Actelion, Ltd., Cephalon, Inc., Eli Lilly and Co., Garda Siochana Inspectorate, Johnson & Johnson, Koninklijke Philips Electronic, NV., Philips Respironics, Portland Trailblazers, Sanofi Aventis, Sepracor, Inc., Sleep Multimedia, Inc., Somnus Therapeutics, Inc., Vanda Pharmaceuticals, Inc., and Zeo, Inc.; has received grants from Cephalon, Inc., Koninklijke Philips Electronic, NV., Philips Respironics, Sanofi Aventis, Sepracor, Inc., ResMed, Tempur-Pedic, Takeda Pharmaceuticals; serves on the Speakers Bureau for Cephalon, Inc., and Sanofi Aventis; serves on the Advisory Board for Cephalon, Inc., and Sleep Multimedia, Inc.; served as an expert witness for Delta Airlines and Global Ground Support; has equity interest in Somnus Therapeutics, Inc., Vanda Pharmaceuticals, Inc., Zeo, Inc., and Lifetrac, Inc.; receives royalties from McGraw Hill and Penguin press; has received gifts or prizes from Gerald E. McGinnis, Sleep Research Society, Boehringer Ingelheim Pharmaceuticals, Inc., George H. Kidder, Esq., GlaxoSmithKline, Herbert Lee, Hypnion, Jazz Pharmaceuticals, Jordan's Furniture, Merck & Co., Inc., Peter C. Farrell, PhD, Sealy, Inc., Simmons, Sleep Health Center LLC, Spring Aire, Catalyst Group, Farrell Family Foundation, Fisher & Paykel Healthcare Corporation, and Select Comfort Corporation; and his spouse is an independent contractor for New Babies at Newton Wellesley and is employed by Dedham Medical Associates.

Derk-Jan Dijk, PhD is an industry funded research/investigator for GlaxoSmithKline, H Lundbeck A/S, Merck&Co Inc, Philips Lighting, and Organon, and is a consultant for GlaxoSmithKline, H Lundbeck A/S, Merck&Co Inc, Philips Lighting, Actelion, and Sanofi-Aventis.

Teofilo Lee-Chiong, Jr., MD (Consulting Editor) is an independent contractor for NIH, Restore, Respironics, Schwarz Pharma, and Takeda, and is a consultant for Elsevier.

Shantha M.W. Rajaratnam, PhD is an industry funded research/investigator for Philips Lighting, Respironics Sleep and Respiratory Research Foundation, ResMed Foundation, Vanda Pharmaceuticals, and Takeda Pharmaceuticals North America.

Naomi L. Rogers, PhD is an independent contractor for Cephalan Inc., and Vanda Pharmaceuticals, and serves on the Speakers Bureau for CSL Biotherapies.

Makoto Uchiyama, MD, PhD is an industry funded research/investigator for Takeda Pharaceuticals, Astellas, Sanofi-Aventis, Tanabe Mitsubishi, Japan Eli Lilly, Nippon Boehringer-Ingelheim, and Janssen Pharmaceutical, serves on the Advisory Committee for Tanabe Mitsubishi and Eisai, and is a consultant for Takeda Pharmaceuticals, Astellas, and Sanofi-Aventis.

Anna Wirz-Justice, PhD is an industry funded research/investigator for Buhlmann Laboratories and Servier France, and is a consultant for Servier France.

Kenneth P. Wright, Jr., PhD (Guest Editor) serves on the Advisory Committee and holds a patent with Zeo, Inc., and is a consultant and industry funded research/investigator with Takeda Pharmaceuticals and Cephalon, Inc.

Phyllis C. Zee, MD, PhD serves on the Advisory Committee for Takeda Pharmaceutical, Sanofi-Aventis, Respironics/Philips, and Cephalon, is a consultant for Takeda Pharmaceutical and Sanofi-Aventis, and is an industry funded research/investigator for Takeda Pharmaceutical.

Disclosure of Discussion of Non-FDA Approved Uses for Pharmaceutical Products and/or Medical Devices.

The University of Virginia School of Medicine, as an ACCME provider, requires that all faculty presenters identify and disclose any off-label uses for pharmaceutical and medical device products. The University of Virginia School of Medicine recommends that each physician fully review all the available data on new products or procedures prior to clinical use.

TO ENROLL

To enroll in the Sleep Clinics of North America Continuing Medical Education program, call customer service at 1-800-654-2452 or visit us online at www.theclinics.com/home/cme. The CME program is available to subscribers for an additional fee of $99.95.

Sleep Medicine Clinics

THE CLINICS ARE NOW AVAILABLE ONLINE!

Access your subscription at:
www.theclinics.com

Contributors

CONSULTING EDITOR

TEOFILO LEE-CHIONG, Jr., MD
Head, Division of Sleep Medicine, National Jewish
Health; Associate Professor of Medicine,
University of Colorado Denver School of Medicine,
Denver, Colorado

GUEST EDITOR

KENNETH P. WRIGHT, Jr., PhD
Associate Professor, Department of Integrative
Physiology; Director, Sleep and Chronobiology
Laboratory, University of Colorado, Boulder,
Colorado

AUTHORS

SABRA M. ABBOTT, MD, PhD
Department of Molecular and Integrative
Physiology and the College of Medicine, University
of Illinois at Urbana-Champaign, Urbana, Illinois;
Clinical Fellow, Department of Medicine, Harvard
Medical School; Medical Resident, Department
of Internal Medicine, Massachusetts General
Hospital, Boston, Massachusetts

TORBJÖRN ÅKERSTEDT, PhD
Professor, Stress Research Institute, Stokholm
University; Clinical Neuroscience, Karolinska
Institutet, Stockholm, Sweden

SIMON N. ARCHER, PhD
Surrey Sleep Research Centre, Faculty of Health
and Medical Sciences, University of Surrey,
Guildford, United Kingdom

R. ROBERT AUGER, MD
Assistant Professor, Department of Psychiatry
and Psychology, and Department of Medicine,
Mayo Clinic College of Medicine; Consultant,
Mayo Center for Sleep Medicine, Rochester,
Minnesota

RICHARD R. BOOTZIN, PhD
Professor, Department of Psychology, University
of Arizona, Tucson, Arizona

VIVIEN BROMUNDT, MSc
Centre for Chronobiology, Psychiatric University
Clinics, Basel, Switzerland

HELEN J. BURGESS, PhD
Associate Professor, Behavioral Sciences
Department; Associate Director, Biological
Rhythms Research Laboratory, Rush University
Medical Center, Chicago, Illinois

TINA M. BURKE, MS
Department of Integrative Physiology; Sleep and
Chronobiology Laboratory, University of Colorado,
Boulder, Colorado

ALLIE BUTI, BS
Sleep and Mood Disorders Laboratory,
Department of Psychiatry, Oregon Health &
Science University, Portland, Oregon

CHRISTIAN CAJOCHEN, PhD
Professor, Centre for Chronobiology, Psychiatric
Hospital of the University of Basel, Basel,
Switzerland

DANIEL A. COHEN, MD
Instructor in Neurology, Harvard Medical School; Associate Physician, Division of Sleep Medicine, Department of Medicine, Brigham and Women's Hospital; Staff Physician, Department of Neurology, Beth Israel Deaconess Medical Center, Boston, Massachusetts

CHARLES A. CZEISLER, PhD, MD
Baldino Professor of Sleep Medicine and Director, Division of Sleep Medicine, Harvard Medical School; Chief, Division of Sleep Medicine, Department of Medicine, Brigham and Women's Hospital, Boston, Massachusetts

DERK-JAN DIJK, PhD
Surrey Sleep Research Centre, Faculty of Health and Medical Sciences, University of Surrey, Guildford, United Kingdom

JEANNE F. DUFFY, MBA, PhD
Assistant Professor, Division of Sleep Medicine, Brigham and Women's Hospital; Harvard Medical School, Boston, Massachusetts

CHARMANE I. EASTMAN, PhD
Professor, Behavioral Sciences Department; Director, Biological Rhythms Research Laboratory, Rush University Medical Center, Chicago, Illinois

JONATHAN S. EMENS, MD
Assistant Professor of Psychiatry, Sleep and Mood Disorders Laboratory, Department of Psychiatry, Oregon Health & Science University, Portland, Oregon

STEVEN C. FIALA, BA
Sleep and Mood Disorders Laboratory, Department of Psychiatry, Oregon Health & Science University, Portland, Oregon

MARTHA U. GILLETTE, PhD
Alumni Professor, Department of Cell and Developmental Biology, Chemistry and Life Sciences Lab; The Neuroscience Program; Department of Molecular and Integrative Physiology and the College of Medicine, University of Illinois at Urbana-Champaign, Urbana, Illinois

LEON C. LACK, PhD
Professor, School of Psychology, Flinders University, Adelaide, South Australia, Australia

AARON D. LAPOSKY, PhD
Program Director, Sleep and Neurobiology, National Center on Sleep Disorders Research, National Institutes of Health, National Heart, Lung, and Blood Institute/Division of Lung Diseases, Bethesda, Maryland

AMBER L. LAURIE, BA
Sleep and Mood Disorders Laboratory, Department of Psychiatry, Oregon Health & Science University, Portland, Oregon

TEOFILO LEE-CHIONG, Jr., MD
Head, Division of Sleep Medicine, National Jewish Health; Associate Professor of Medicine, University of Colorado Denver School of Medicine, Denver, Colorado

ALFRED J. LEWY, MD, PhD
Philips Professor of Biological Psychiatry, Sleep and Mood Disorders Laboratory, Department of Psychiatry, Oregon Health & Science University, Portland, Oregon

MIKHAIL LITINSKI, MD
Clinical Fellow, Division of Sleep Medicine, Brigham & Women's Hospital, Boston, Massachusetts

STEVEN W. LOCKLEY, PhD
Associate Neuroscientist, Division of Sleep Medicine, Brigham and Women's Hospital; Assistant Professor of Medicine, Harvard Medical School, Boston, Massachusetts

SHANTHA M.W. RAJARATNAM, PhD
Associate Professor, School of Psychology, Psychiatry and Psychological Medicine, Monash University, Clayton, Victoria, Australia; Associate Neuroscientist, Division of Sleep Medicine, Department of Medicine, Brigham and Women's Hospital; Lecturer in Medicine, Division of Sleep Medicine, Harvard Medical School, Boston Massachusetts

NAOMI L. ROGERS, PhD
Associate Professor and Director, Chronobiology and Sleep Group, Brain and Mind Research Institute, University of Sydney, Camperdown, New South Wales, Australia

FRANK AJL SCHEER, PhD
Instructor in Medicine, Harvard Medical School
and Division of Sleep Medicine, Brigham &
Women's Hospital, Boston, Massachusetts

STEVEN A SHEA, PhD
Associate Professor of Medicine, Harvard Medical
School and Division of Sleep Medicine, Brigham &
Women's Hospital, Boston, Massachusetts

NEELAM SIMS, BS
Sleep and Mood Disorders Laboratory,
Department of Psychiatry, Oregon Health &
Science University, Portland, Oregon

JEANNIE B. SONGER, BA
Sleep and Mood Disorders Laboratory,
Department of Psychiatry, Oregon Health &
Science University, Portland, Oregon

FRED W. TUREK, PhD
Charles E. & Emma H. Morrison Professor
of Biology and Director, Northwestern University,
Evanston, Illinois

MAKOTO UCHIYAMA, MD, PhD
Professor and Chair, Department of Psychiatry,
Nihon University School of Medicine, Tokyo, Japan

MICHAEL V. VITIELLO, PhD
Professor, Department of Psychiatry and
Behavioral Sciences, University of Washington
School of Medicine, Seattle, Washington

ANNA WIRZ-JUSTICE, PhD
Professor, Centre for Chronobiology, Psychiatric
Hospital of the University of Basel, Basel,
Switzerland

HELEN R. WRIGHT, PhD
Research Fellow, School of Psychology,
Flinders University, Adelaide, South Australia,
Australia

KENNETH P. WRIGHT, Jr., PhD
Associate Professor, Department of Integrative
Physiology; Director, Sleep and Chronobiology
Laboratory, University of Colorado, Boulder,
Colorado

PHYLLIS C. ZEE, MD, PhD
Professor, Department of Neurology,
Northwestern University Medical School, Chicago,
Illinois

Contents

> This article explains the neurobiology of circadian timekeeping, describing what is known about the master pacemaker for circadian rhythmicity, how various biological systems can provide input to the endogenous biological timing, and how the pacemaker can influence the physiology and behavior of the individual. It discusses how the circadian system can adapt to a changing environment by resetting the circadian clock in the face of various inputs, including changes in light, activity, and the sleep–wake cycle. Finally, the article discusses the genetics of circadian time keeping, highlighting what is known about heritable disorders in circadian timing.

> Sleep physiology and waking performance are regulated through the interaction of an endogenous circadian process and a sleep-wake–dependent homeostatic process. The two processes are not independent: the observed circadian amplitude of waking performance depends on homeostatic sleep pressure, so that the negative effects of sleep loss are most pronounced in the early morning if homeostatic sleep pressure is high. These findings underscore the close interrelations between sleep, circadian rhythmicity, and waking performance and suggest that some circadian phenotypes are related to changes in sleep-regulatory processes. Understanding the effects of these alterations in clock genes, such as *PER3*, at the cellular and biochemical level may provide insights into the nature of the sleep homeostat and its interaction with circadian rhythmicity in the regulation of waking performance.

> The circadian clock has evolved over millions of years to optimize the coordination of the organism with its environment and to maintain internal coordination among multiple physiologic and molecular processes. Tremendous progress has been made in elucidating the molecular mechanisms that underlie circadian function and in detecting cell-autonomous, self-sustaining circadian clocks in tissues/organs throughout the body. The circadian research field is now in a position to move these discoveries into translational-level research and to define how circadian function is an integral component of health and disease processes. This article provides an overview of animal studies that have examined behavioral and molecular links between the circadian clock and various physiologic processes, with a focus on energy metabolism.

patients who have non–24-hour sleep–wake syndrome, discusses the biologic mechanisms that may underlie its development, and describes potential treatment strategies.

Circadian Rhythm Sleep Disorder: Irregular Sleep Wake Rhythm   213

Phyllis C. Zee and Michael V. Vitiello

Irregular sleep–wake rhythm disorder (ISWRD) is characterized by the relative absence of a circadian pattern in an individual's sleep–wake cycle. ISWRD is thought to result from some combination of degeneration or decreased neuronal activity of suprachiasmatic nucleus neurons, decreased responsiveness of the circadian clock to entraining agents such as light and activity, and decreased exposure to bright light and structured social and physical activity during the day. Studies of the effectiveness of pharmacologic treatments for ISWRD generally have yielded negative or inconsistent results. In general multimodal nonpharmacologic approaches involving increased exposure to light, increased physical and social activities, and improved sleep hygiene have been the most successful therapeutic approaches.

Advance-Related Sleep Complaints and Advanced Sleep Phase Disorder   219

R. Robert Auger

Patients with pathologic advance-related sleep complaints live at a circadian phase that is incompatible with their personal and social obligations. Pathophysiologic research is in its early stages, but mutations in various clock genes have been identified among those with familial advanced sleep phase disorder. Various assessment tools, including actigraphic monitoring and morningness-eveningness questionnaires, can complement a thorough clinical history and assist in the attribution of a sleep complaint to a circadian-based entity. Research protocols have demonstrated efficacy with evening phototherapy, which has proven difficult to translate into the clinical arena. Other treatment options include exogenous melatonin, chronotherapy, hypnotics, and, in rare instances, stimulant medications. Proper recommendations regarding avoidance and receipt of light should be provided in all instances.

Delayed Sleep-Phase Disorder   229

Leon C. Lack, Helen R. Wright, and Richard R. Bootzin

Delayed sleep-phase disorder (DSPD) can range from mild to severe and affects not only an individual's sleep but also daytime functioning. A comprehensive assessment is necessary to reliably estimate the degree of circadian-phase delay and thus determine the most effective treatment (morning bright light or chronotherapy). For phase advancing the circadian rhythms and sleep-wake cycle, the recommendation is a schedule of incremental advances of wake-up time and morning bright light as well as low-dose early-evening melatonin administration. It is also important to treat any psychophysiological insomnia with cognitive/behavior therapy. For the more extremely delayed DSPD individual, chronotherapy involving delays of scheduled sleep periods in increments of 2 hours is recommended. Following either type of therapy, maintenance of consistent wake times, exposure to morning light, changes in lifestyle, and improvement of attitudes about morning times are also recommended to help prevent relapse.

This article describes in detail how melatonin, bright light, and sleep schedules can be used in conjunction with currently available flight times to reduce or eliminate jet lag. The goal is to educate circadian rhythm researchers and sleep clinicians about the principles involved so that they can make similar jet travel schedules customized for individuals traveling in any direction across multiple time zones.

Shift work is highly prevalent in industrialized societies. When it includes night work, it has pronounced negative effects on sleep, subjective and physiologic sleepiness, performance, accident risk, and health outcomes such as cardiovascular disease and certain forms of cancer. The reason is the conflict between the day-oriented circadian physiology and the requirement for work and sleep at the "wrong" biologic time of day. Although some countermeasures may be used to ameliorate the negative impact of shift work on nighttime sleepiness and daytime insomnia (combined countermeasures may be the best available), there seems to be no way to eliminate most of the negative effects of shift work on human physiology and cognition.

Strong evidence for an involvement of the circadian clock in psychiatric disorders has emerged. Indeed, some of the major hallmarks of diseases such as major depressive disorder, bipolar disorder, Alzheimer's disease, and schizophrenia are abnormal sleep–wake, appetite, and social rhythms. In addition, many of the successful treatments in psychiatry affect circadian rhythms, and it appears that the phase shifts, resetting and stabilization of rhythms produced by these treatments are important for therapeutic efficacy. Psychiatric disorders account for more than 25% of inpatient hospital beds worldwide, and disturbed sleep–wake cycles in patients are a top-cited reason for the choice of inpatient care. Thus, the relationship between circadian disruption and psychiatric disorders is a topic of great medical relevance.

The phase-shift hypothesis (PSH) states that most patients who have seasonal affective disorder become depressed in the winter because of a delay in circadian rhythms with respect to the sleep/wake cycle. According to the PSH, these patients should respond preferentially to the antidepressant effects of bright light exposure when it is scheduled in the morning to provide a corrective phase advance and restore optimum alignment between the circadian rhythms tightly coupled to the endogenous circadian pacemaker and the rhythms that are related to the sleep/wake cycle. Recent support for the PSH has come from studies in which symptom severity was shown to correlate with the degree of circadian misalignment. This article includes a review of resolved and unresolved issues related to circadian rhythms.

This glossary defines key terms used in basic and applied circadian science. The glossary is designed to enhance knowledge of basic concepts and assist with the translation of circadian principles to improve understanding of the pathophysiology and treatment of circadian sleep disorders. Definitions should be useful as a resource for researchers and clinicians with an interest in circadian research and circadian and sleep medicine. This glossary complements articles included in this issue devoted to circadian rhythm sleep disorders.

Foreword

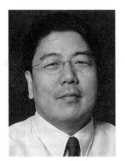

Teofilo Lee-Chiong, Jr., MD
Consulting Editor

Try to imagine a world inhabited by organisms whose biological activities are *not* governed by circadian rhythms. The first thing that comes to mind is, most likely, chaos—wherein physiologic processes, unencumbered by regulatory rhythms and synchronized to neither the environment or each other, either proceed relentlessly at maximal intensity until exhaustion eventually overcomes the organism and kills it or operate at such perpetually low levels that it would be tricky to distinguish living organisms from inanimate objects.

It can be argued that, in such a world, there would be no mammals, reptiles, birds, or amphibians; no trees or grasses; and definitely nothing that can be clearly visible to the unaided eye. Organisms, if they exist at all, might have to be extremely small, perhaps no more than several cells interacting with each other, for it will be nearly impossible to sustain the energy needs of larger, more complex, organisms. Existence will most likely be brief, and the ability to procreate and perpetuate the species limited. On a cellular level, organelles also would be rudimentary and not possess the intricate specialization that characterizes the functions of the mitochondria or Golgi bodies; rather, nutrients will passively enter the cells by osmosis. Locomotion is unlikely, and, thus, organisms will have to live in the ocean or in small crevices or fissures in the narrow strip of land immediately adjacent to bodies of water, lest they succumb to the harsh heat of the day or the frigid cold of the evening that they will be incapable of escaping or surviving. In short, the surface of this world will be barren.

Undoubtedly, rhythmicity in biological processes is fundamental to life or, more specifically, to complex life-forms. There is simply insufficient cellular energy to enable organisms to perform every function at the same constant "steady state," and *all* at the same time. Thus, biological rhythms are ubiquitous and are present in prokaryotic and eukaryotic microbes, plants, insects, and animals, including humans. In earth-bound organisms, different physiologic variables attain peak levels of activity at different points in time throughout a specific period corresponding closely to the 24-hour day dictated by the planet's rotation on its axis; thus, the term "circadian" rhythm was coined from the Latin words "*circa*," which means "about," and "*diem*," referring to "day". Some biological rhythms peak during the day, whereas others have their highest levels of activity at night. Still, other rhythms are influenced by both circadian rhythms and sleep-wake patterns; the latter, by the way, is also controlled by the circadian neurosystem.

It is propitious that circadian rhythms—although not always having frequencies of exactly 24 hours but rather ranging from slightly under or, more frequently, over 24 hours—are commonly about 24.2 hours, referred to as "*tau*," as it is this close concordance with the environmental day that bestows a survival benefit to the organism. Neither a markedly ultradian (one oscillation lasting less than 24 hours) nor an exceedingly infradian (one oscillation lasting greater than 24 hours) rhythm confers a similar advantage. Indeed, any deviation from the external 24-hour world is rapidly restored into synchrony each day by zeitgebers (from the German word "time-giver") through the process of entrainment.

Circadian rhythms are, for the most part, genetically determined. Oscillations in biochemical and physiological variables have distinct

Sleep Med Clin 4 (2009) xv–xvi
doi:10.1016/j.jsmc.2009.03.003

frequencies, period lengths, amplitudes, peak, trough, and phases that are autoregulated by transcription–translation-positive and -negative feedback loops involving clock genes and other regulatory factors. There is a high degree of similarity in the circadian rhythm-related genes found in the fruit fly, *Drosophila melanogaster*, and in mammals, such as mice. If phylogeny is indeed but a snapshot of evolution, one has to assume that similar genes exist in ancient, and now extinct, organisms.

It has been estimated that life started on earth three-and-a-half billion years ago. It was very much later, about 220 million years ago, that dinosaurs began to appear. Humans were latecomers, only having evolved from ape-like species a quarter of a million years ago. Therefore, when life began, the earth day was much shorter than our current 24 hours. Were circadian rhythms correspondingly shorter as well? And if circadian rhythmicity is genetically determined by the transcription–translation and natural decay of circadian-related proteins, were there different circadian genes and proteins then? Is extinction the inevitable outcome of organisms whose circadian rhythms deviated so much from the slowly lengthening global day that entrainment became impossible?

It is, therefore, probable that circadian rhythms are not merely fundamental to life but that they directly dictate what form life takes across the eons of time and expanse of space.

Teofilo Lee-Chiong, Jr., MD
Division of Sleep Medicine
National Jewish Health
University of Colorado Denver School of Medicine
1400 Jackson Street
Room J221
Denver, CO 60206, USA

E-mail address:
Lee-ChiongT@NJC.ORG (T. Lee-Chiong)

Preface

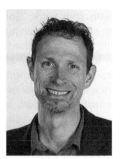

Kenneth P. Wright, Jr., PhD
Guest Editor

This issue of *Sleep Medicine Clinics* provides state-of-the-art reviews by physiologists, geneticists, molecular biologists, neuroscientists, psychologists, psychiatrists, and physicians on the basics of circadian physiology and circadian rhythm sleep disorders (CRSDs). Circadian biology is a rapidly changing field at the cutting edge of the molecular regulation of complex behaviors and disorders. Circadian clock genes are present in many tissues throughout the body, and disruption of these clock genes may be involved in impaired physiological function. Circadian rhythm sleep disorders (CRDSs) are a specialized class of sleep disorders associated with disruption of internal circadian physiology and/or a misalignment between internal biological time and environmental time. There are six CRSDs currently recognized in the International Classification of Sleep Disorders (ICSD-2): non-24-hour disorder (free-running type); irregular sleep–wake phase disorder (irregular sleep–wake type); advanced sleep phase disorder (advanced sleep phase type); delayed sleep phase disorder (delayed sleep phase type); jet lag (jet lag type); and shift–work disorder (shift–work type). The ICSD-2 also recognizes CRSDs secondary to medical conditions and drug or substance abuse, as well as a general category: CRSD Not Otherwise Specified (NOS).

The authors have made this issue a success. It was a great pleasure to work with my colleagues involved in writing articles for this issue. They are among the most influential and widely respected researchers and clinicians in their respective fields. I am grateful for the time and effort they devoted to the reviews in this issue. The articles provide synthesis and well balanced views on the state of the art in circadian biology and treatment of CRSDs.

The internal circadian timekeeping system evolved to regulate and modulate physiological and behavioral processes across the 24-hour solar day–night cycle so that a multitude of the organism's physiological and behavioral processes occur at an appropriate environmental time. Drs. Gillette and Abbott review the neurophysiology of the circadian timekeeping system in mammals, including inputs to the master internal circadian clock located in the suprachiasmatic nuclei (SCN) of the hypothalamus and the outputs from the SCN that influence physiology and behavior. Drs. Dijk and Archer provide an overview of how sleep and circadian systems interact to influence human physiology and behavior and discuss cutting-edge research on the role of circadian clock genes in sleep physiology and cognitive function during sleep deprivation. Drs. Laposky and Turek cover recent advances in circadian biology using animal models, providing evidence that misalignment and disruption of circadian rhythms lead to adverse health consequences. The articles by Drs. Gillette and Abbott; Dijk and Archer; and Laposky and Turek provide the fundamentals of circadian rhythms to improve understanding of mechanisms underlying CRSDs.

The influence of internal circadian phase on disease severity and the consequences of circadian misalignment on cardiovascular disease, asthma, cancer, epilepsy, diabetes, and obesity are reviewed by Dr. Litinski and colleagues. Dr. Litinski and coauthors also discuss chronotherapy, which is the application of circadian principles to time treatment according to internal biological time to maximize the effectiveness of

Sleep Med Clin 4 (2009) xvii–xviii
doi:10.1016/j.jsmc.2009.03.004

treatment outcomes and/or minimize side effects. Drs. Duffy and Czeisler provide an update on how environmental light exposure influences the human circadian timing system, highlighting the importance of biological timing, duration, intensity, wavelength, and prior history of light exposure for resetting the timing of the internal circadian clock. Dr. Rajaratnam and colleagues discuss the role of the endogenous melatonin rhythm in human physiology, as well as the use of exogenous melatonin and melatonin analogs to influence circadian physiology. The articles by Drs. Duffy and Czeisler and Rajaratnam and coauthors provide circadian principles upon which current treatments of CRSDs are based. The remaining reviews provide insight into the pathophysiology and treatment of CRSDs. Drs. Uchiyama and Lockley provide a perspective on non-24-hour disorder in sighted and blind individuals, which results in chronic circadian misalignment akin to non-affected healthy humans experiencing chronic jet lag. As the number of older adults continues to increase, so does the prevalence of neurological disorders associated with CRSDs. Drs. Zee and Vitiello review what is known about irregular sleep–wake rhythm disorder, a condition that results in sleep and wakefulness episodes that occur across the 24-hour day and lead not only to sleep and wakefulness impairments in the individuals inflicted but also their caregivers. Dr. Auger provides a synthesis of advance sleep phase disorder, which is most common in older adults and results in bed and wake times earlier than desired; whereas Dr. Lack and coauthors provide insight into delayed sleep phase disorder, which is most common in adolescence and young adults and often results in bed and wake times later than desired. Delayed sleep phase can also result in shortened sleep duration and lead to impaired school and work performance. Drs. Eastman and Burgess discuss the negative impact of jet lag, which afflicts millions of jet-setters worldwide, and ways to make jet travel easier. Drs. Akerstedt and Wright review the consequences of schedule-induced sleepiness and insomnia associated with shift work. Some individuals appear to have clinically meaningful impairments associated with their work schedule that require intervention to improve safety and, perhaps, health. Drs. Wirz-Justice, Bromundt, and Cajochen review evidence for the influence of circadian disruption in psychiatric disorders and suggest that stabilizing biological timing and sleep may improve treatment outcomes. Lastly, Dr. Lewy and colleagues provide a historical perspective of winter depression and discuss a model for understanding the pathophysiology and treatment of this cyclic psychiatric disorder that negatively impacts individuals especially at latitudes far from the equator.

Recognition of CRSDs and their treatment options is required for reducing the negative impact of circadian disruption and circadian misalignment common in modern society. Available treatments for CRSDs are based primarily on principles learned from laboratory-based circadian science. The challenge for circadian science and medicine is to translate these basic circadian principles into more effective treatments, not only for CRSDs but also for other conditions where circadian disruption contributes to disease processes and symptoms. Future implementation of circadian medicine requires large-scale clinical trials and the implementation of circadian assessment tools to improve the understanding of disease processes and the most effective treatments.

Kenneth P. Wright, Jr., PhD
Department of Integrative Physiology
Sleep and Chronobiology Laboratory
University of Colorado at Boulder
1725 Pleasant Street, Clare Small 114
Boulder, CO 80309, USA

Biological Timekeeping

Martha U. Gillette, PhD[a,b,c,*], Sabra M. Abbott, MD, PhD[c,d,e]

KEYWORDS

- Biological rhythms • Sleep • Circadian
- Suprachiasmatic nucleus • Acetylcholine
- Advanced Sleep Phase Syndrome • Glutamate • Melatonin

The daily transition from light to darkness has shaped the evolution of most living species, from unicellular organisms to mammals. Adaptation to this environmental constraint occurred through the emergence of a circadian system capable of adjusting behavioral and physiological processes to this light-dark cycle. Superimposed upon the daily light–dark cycle is a seasonal influence that modifies the relative durations of day and night over the course of a year. Be they day-active or night-active, all organisms need a means of keeping time in a 24-hour world in order to adapt to the availability of food, and to avoid predators. In addition, they require a means of adjusting to changes in day length or transition times that may occur.

Interestingly, rather than simply reflecting the external day–night cycle, these rhythms in behaviors persist in the absence of exogenous timing cues such as light, food availability, or social cues. Every organism expresses an endogenous rhythm that varies slightly from 24 hours, making it circadian, or about a day. Uninterrupted, this circadian rhythm persists.

These circadian rhythms can be observed in outputs such as the patterning of the sleep–wake cycle, and in people, core body temperature often is used as a marker of circadian phase. In addition, numerous endogenous hormones can be used as markers.[1] Although hormonal rhythms exhibit complex waveforms because of combined effects of the circadian pacemaker; organismic state, such as activity level, sleep and feeding; and the pulsatile nature of secretion, clear diurnal patterns of secretion have been reported.[2] Plasma melatonin,[3,4] growth hormone,[5] prolactin,[6] thyrotropin-releasing hormone,[7] luteinizing hormone,[8] and leptin[9,10,11] are elevated during the night, in antiphase to adrenocorticotropic hormone and cortisol.[12,13] These oscillations in hormone secretion continue in a constant environment, and therefore, are clock-regulated. Circadian rhythmicity appears to be present at virtually every level of functioning studied. In fact, maintenance of a constant milieu interior may be a consequence of a balance among rhythmic, mutually opposed control mechanisms.[2]

This article explains the neurobiology of circadian timekeeping, describing what is known about the master pacemaker for circadian rhythmicity, how various biological systems can provide input to the endogenous biological timing, and how the pacemaker can in influence the physiology and behavior of the individual. It discusses how the circadian system can adapt to a changing environment by resetting the circadian clock in the face of various inputs, including changes in light, activity, and the sleep–wake cycle. Finally, the article

This work was supported by the following past and present grants from the National Institutes of Health: HL08670, HL67007, NS22155, and NS35859 (MUG), and F30 NS047802, and GM07143 (SMA).

a Department of Cell and Developmental Biology, Chemistry and Life Sciences Laboratory, University of Illinois at Urbana-Champaign, 601 South Goodwin Avenue, Urbana, IL 61801, USA
b The Neuroscience Program, University of Illinois at Urbana-Champaign, Urbana, IL 61801, USA
c Department of Molecular and Integrative Physiology and the College of Medicine, University of Illinois at Urbana-Champaign, Urbana, IL 61801, USA
d Department of Medicine, Harvard Medical School, Boston, MA 02115, USA
e Department of Internal Medicine, Massachusetts General Hospital, 55 Fruit Street, Boston, MA 02114, USA
* Corresponding author. Department of Cell and Developmental Biology, Chemistry and Life Sciences Laboratory, University of Illinois at Urbana-Champaign, 601 South Goodwin Avenue, Urbana, IL 61801.
E-mail address: mgillett@life.illinois.edu (M.U. Gillette).

discusses the genetics of circadian time keeping, highlighting what is known about heritable disorders in circadian timing.

THE CIRCADIAN CLOCK

In mammals, circadian rhythms are regulated by a paired set of nuclei located at the base of the hypothalamus, directly above the optic chiasm, hence their name, the suprachiasmatic nuclei (SCN) (**Fig. 1**). Multiple experiments have demonstrated the role of the SCN as a central pacemaker for circadian rhythms. Lesioning studies found that damage to the SCN disrupts rhythmicity in corticosterone levels, drinking, and wheel-running behavior.[14,15] This provided the initial evidence that the central pacemaker for the mammalian clock lay within the SCN.

In later work, it was found that transplanting fetal SCN tissue into the third ventricle of animals in which the SCN had been lesioned could restore rhythmicity.[16] Furthermore, if fetal SCN tissue from a wild-type hamster was implanted into a hamster with a genetic alteration that shortened the free-running period, the new free-running period resembled that of the SCN donor rather than the host animal. This evidence suggested that not only was the SCN necessary for

generating rhythms, but also that this rhythmicity was an intrinsic property of the SCN cells, which could drive the rhythms for the entire animal.[17]

In the mouse, each SCN measures approximately 300 μm medial to lateral, 350 μm dorsal to ventral, and spans approximately 600 μm from rostral to caudal end. One SCN contains approximately 10,500 cells.[18] Based on peptide localization, it is common to divide the rodent SCN into a ventrolateral or core region, and a dorsomedial or shell region (see **Fig. 1**). The core neurons are small and contain vasoactive intestinal peptide (VIP), calretinin (CALR), and gastrin-releasing peptide (GRP) colocalized with γ-amino butyric acid (GABA), while the shell neurons are larger and contain arginine vasopressin (AVP), met-enkephalin (mENK), and angiotensin II (AII).[18] There are topographic connections between the contralateral shells and the contralateral cores, and a unidirectional connection between the core and shell within each nucleus.[19]

The human SCN is not as compact as the rodent but contains many of the same subdivisions. The dorsal and medial regions contain neurophysin/vasopressin neurons. The core region contains calbindin, synaptophysin, and VIP neurons, while the ventral and rostral regions contains synaptophysin, calbindin, and substance P.[20]

Inputs

In conjunction with its ability to regulate circadian timing, the SCN also is positioned to receive information about the behavioral and environmental state of the animal in order to ensure proper setting of the circadian clock. This information is conveyed to the SCN by projections from various different brain regions.

One of the most extensively studied inputs to the SCN comes from a subpopulation of retinal ganglion cells whose central projections form the retinohypothalamic tract (RHT). Lesions of the SCN disrupt the development of these neurons,[21] and disruption of the RHT results in an inability to respond to resetting light signals.[22,23] Recent work has found that many of the retinal ganglion cells that comprise the RHT contain a photopigment, melanopsin.[24] These melanopsin-containing cells are photosensitive at the same wavelengths that are most effective for circadian resetting.[25] Additionally, the terminals of the melanopsin-positive retinal ganglion cells collocalize glutamate (GLU) and pituitary adenylate cyclase-activating polypeptide (PACAP),[26] the putative neurotransmitters of the RHT.

The RHT also sends projections to the thalamic intergeniculate leaflet (IGL), which in turn sends

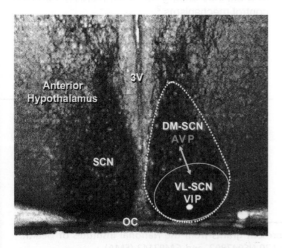

Fig. 1. Anatomy of the mammalian suprachiasmatic nucleus (SCN). This medial, transverse section of the rat anterior hypothalamus shows the bilateral SCN stained darkly with an antibody to an endogenous peptide. The paired SCNs are at the base of the brain, flanking the third ventricle (V3) and positioned directly above the optic chaism (OC). The two major subdivisions of the SCN are delineated. The dorsomedial SCN (DM-SCN) is marked by neurons expressing arginine vasopressin (AVP), whereas neurons of the ventrolateral SCN (VL-SCN) express vasoactive intestinal peptide (VIP).

projections back to the SCN through the geniculo-hypothalamic tract (GHT). The GHT contains neuropeptide Y (NPY) and GABA. NPY is believed to be involved in activity-induced phase shifts during the daytime in nocturnal animals, but also appears to be able to modulate light-induced phase shifts.[27,28] However, while the GHT pathway can transmit photic signals, disruption of this pathway does not prevent entrainment.[29]

The SCN also receives serotonergic input, primarily from the median raphe, that primarily is involved in activity-induced phase shifts during the daytime. Activation of the median raphe results in an increase in serotonin (5-HT) release at the SCN.[30,31,32] 5-HT release also shows a strong circadian release pattern in the SCN, with 5-HT release peaking at CT 14, and 5-hydroxyindole acetic acid (5-HIAA), the major metabolite of 5-HT, peaking at CT 16.[33] SCN sensitivity is similar to NPY. 5-HT causes daytime phase shifts in nocturnal animals and modulates the response to light signals at night.[34,35]

Cholinergic projections to the SCN originate in the brainstem and basal forebrain in brain nuclei, with identified roles in sleep and arousal,[36] and they recently were demonstrated to also be present in diurnal animals.[37] Within the brainstem, these cholinergic projections arise from three nuclei. The parabigeminal nucleus (PBg) is considered a satellite region of the superior colliculus, which appears to play a role in generating target location information as part of saccadic eye movements,[38] while the laterodorsal tegmental (LDTg) and pedunculopontine tegmental (PPTg) nuclei are important for regulating the sleep–wake cycle.[39] In the basal forebrain, the substantia innominata (SI) within the nucleus basalis magnocellularis (NBM) in the basal forebrain contributes to arousal and focused attention.[40] The LDTg, PPTg, and NBM are interconnected, and all play roles in regulating the sleep and arousal states of the animal. This would suggest that the cholinergic input to the SCN is providing a signal regarding the sleep and arousal states of the animal, and may provide a link between the sleep–wake cycle and circadian rhythms.

Additional sleep–wake input to the SCN may come from tuberomammillary nucleus (TMN). Studies have shown histaminergic input to the SCN from the TMN.[41] Histamine is a regulator of the sleep–wake cycle, primarily providing a signal of wakefulness.

Outputs

The SCN exerts its influence on the rest of the body primarily by sending projections to the rest

of the hypothalamus. Neurons from the core region project to the lateral region of the subparaventricular zone (sPVHz), the peri-suprachiasmatic area (PSCN), and the ventral tuberal area (VTU), all within the hypothalamus. The shell projects to medial preoptic area (MPOA), medial sPVHz, dorsal parvocellular paraventricular nucleus (dPVN), and the dorsal medial hypothalamus (DMH), also all within the hypothalamus.[42] The targets of efferents to the dPVN consist of either endocrine neurons, autonomic neurons, or intermediate neurons that potentially serve to integrate numerous hypothalamic signals.[43] The DMH projections are particularly interesting, as many of these neurons appear to be projecting to neurons containing hypocretin/orexin, a peptide known for its role in arousal.[44,45] In addition, evidence exists for a multisynaptic pathway between the SCN and locus coeruleus (LC), an important arousal center in the brain, mediated by orexin,[46] with the DMH as a relay.[47] The SCN also contains a minor set of efferents to the ventrolateral preoptic nucleus (VLPO), a region that if lesioned produces prolonged reduction in sleep duration and amplitude.[48] In addition, the SCN contains projections to the paraventricular nucleus (PVT) and intergeniculate leaflet (IGL) of the thalamus. Both nuclei project back to the SCN. The PVT loop is proposed to provide assessment of sleep/arousal states and SCN modulation, whereas the IGL loop is thought to provide the SCN with information from higher, integratative visual centers.[49,50,51] The PVN appears to act as a relay between the SCN and the amygdala, which may provide a link between the circadian system and affective disorders.[52] Overall, the SCN appears to be situated uniquely within a network that allows it to interact closely with the regions controlling sleep and arousal states.

One of the major output roles of the SCN appears to be to provide an inhibitory signal for activity. Two recently discovered candidate factors for communicating such signals include transforming growth factor-α (TGF-α) and prokineticin 2 (PK2). Under normal conditions, TGF-α peptide is expressed rhythmically in the SCN with a peak during the animal's inactive period, and a trough during the active period. When infused continuously into the ventricles, TGF-α inhibits locomotor activity. Conversely, mice lacking the epidermal growth factor (EGF) receptor, making them unable to respond to TGF-α, show an excessive amount of daytime activity.[53] PK2 also is expressed rhythmically in the SCN, again showing peak expression during the animal's inactive period, and it can inhibit locomotor activity when infused continuously.[54] This suggests a role for the output signal of the SCN in promoting an inactive state that would be permissive for sleep.

CIRCADIAN RESETTING

Within such a complex neuronal clock structure, there is a consensus that timekeeping is a cellular process. Indeed, the expression of independently phased circadian firing rhythms from individual neurons dissociated from neonatal rat SCN cultured on an electrode array provides compelling evidence for the cellular nature of this clock.[55] It follows that gating of sensitivity to resetting stimuli and phase resetting must be cellular properties. Moreover, the clock must be able to restrict the range of responses in the cellular repertoire so that activation of select signaling pathways can occur only at the appropriate time in the circadian cycle. The authors have endeavored to determine how the clock temporally regulates the responsiveness of specific signaling pathways.

In an attempt to define and understand the underlying control mechanisms subserving clock-gated windows of sensitivity, the authors exposed the SCN-bearing brain slices in vitro to treatments that activate elements of specific signaling pathways. Treatments were administered at various discrete points in the circadian cycle, and the time of the peak in the spontaneous rhythm of neuronal activity was assessed over the next one or two circadian cycles in vitro. If the time of peak appeared earlier during cycle(s) after treatment compared with controls, the phase of the rhythm had been advanced. If the time of peak appeared later than in controls, then the phase had been delayed by the treatment. By assessing the changing relationship between the circadian time of treatment and its effect on phase, a phase–response curve (PRC) was generated. This relationship graphically presents the temporal pattern of SCN sensitivity to activation of specific signaling pathways and, in fact, defines the window of sensitivity to phase resetting by means of this pathway. The permanence of the phase shift was examined by evaluating the time of the peak in neuronal activity over 1 or 2 days after a treatment. Timing of the peak after experimental reagents had been administered at the maximal point of sensitivity was compared with the time of the peak in media-treated controls.

Temporal spheres identified as sensitive to phase resetting by means of specific first and second messenger pathways coincide with discrete portions of the circadian cycle. In terms of these temporal restrictions, the circadian cycle can be divided into several discrete temporal

states, or domains, of the clock: day, night, dusk, and dawn.[56] The authors' studies not only contribute to defining the properties of the clock's temporal domains, they emphasize the complexity of control that the clock exerts over signal integration and phase resetting within the SCN. These properties have been incorporated into putative clock-gated regulatory pathways. Each will be discussed in the context of the clock domain that is regulated.

Subjective day and night are distinct with respect to their sensitivities and response characteristics. Furthermore, each correlates with discrete periods of sensitivity to specific neurotransmitter systems that are demonstrated to impinge upon this hypothalamic site as evidenced by a large body of neuroanatomical studies.[57] This permits speculation regarding the nature of pathways that gain access to and regulate the biological clock at different points in the circadian cycle. This article now considers, in turn, the major identified domains of clock sensitivity.

Circadian Clock Regulators

Daytime
Several signaling molecules appear to be important in resetting circadian rhythms during the daytime, including 5-HT, PACAP, NPY, and GABA (**Fig. 2**). Most of these experiments have been performed in nocturnal rodents, so daytime is defined as the time in which the lights are on, or the animal is inactive. As a result, the functional context of this regulation seems to be tied to

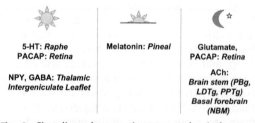

| 5-HT: *Raphe*
PACAP: *Retina*

NPY, GABA: *Thalamic*
Intergeniculate Leaflet | Melatonin: *Pineal* | Glutamate,
PACAP: *Retina*

ACh:
Brain stem (*PBg,*
LDTg, PPTg)
Basal forebrain
(*NBM*) |

Fig. 2. Circadian changes in temporal windows of suprachiasmatic nucleus (SCN) sensitivity to phase-resetting signals transmitted from various brain sites. Time of day-specific signals are presented together with the major sources of SCN innervation by projections bearing these neurotransmitters and neuropeptides. Daytime is marked by sensitivity to serotonin (5-HT), pituitary adenylate cyclase-activating peptide (PACAP), neuropeptide Y (NYP), and γ-aminobutyric acid (GABA). During dusk and dawn, the pineal hormone melatonin can stimulate resetting of the SCN clock. At night, the SCN is sensitive to phase adjustment by glutamate and PACAP from the eye, and by cholinergic inputs from brain regions that regulate sleep and wakefulness.

arousal-induced resetting, often referred to as nonphotic resetting. Nonphotic signals cover various phenomenon, including sleep deprivation, activity associated with exposure to a novel wheel, or even cage changes. The unifying factor in non-photic signals is that they involve arousal during a time when the animal normally would be inactive.

Although 5-HT is believed to play a role in activity-induced or nonphotic phase shifts during the day, there is some question about whether this form of phase shifting is due entirely to 5-HT. If serotonergic agonists are applied to the hypo-thalamic brain slice during the daytime, the peak in electrical firing activity advances, but no change in peak firing rate is seen if the agonists are applied during the night.[34] Similar results are seen in vivo if the dorsal or medial raphe is stimulated,[32] a para-digm that has been shown by microdialysis to increase 5-HT release at the level of the SCN.[58] During forced wheel running or sleep deprivation during the daytime, there is also an increase in 5-HT release at the SCN.[59,60] This suggests a possible link between 5-HT and nonphotic phase shifting, but evidence also exists to complicate this assertion. If 85% to 95% of the serotonin is depleted from the raphe projections to the SCN, animals still are capable of phase shifting in response to daytime forced activity.[61] In addition, these activity-induced phase shifts are not attenu-ated significantly following injection of seroto-nergic antagonists.[62] These data suggest that although 5-HT may play a role in nonphotic reset-ting, the full resetting response depends on addi-tional modulatory neurotransmitters, possibly neuropeptides.

PACAP appears to play a dual role in the SCN, producing effects both during the daytime by itself and at night by acting in conjunction with GLU. PACAP is not intrinsic to the SCN; it is released from the RHT, where it is colocalized with GLU.[63] Examining levels of PACAP in tissue samples collected throughout the 24-hour cycle revealed that PACAP exhibits a significant oscillation in the SCN, but not in other brain regions, and it is lower during the light period than the dark period.[64] If PACAP is applied to the brain slice at different times of day, micromolar quantities will cause an advance in neuronal firing activity during the daytime, but have relatively little effect during the night.[26] The in vivo response, however, is more complicated. When PACAP is injected into the SCN of the hamster between CT 4-8, transient phase advances in wheel-running activity are seen during the first day after treatment, paralleling the results seen with the brain slice, but the long-term effects of a PACAP injection appear to produce a delay in wheel-running activity.[65] This

suggests that although PACAP has an effect on circadian rhythms during the daytime, further work is needed to determine the precise nature of this signal.

NPY also appears to play a dual role in the SCN, resetting the circadian clock both during the daytime and at night. NPY is released from the GHT, the projection from the IGL to the SCN. Studies have examined the effects of either inject-ing NPY into the SCN region of the intact animal and monitoring wheel-running behavior[66,67] or applying NPY directly to the hypothalamic brain slice and examining the peak in neuronal firing activity.[27] In both cases, it was found that when NPY was applied during the daytime, it induced a phase advance. Additional in vivo studies stimu-lated the IGL, presumably inducing the release of NPY at the SCN. These stimulations also produced advances in wheel-running behavior during the daytime.[68] Interestingly, it has been found that exposing an animal to light[69] or applying GLU to the brain slice[70] were both capable of blocking the response to daytime appli-cation of NPY. The addition of the GABA$_A$ antago-nist, bicuculline, is also capable of inhibiting the effects of NPY,[71] suggesting that the effects of NPY are linked to GABAergic signaling.

One factor that daytime signaling pathways hold in common is that they all appear to be mediated by cyclic adenosine monophosphate (cAMP). In the hypothalamic brain slice, cAMP or a cAMP analog applied during the daytime induces phase advances in the circadian clock, while at night they have little effect.[72,73] In addition, endogenous cAMP is high during late day, and late night,[74] sug-gesting a role for cAMP in the transition periods between day and night. It can be hypothesized that by increasing cAMP, these daytime resetting signals are moving the animal to a state that resembles late day, thus resetting the clock.

Dawn and dusk
The primary resetting signal associated with dawn and dusk is melatonin (see **Fig. 2**). This hormone of darkness is produced at night in the absence of light, providing a means by which the animal can measure night length. Photoperiod is an important measure for animals, such as the hamster, which are seasonally reproductive. Mela-tonin is produced by the pineal gland, and in many vertebrates, the pineal is actually the primary regu-lator of circadian rhythms, rather than the SCN. In mammals, however, this timekeeping mechanism has moved to the SCN, as demonstrated by the fact that removal of the pineal does not disrupt circadian rhythms of rats significantly.[75]

Although the pineal is not necessary for maintenance of mammalian circadian rhythms, it is possible to entrain free-running rats with daily injections of melatonin. Entrainment appears to work best if the melatonin injections are timed to occur shortly before the onset of the animal's active period. This entrainment appears to be working through the SCN, as lesioning the SCN, but not the pineal, abolishes the ability of a rat to entrain to melatonin injections.[76]

Evidence that melatonin can entrain circadian rhythms led to several studies looking at the direct effect of melatonin on the SCN. Using either 2-deoxy-[1-^{14}C]glucose (2-DG) or neuronal activity as a marker of SCN activity, melatonin decreases 2-DG uptake and neuronal firing activity in the rat or hamster most significantly when applied right before dusk.[77,78,79] By examining electrophysiological activity in vitro in the SCN, melatonin applied at either dawn or dusk advances the peak in neuronal firing, but produces no effects when applied at other times of day.[80,81] This resetting pattern mimics that seen in response to activation of protein kinase C (PKC), and was blocked by inhibitors of PKC, suggesting that PKC is a downstream component of this resetting pathway.[81] In addition, this resetting could be inhibited with antagonists specific for the MT-2 type melatonin receptor.[82] In people, circadian sensitivity to melatonin also occurs at dawn and dusk, but the effect is to advance the circadian system at dusk but to delay it at dawn.

Nighttime

In the nighttime domain there are two known key players, GLU and acetylcholine (ACh), and several modulatory substances associated with these signals (see **Fig. 2**). As was discussed previously, considerable evidence supports GLU as the neurochemical signal transmitting photic stimuli from the retina to the SCN, but the functional context of the cholinergic resetting signal remains unknown.

The GLU signaling pathway is similar to many of the pathways that have been discussed in that it resets the circadian clock at a discrete time of day and in a specific direction. The GLU signaling pathway can advance or delay the clock, depending on what time of day the signal is presented.[83,84] The GLU resetting pathway has been demonstrated in vitro and in vivo to be mediated through an N-methyl-D-aspartate (NMDA) receptor-mediated rise in intracellular calcium, followed by nitric oxide synthase (NOS) induction and resultant production of nitric oxide (NO).[83,85,86,87,88] Beyond this point, the early and late night pathways diverge. During the early

night, GLU induces delays in the circadian clock through ryanodine receptor (RyR)-mediated calcium release.[89] GLU exposure during the late night, however, advances the circadian clock through a cyclic guanosine monophosphate/protein kinase G (cGMP/PKG) signaling cascade followed by cAMP response element-binding protein (CREB)-activated transcription.[89,90,91]

Although GLU alone is capable of resetting circadian rhythms, there are many substances that modulate this resetting. These can be divided into two categories: those that decrease the phase-resetting effect of GLU during both the early and late night, which include NPY and GABA,[34,35] and those that have differing effects on GLU-induced phase shifts, depending on what time of night they are applied.

This second category of time-dependent modulators includes 5-HT and PACAP. If animals are depleted of 5-HT, they show increased phase delays in response to light.[92,93] Co-application of a PACAP antagonist, however, either in vitro or in vivo, decreases the phase delay seen in early night, and increases the late night phase advance in both rat and hamster.[94,95] When PACAP is administered in conjunction with GLU, it increases the early night phase delays, but decreases the late night phase advances. This is similar to the effects seen following application of cAMP analogs to the hypothalamic brain slice, suggesting that the effects of PACAP may be mediated by a cAMP pathway.[96]

The role of ACh in resetting circadian rhythms has been unclear, with much of the confusion arising from the fact that its effects vary depending on the site of application. The first evidence that ACh might play a role in resetting the circadian clock came in 1979, when Zatz and Brownstein examined whether pharmacological manipulation of the SCN could affect circadian rhythms, using serotonin N-acetyltransferase (SNAT) activity in the pineal as a marker of circadian phase. SNAT activity has an endogenous rhythm in the pineal that is higher during the night than during the day, and this rhythm previously was found to be reset by light. It was found that injections of carbachol into the lateral ventricle of Sprague-Dawley rats at CT 15 caused phase delays in SNAT activity that were similar to, but not as large as, the phase delays produced by light.[97] Carbachol injections into the lateral ventricle also were repeated later in mice[98] and hamsters,[99] where it was found that administration of carbachol during early night caused phase delays, while late night administration caused phase advances.

This pattern of sensitivity and response is similar to that previously demonstrated in response to light or GLU. Support for the involvement of ACh in the light response came from studies looking at ACh levels in the rat SCN using a radioimmunoassay (RIA).[100] Using this technique, no significant oscillation in ACh levels was found under constant conditions, but light pulses administered at CT 14 were found to increase ACh levels in the SCN. Only one time point was examined, however, so it is not known whether this increase was simply a response to exposure to light or if there was actually a circadian pattern to the light-stimulated release. The implication of these studies, however, is that ACh might be the primary neurotransmitter providing the signal of light to the clock.

Significant evidence, however, began to emerge indicating that ACh was not likely to be the primary signal of light. First, whereas it previously had been determined that the RHT transmitted the signal of light from the eye to the SCN, it was found that choline acetyltransferase (ChAT) was not present in this projection,[101] making it anatomically unlikely that ACh was the primary neurotransmitter involved in this signal. This evidence might need to be reconsidered, however, as recent studies have found an alternative splice variant of ChAT present in ganglion cells that was not picked up using previous antibodies.[102] Experiments have not yet been published looking at whether this alternative form of ChAT is present in the RHT.

Additional evidence against ACh being the signal of light came from experiments that found intracerebroventricular (icv) injections of hemicholinium, which significantly depletes ACh stores in the brain, did not block the ability of the animal to phase shift in response to light.[103] There was also evidence that injecting NMDA receptor antagonists could block carbachol-induced phase shifts, suggesting that although ACh may play a role in the light response, it was upstream of a glutamatergic signal.[104] Finally, Liu and Gillette,[105] using extracellular recording in vitro, found that microdrop applications of carbachol directly to the SCN caused only phase advances, regardless of whether the carbachol was applied early or late in the evening.

In an attempt to explain these contradicting data, it was hypothesized by the authors' laboratory that the dual response pattern of the SCN to cholinergic stimulation was a result of the location of application. Note that in the initial in vivo studies, carbachol was injected into the lateral or third ventricle, where the drug could have a diffuse effect, while in the in vitro studies carbachol was applied in microdrops directly to the SCN. As was predicted, if the in vivo experiments were performed by injecting carbachol directly into the SCN rather than into the ventricle, a similar phase response pattern to that observed in the in vitro experiments using microdrop applications resulted.[106] Furthermore, it was found that mice lacking the M_1-type muscarinic receptor (M_1AChR) do not respond to intra-SCN carbachol injections,[107] but still exhibit biphasic responses to light and icv injections of carbachol.[108] Together this evidence suggests that ACh has at least two different effects on the circadian clock, depending upon the site of application. There is an indirect response, working through the ventricles, that is likely upstream of a glutamatergic signal, and a direct response that is mediated by the M_1AChR. Based on the anatomical studies looking at cholinergic projections to the SCN that originate in the LDTg and PPTg, and the NBM, the current hypothesis is that this cholinergic signal may be involved in linking the sleep–wake and circadian cycles together.

GENETICS OF CIRCADIAN RHYTHMS

Much research effort has focused on determining how a biological system keeps 24-hour time. With the discovery that single, dispersed cells can exhibit circadian rhythms, the focus turned towards understanding cellular processes that generate a near 24-hour timebase. A molecular clockwork appears to generate an approximately 24-hour rhythm through a feedback cycle involving a set of core clock genes, their mRNAs, and proteins. Together they form the molecular clockwork. This cycle consists of a set of interconnected positive and negative feedback loops and their regulatory elements. Positive elements, which include Clock and Bmal1, are transcribed into mRNA, which is translated into proteins that heterodimerize and are translocated into the nucleus. In the nucleus, they activate continued transcription of their own genes, and activate transcription of negative elements. The negative elements, which include Period, Cryptochrome and Rev-erbα, then are transcribed and translated. Proteins of the negative elements also associate in complexes and are translocated to the nucleus, where they feed back to inhibit transcription of the positive elements. Additional genes that have been proposed to be involved in the circadian clock include Rorα,[109] Timeless (Tim),[110] Dec1 and Dec2,[111] and most recently SIRT1.[31,112,113] These feedback loops are affected further by regulatory enzymes, including casein kinase 1 epsilon (CKIε) and glycogen synthase kinase (GSK)[114,115,116] and small intracellular regulatory molecules with established roles in signal transduction.[31,117] The cycle of these feedback loops takes approximately 24 hours to complete, providing a means by which cells within the SCN can maintain a circadian rhythm.

Core clock elements have been found to play a critical role in human sleep disorders. For example, inherited forms of advanced sleep phase syndrome (ASPS) have been associated with either a mutation in the Per2 gene that interferes with a normal phosphorylation site of $CKI\delta/\epsilon$[118] or with a mutation in $CKI\delta$.[119] Delayed sleep phase syndrome (DSPS) on the other hand has been found in some cases to be associated with a specific polymorphism of hPER3.[31,120,121] Recently PER3 expression patterns in human leukocytes were found to correlate with sleep–wake timing, particularly in those individuals who have a morningness preference.[122] Finally, morningness/eveningness preference has been associated with a polymorphism of the human Clock gene.[31,123,124]

SUMMARY

Circadian rhythms are the near 24-hour oscillations brain and body functions, such as core body temperature, hormone release, and the sleep–wake cycle. The master pacemaker regulating these rhythms is located in the SCN in the hypothalamus. The SCN is situated ideally to receive input about environmental light, sleep–wake state, and activity status. It can be reset in response to these stimuli and, in turn, provide output signals to regulate the timing of activity and behavior. The core mechanisms providing this timekeeping ability are still being elucidated, but appear to be provided by through transcription/translation feedback loops, consisting of both positive and negative elements, coupled with other intracellular elements associated with signaling events. Interestingly, circadian rhythm sleep disorders and sleep phenotypes are beginning to be correlated with abnormalities in the genes regulating circadian rhythms.

REFERENCES

1. Van Cauter E. Diurnal and ultradian rhythms in human endocrine function: a minireview. Horm Res 1990;34(2):45–53.
2. Schwartz WJ. A clinicians primer on the circadian clock: its localization, function, and resetting. Adv Intern Med 1993;38:81–106.
3. Arendt J, Minors D, Waterhouse J, editors. Biological rhythms in clinical practice. Bristol (England): John Wright; 1989.
4. Van Cauter E, Turek FW. In: DeGroot JL, editor. Endocrinology. Philadelphia: WB Saunders; 1995.
5. Takahashi Y, Kipnis D, Daughaday W. Growth hormone secretion during sleep. J Clin Invest 1968;47(9):2079–90.
6. Van Cauter E, L'Hermite M, Copinschi G, et al. Quantitative analysis of spontaneous variations of plasma prolactin in normal man. Am J Physiol 1981;241(5):E355–63.
7. van Coevorden A, Laurent E, Decoster C, et al. Decreased basal and stimulated thyrotropin secretion in healthy elderly men. J Clin Endocrinol Metab 1989;69(1):177–85.
8. Kapen S, Boyar R, Hellman L, et al. The relationship of luteinizing hormone secretion to sleep in women during the early follicular phase: effects of sleep reversal and a prolonged three-hour sleep–wake schedule. J Clin Endocrinol Metab 1976;42(6):1031–40.
9. Sinha M, Ohannesian J, Heiman M, et al. Nocturnal rise of leptin in lean, obese, and noninsulin-dependent diabetes mellitus subjects. J Clin Invest 1996;97(5):1344–7.
10. Licinio J, Mantzoros C, Negrao A, et al. Human leptin levels are pulsatile and inversely related to pituitary–adrenal function. Nat Med 1997;3(5):575–9.
11. Licinio J, Negrao A, Mantzoros C, et al. Synchronicity of frequently sampled, 24-h concentrations of circulating leptin, luteinizing hormone, and estradiol in healthy women. Proc Natl Acad Sci U S A 1998;95(5):2541–6.
12. Weitzman E, Zimmerman J, Czeisler C, et al. Cortisol secretion is inhibited during sleep in normal man. J Clin Endocrinol Metab 1983;56(2):352–8.
13. Lejeune-Lenain C, Van Cauter E, Desir D, et al. Control of circadian and episodic variations of adrenal androgens secretion in man. J Endocrinol Invest 1987;10(3):267–76.
14. Stephan FK, Zucker I. Circadian rhythms in drinking behavior and locomotor activity of rats are eliminated by hypothalamic leions. Proc Natl Acad Sci U S A 1972;69:1583–6.
15. Moore RY, Eichler VB. Loss of a circadian adrenal corticosterone rhythm following suprachiasmatic lesions in the rat. Brain Res 1972;42:201–6.
16. Drucker-Colin R, Aguilar-Roblero R, Garcia-Hernandez F, et al. Fetal suprachiasmatic nucleus transplants: diurnal rhythm recovery of lesioned rats. Brain Res 1984;311:353–7.
17. Ralph MR, Foster RG, Davis FC, et al. Transplanted suprachiasmatic nucleus determines circadian period. Science 1990;247:975–8.
18. Abrahamson EE, Moore RY. Suprachiasmatic nucleus in the mouse: retinal innervation, intrinsic organization, and efferent projections. Brain Res 2001;916:172–91.

19. Moore RY, Speh JC, Leak RK. Suprachiasmatic nucleus organization. Cell Tissue Res 2002;309: 89–98.

20. Mai J, Kedziora O, Teckhaus L, et al. Evidence for subdivisions in the human suprachiasmatic nucleus. J Comp Neurol 1991;305(3):508–25.

21. Mosko S, Moore R. Retinohypothalamic tract development: alteration by suprachiasmatic lesions in the neonatal rat. Brain Res 1979;1979(164):1–15.

22. Rusak B. Neural mechanisms for entrainment and generation of mammalian circadian rhythms. Fed Proc 1979;38(12):2589–95.

23. Johnson RF, Moore RY, Morin LP. Loss of entrainment and anatomical plasticity after lesions of the hamster retinohypothalamic tract. Brain Res 1988; 460:297–313.

24. Hattar S, Lucas RJ, Mrosovsky N, et al. Melanopsin and rod–cone photoreceptive systems account for all major accessory visual functions in mice. Nature 2003;424:76–81.

25. Berson DM, Dunn FA, Takao M. Phototransduction by retinal ganglion cells that set the circadian clock. Science 2002;295:1070–3.

26. Hannibal J, Ding JM, Chen D, et al. Pituitary adenylate cyclase-activating peptide (PACAP) in the retinohypothalamic tract: a potential daytime regulator of the biological clock. J Neurosci 1997;17: 2637–44.

27. Medanic M, Gillette MU. Suprachiasmatic circadian pacemaker of rat shows two windows of sensitivity to neuropeptide Y in vitro. Brain Res 1993;620: 281–6.

28. Yannielli PC, Harrington ME. The neuropeptide Y Y5 receptor mediates the blockade of "photic-like" NMDA-induced phase shifts in the golden hamster. J Neurosci 2001;21(14):5367–73.

29. Reghunandanan V, Reghunandanan R, Singh PI. Neurotransmitters of the suprachiasmatic nucleus: role in the regulation of circadian rhythms. Prog Neurobiol 1993;41:647–55.

30. van den Pol AN, Tsujimoto KL. Neurotransmitters of the hypothalamic suprachiasmatic nucleus: immunocytochemical analysis of 25 neuronal antigens. Neuroscience 1985;15:1049–86.

31. Imaizumi T, Kay S, Schroeder J. Circadian rhythms. Daily watch on metabolism. Science 2007; 318(5857):1730–1.

32. Glass JD, DiNardo LA, Ehlen JC. Dorsal raphe nuclear stimulation of SCN serotonin release and circadian phase-resetting. Brain Res 2000;859: 224–32.

33. Barassin S, Raison S, Saboureau M, et al. Circadian tryptophan hydroxylase levels and serotonin release in the suprachiasmatic nucleus of the rat. Eur J Neurosci 2002;15:833–40.

34. Medanic M, Gillette MU. Serotonin regulates the phase of the rat suprachiasmatic circadian pacemaker in vitro only during the subjective day. J Physiol 1992;450:629–42.

35. Yannielli PC, Harrington ME. Neuropeptide Y applied in vitro can block the phase shifts induced by light in vivo. Neuroreport 2000;11(7):1587–91.

36. Bina KG, Rusak B, Semba K. Localization of cholinergic neurons in the forebrain and brainstem that project to the suprachiasmatic nucleus of the hypothalamus in rat. J Comp Neurol 1993;335:295–307.

37. Castillo-Ruiz A, Nunez A. Cholinergic projections to the suprachiasmatic nucleus and lower subparaventricular zone of diurnal and nocturnal rodents. Brain Res 2007;1151:91–101.

38. Cui H, Malpeli JG. Activity in the parabigeminal nucleus during eye movements directed at moving and stationary targets. J Neurophysiol 2003;89: 3128–42.

39. Deurveilher S, Hennevin E. Lesions of the pedunculopontine tegmental nucleus reduce paradoxical sleep (PS) propensity: evidence from a short-term PS deprivation study in rats. Eur J Neurosci 2001; 13:1963–76.

40. Semba K. Multiple output pathways of the basal forebrain: organization, chemical heterogeneity, and roles in vigilance. Behav Brain Res 2000;115:117–41.

41. Michelsen Ka, Lozada A, Kaslin J, et al. Histamine-immunoreactive neurons in the mouse and rat suprachiasmatic nucleus. Eur J Neurosci 2005; 22(8):1997–2004.

42. Leak RK, Moore RY. Topographic organization of suprachiasmatic nucleus projection neurons. J Comp Neurol 2001;433:312–34.

43. Kalsbeek A, Buijs RM. Output pathways of the mammalian suprachiasmatic nucleus: coding circadian time by transmitter selection and specific targeting. Cell Tissue Res 2002;309:109–18.

44. Abrahamson E, Leak RK, Moore RY. The suprachiasmatic nucleus projects to posterior hypothalamic arousal systems. Neuroreport 2001;12(2): 435–40.

45. de Lecea L, Kilduff TS, Peyron C, et al. The hypocretins: hypothalamus-specific peptides with neuroexcitatory activity. Proc Natl Acad Sci U S A 1998;95:322–7.

46. Gompf HS, Aston-Jones G. Role of orexin input in the diurnal rhythm of locus coeruleus impulse activity. Brain Res 2008;11(1224):43–52.

47. Aston-Jones G, Chen S, Zhu Y, et al. A neural circuit for circadian regulation of arousal. Nat Neurosci 2001;4(7):732–8.

48. Chou TC, Bjorkum AA, Gaus SE, et al. Afferents to the ventrolateral preoptic nucleus. J Neurosci 2002; 22(3):977–90.

49. Buijs R, Hou Y, Shinn S, et al. Ultrastructural evidence for intra- and extranuclear projections of GABAergic neurons of the suprachiasmatic nucleus. J Comp Neurol 1994;340(3):381–91.

50. Morin LP. The circadian visual system. Brain Res Brain Res Rev 1994;19(1):102–27.

51. Moga M, Weis R, Moore RY. Efferent projections of the paraventricular thalamic nucleus in the rat. J Comp Neurol 1995;359(2):221–38.

52. Peng Z-C, Bentivoglio M. The thalamic paraventricular nucleus relays information from the suprachiasmatic nucleus to the amygdala: a combined anterograde and retrograde tracing study in the rat at the light and electron microscopic levels. J Neurocytol 2004;33(1):101–16.

53. Kramer A, Yang F-C, Snodgrass P, et al. Regulation of daily locomotor activity and sleep by hypothalamic EGF receptor signaling. Science 2001;294: 2511–5.

54. Cheng MY, Bullock CM, Li C, et al. Prokineticin 2 transmits the behavioural circadian rhythm of the suprachiasmatic nucleus. Nature 2002;417: 405–10.

55. Walsh I, van den Berg R, Rietveld W. Ionic currents in cultured rat suprachiasmatic neurons. Neuroscience 1995;69(3):915–29.

56. Gillette MU. Regulation of entrainment pathways by the suprachiasmatic circadian clock: sensitivities to second messengers. Prog Brain Res 1996;111: 121–32.

57. Moga M, Moore RY. Putative excitatory amino acid projections to the suprachiasmatic nucleus in the rat. Brain Res 1996;743(1–2):171–7.

58. Dudley TE, Dinardo LA, Glass JD. In vivo assessment of the midbrain raphe nuclear regulation of serotonin release in the hamster suprachiasmatic nucleus. J Neurophysiol 1999;81(4):1469–77.

59. Dudley TE, DiNardo LA, Glass JD. Endogenous regulation of serotonin release in the hamster suprachiasmatic nucleus. J Neurosci 1998;18(13): 5045–52.

60. Grossman GH, Mistlberger RE, Antle MC, et al. Sleep deprivation stimulates serotonin release in the suprachiasmatic nucleus. Neuroreport 2000; 11(9):1929–32.

61. Bobrzynska KJ, Vrang N, Mrosovsky N. Persistence of nonphotic phase shifts in hamsters after serotonin depletion in the suprachiasmatic nucleus. Brain Res 1996;741(1–2):205–14.

62. Antle MC, Marchant EG, Niel L, et al. Serotonin antagonists do not attenuate activity-induced phase shifts of circadian rhythms in the Syrian hamster. Brain Res 1998;813:139–49.

63. Hannibal J, Moller M, Ottersen OP, et al. PACAP and glutamate are co-stored in the retinohypothalamic tract. J Comp Neurol 2000;418:147–55.

64. Fukuhara C, Suzuki N, Matsumoto Y, et al. Day–night variation of pituitary adenylate cyclase-activating polypeptide (PACAP) level in the rat suprachiasmatic nucleus. Neurosci Lett 1997; 229:49–52.

65. Piggins HD, Marchant EG, Goguen D, et al. Phase-shifting effects of pituitary adenylate cyclase activating polypeptide on hamster wheel-running rhythms. Neurosci Lett 2001;305:25–8.

66. Albers HE, Ferris CF. Neuropeptide Y: role in light-dark cycle entrainment of hamster circadian rhythms. Neurosci Lett 1984;50:163–8.

67. Huhman KL, Albers HE. Neuropeptide Y microinjected into the suprachiasmatic region phase shifts circadian rhythms in constant darkness. Peptides 1994;15(8):1475–8.

68. Rusak B, Meijer JH, Harrington ME. Hamster circadian rhythms are phase-shifted by electrical stimulation of the geniculo–hypothalamic tract. Brain Res 1989;493:283–91.

69. Biello SM, Mrosovsky N. Blocking the phase-shifting effect of neuropeptide Y with light. Proc Biol Sci 1995;259:179–87.

70. Biello SM, Golombek DA, Harrington ME. Neuropeptide Y and glutamate block each other's phase shifts in the suprachiasmatic nucleus in vitro. Neuroscience 1997;77(4):1049–57.

71. Huhman KL, Babagbemi TO, Albers HE. Bicuculline blocks neuropeptide Y-induced phase advances when microinjected in the suprachiasmatic nucleus of syrian hamsters. Brain Res 1995; 675:333–6.

72. Gillette MU, Prosser RA. Circadian rhythm of the rat suprachiasmatic brain slice is rapidly reset by daytime application of cAMP analogs. Brain Res 1988;474:348–52.

73. Prosser RA, Gillette MU. The mammalian circadian clock in the suprachiasmatic nuclei is reset in vitro by cAMP. J Neurosci 1989;9(3):1073–81.

74. Prosser RA, Gillette MU. Cyclic changes in cAMP concentration and phosphodiesterase activity in a mammalian circadian clock studied in vitro. Brain Res 1991;568:185–92.

75. Cheung PW, McCormick CE. Failure of pinealectomy or melatonin to alter circadian activity rhythm of the rat. Am J Physiol 1982;242:R261–4.

76. Cassone VM, Chesworth MJ, Armstrong SM. Entrainment of rat circadian rhythms by daily injection of melatonin depends upon the hypothalamic suprachiasmatic nuclei. Physiol Behav 1986;36: 1111–21.

77. Cassone VM, Roberts MH, Moore RY. Effects of melatonin on 2-deoxy-[1-^{14}C]glucose uptake within rat suprachiasmatic nucleus. Am J Physiol 1988; 255(2):R332–7.

78. Shibata S, Cassone VM, Moore RY. Effects of melatonin on neuronal activity in the rat suprachiasmatic nucleus in vitro. Neurosci Lett 1989;97:140–4.

79. Margraf RR, Lynch GR. An in vitro circadian rhythm of melatonin sensitivity in the suprachiasmatic nucleus of the djungarian hamster, *Phodopus sungorus*. Brain Res 1993;609:45–50.

80. McArthur AJ, Gillette MU, Prosser RA. Melatonin directly resets the rat suprachiasmatic circadian clock in vitro. Brain Res 1991;565:158–61.

81. McArthur AJ, Hunt AE, Gillette MU. Melatonin action and signal transduction in the rat suprachiasmatic circadian clock: activation of protein kinase C at dusk and dawn. Endocrinology 1997; 138(2):627–34.

82. Hunt AE, Al-Ghoul WM, Gillette MU, et al. Activation of MT2 melatonin receptors in rat suprachiasmatic nucleus phase advances the circadian clock. Am J Physiol 2001;280:C110–8.

83. Ding JM, Chen D, Weber ET, et al. Resetting the biological clock: mediation of nocturnal circadian shifts by glutamate and NO. Science 1994;266: 1713–7.

84. Shirakawa T, Moore RY. Glutamate shifts the phase of the circadian neuronal firing rhythm in the rat suprachiasmatic nucleus in vitro. Neurosci Lett 1994;178:47–50.

85. Shibata S, Watanabe A, Hamada T, et al. N-methyl-D-aspartate induces phase shifts in circadian rhythm of neuronal activity of rat SCN in vitro. Am J Physiol 1994;267(2):R360–4.

86. Watanabe A, Hamada T, Shibata S, et al. Effects of nitric oxide synthase inhibitors on N-methyl-D-aspartate-induced phase delay of circadian rhythm of neuronal activity in the rat suprachiasmatic nucleus in vitro. Brain Res 1994;646:161–4.

87. Watanabe A, Ono M, Shibata S, et al. Effect of a nitric oxide synthase inhibitor, N-nitro-L-arginine methylester, on light-induced phase delay of circadian rhythm of wheel-running activity in golden hamsters. Neurosci Lett 1995;192:25–8.

88. Weber ET, Gannon RL, Michel AM, et al. Nitric oxide synthase inhibitor blocks light-induced phase shifts of the circadian activity rhythm, but no c-fos expression in the suprachiasmatic nucleus of the Syrian hamster. Brain Res 1995; 692:137–42.

89. Ding JM, Buchanan GF, Tischkau SA, et al. A neuronal ryanodine receptor mediates light-induced phase delays of the circadian clock. Nature 1998;394:381–4.

90. Ding JM, Faiman LE, Hurst WJ, et al. Resetting the biological clock: mediation of nocturnal CREB phosphorylation via light, glutamate, and nitric oxide. J Neurosci 1997;17(2):667–75.

91. Tischkau SA, Mitchell JW, Tyan SH, et al. Ca2+/cAMP response element-binding protein (CREB)-dependent activation of Per1 is required for light-induced signaling in the suprachiasmatic nucleus circadian clock. J Biol Chem 2003;278(2):718–23.

92. Mintz EM, Jasnow AM, Gillespie CF, et al. GABA interacts with photic signaling in the suprachiasmatic nucleus to regulate circadian phase shifts. Neuroscience 2002;109(4):773–8.

93. Bradbury MJ, Dement WC, Edgar DM. Serotonin-containing fibers in the suprachiasmatic hypothalamus attenuate light-induced phase delays in mice. Brain Res 1997;768:125–34.

94. Bergstrom AL, Hannibal J, Hindersson P, et al. Light-induced phase shift in the Syrian hamster (Mesocricetus auratus) is attenuated by the PACAP receptor antagonist PACAP6-38 or PACAP immunoneutralization. Eur J Neurosci 2003;18: 2552–62.

95. Chen D, Buchanan GF, Ding JM, et al. Pituitary adenylyl cyclase-activating peptide: a pivotal modulator of glutamatergic regulation of the suprachiasmatic circadian clock. Proc Natl Acad Sci U S A 1999;96:13468–73.

96. Tischkau SA, Gallman EA, Buchanan GF, et al. Differential cAMP gating of glutamatergic signaling regulates long-term state changes in the suprachiasmatic circadian clock. J Neurosci 2000; 20(20):7830–7.

97. Zatz M, Brownstein MJ. Intraventricular carbachol mimics the effects of light on the circadian rhythm in the rat pineal gland. Science 1979;203:358–60.

98. Zatz M, Herkenham MA. Intraventricular carbachol mimics the phase-shifting effect of light on the circadian rhythm of wheel-running activity. Brain Res 1981;212:234–8.

99. Earnest DJ, Turek FW. Role for acetylcholine in mediating effects of light on reproduction. Science 1983;219:77–9.

100. Murakami N, Takahashi K, Kawashima K. Effect of light on the acetylcholine concentrations of the suprachiasmatic nucleus in the rat. Brain Res 1984;311:358–60.

101. Wenthold RJ. Glutamate and aspartate as neurotransmitters for the auditory nerve. In: Gessa GL, editor. Glutamate as a neurotransmitter. New York: Raven Press; 1981. p. 69–78.

102. Yasuhara O, Tooyama I, Aimi Y, et al. Demonstration of choinergic ganglion cells in rat retina: expression of an alternative splice variant of choline acetyltransferase. J Neurosci 2003;23(7): 2872–81.

103. Pauly JR, Horseman ND. Anticholinergic agents do not block light-induced circadian phase shifts. Brain Res 1985;348:163–7.

104. Colwell CS, Kaufman CM, Menaker M. Phase-shifting mechanisms in the mammalian circadian system: new light on the carbachol paradox. J Neurosci 1993;13(4):1454–9.

105. Liu C, Gillette MU. Cholinergic regulation of the suprachiasmatic nucleus circadian rhythm via a muscarinic mechanism at night. J Neurosci 1996;16(2):744–51.

106. Buchanan GF, Gillette MU. New light on an old paradox: site-dependent effects of carbachol on circadian rhythms. Exp Neurol 2005;193:489–96.

107. Buchanan GF, Artinian LR, Hamilton SE, et al. The M1 muscarinic acetylcholine receptor is a necessary component in cholinergic circadian signaling. Proceedings of the Society for Neuroscience. 2000.

108. Buchanan GF. Cholinergic regulation of the mammalian circadian system: analysis of cholinergic-induced phase shifting in vivo and in vitro in wildtype and M1 knockout mice. Urbana (IL): Molecular and Integrative Physiology, University of Illinois at Urbana-Champaign; 2002.

109. Sato T, Panda S, Miraglia L, et al. A functional genomics strategy reveals Rora as a component of the mammalian circadian clock. Neuron 2004; 43(4):527–37.

110. Barnes J, Tischkau S, Barnes J, et al. Requirement of mammalian timeless for circadian rhythmicity. Science 2003;302:439–42.

111. Honma S, Kawamoto T, Takagi Y, et al. Dec1 and Dec2 are regulators of the mammalian molecular clock. Nature 2002;419(6909):841–4.

112. Asher G, Gatfield D, Stratmann M, et al. SIRT1 regulates circadian clock gene expression through PER2 deacetylation. Cell 2008;134:317–28.

113. Nakahata Y, Kaluzova M, Grimaldi B, et al. The NAD+-dependent deacetylase SIRT1 modulates CLOCK-mediated chromatin remodeling and circadian control. Cell 2008;134:329–40.

114. Harms E, Young M, Saez L. CK1 and GSK3 in the Drosophila and mammalian circadian clock. Novartis Found Symp 2003;253:267–77.

115. Martinek S, Inonog S, Manoukian A, et al. A role for the segment polarity gene shaggy/GSK-3 in the Drosophila circadian clock. Cell 2001;105(6):769–79.

116. Virshup D, Eide E, Forger D, et al. Reversible protein phosphorylation regulates circadian rhythms. Cold Spring Harb Symp Quant Biol 2007;72:413–20.

117. Harrisingh M, Nitabach M. Circadian rhythms. Integrating circadian timekeeping with cellular physiology. Science 2008;320(5878):879–80.

118. Toh K, Jones C, He Y, et al. An hPer2 phosphorylation site mutation in familial advanced sleep phase syndrom. Science 2001;291(5506):1040–3.

119. Xu Y, Padiath Q, Shapiro R, et al. Functional consequences of a CKIdelta mutation causing familial advanced sleep phase syndrome. Nature 2005; 434(7033):640–4.

120. Ebisawa T, Uchiyama M, Kajimura N, et al. Association of structural polymorphisms in the human period 3 gene with delayed sleep phase syndrome. EMBO Rep 2001;2(4):342–6.

121. Archer S, Robilliard D, Skene D, et al. A length polymorphism in the circadian clock gene Per3 is linked to delayed sleep phase syndrome and extreme diurnal preference. Sleep 2003;26(4): 413–5.

122. Archer S, Viola A, Kyriakopoulou V, et al. Dijk D-J. Inter-individual differences in habitual sleep timing and entrained phase of endogenous circadian rhythms of BMAL1, PER2 and PER3 mRNA in human leukocytes. Sleep 2008;31(5): 808–17.

123. Katzenberg D, Young T, Finn L, et al. A CLOCK polymorphism associated with human diurnal preference. Sleep 1998;21(6):569–76.

124. Mishima K, Tozawa T, Satoh K, et al. The 3111T/C polymorphism of hClock is associated with evening preference and delayed sleep timing in a Japanese population sample. Am J Med Genet B Neuropsychiatr Genet 2005;133:101–4.

Circadian and Homeostatic Regulation of Human Sleep and Cognitive Performance and Its Modulation by *PERIOD3*

Derk-Jan Dijk, PhD*, Simon N. Archer, PhD

KEYWORDS

- Sleep • Circadian rhythms • Clock genes
- *PERIOD3* • SWS • Cognition

Humans experience the sleep/wake cycle as an alternation between a state of rest, during which consciousness is absent or altered, and a state of active interaction with the social and physical environment, during which the brain engages in many cognitive and other activities. Appropriate timing and adequate quality of the sleep/wake cycle are of paramount importance for successful functioning within roles at home and at work. According to the conceptual framework of the circadian and homeostatic regulation of the sleep/wake cycle, the timing of sleep and waking is achieved through the interaction of two endogenous oscillatory processes and external factors, such as the light/dark cycle and social constraints. This article describes recent progress in the understanding of this interaction of the two endogenous oscillatory processes, the role of clock genes in regulating these oscillatory processes, and individual differences in the preferences for the timing of waking activities and sleep. It lists core and recent references and also refers to three previous reviews.[1–3]

CIRCADIAN AND HOMEOSTATIC REGULATION OF SLEEP AND COGNITION

Timing of Sleep and Waking Activities: Contribution of Environmental, Social, and Internal Biologic Factors

Bedtime and wake time are directly observable markers of the sleep/wake cycle; from these markers the duration of sleep and its phase relationship with clock time and social and geophysical cycles can be computed. There is ample evidence demonstrating the impact of social factors on sleep timing. Most persons wake up to meet social requirements, such as work schedules, and the timing and duration of sleep differ markedly between weekdays and weekends. Evidence for the important role of light (ie, the combined contribution of natural and artificial light) in the regulation of sleep and wakefulness comes from multiple sources, including blind individuals who often experience chronic sleep disturbances associated with nonsynchronized circadian rhythms.[4] The impact of the geophysical light/

This work was supported by grants from the National Institutes of Health/National Institute on Aging (P01 AG09975); the Biotechnology Biological Sciences Research Council (BB/F022883/1; BB/E003672/1), the Wellcome Trust (069714/Z/02/Z and 0760667/Z04/Z), and the Air Force Office of Scientific Research (FA9550-08-1-0080). The opinions, findings, conclusions, and recommendations expressed in this article are those of the authors and do not necessarily reflect the views of the Office of Naval Research, the Biotechnology Biological Sciences Research Council, or the Wellcome Trust.

Surrey Sleep Research Centre, Faculty of Health and Medical Sciences, University of Surrey, Egerton Road, Guildford GU2 7XP, UK
* Corresponding author.
E-mail address: d.j.dijk@surrey.ac.uk (D-J. Dijk).

Sleep Med Clin 4 (2009) 111–125
doi:10.1016/j.jsmc.2009.02.001

dark cycle (as opposed to the light/dark cycle to which individuals are exposed) on the regulation of sleep is less profound in industrialized societies. Sleep timing with respect to clock time and sleep duration are nearly constant across the seasons, even though in many highly populated areas the timing of dawn and dusk may change by several hours relative to local clock time (eg, approximately 4 hours in London, United Kingdom). Furthermore, for most people, the sleep/wake cycle remains synchronized with clock time even when the phase relationship between clock time and the geophysical light/dark cycle is changed abruptly, as occurs during the change to and from daylight savings time. The residual impact of the geophysical light/dark cycle on the timing of the sleep/wake cycle has been observed, however, in analyses of the timing of sleep relative to clock time in people living at similar latitudes but different longitudes within one time zone.[5]

Evidence for the impact of endogenous biologic factors on sleep–wake timing is plentiful. In fact, the magnitude of the effects of endogenous biologic factors seems to be much larger than the impact of external environmental factors and is comparable to the impacts of social factors, even though the profound effects of local environmental factors, such as traffic noise and ambient temperature, should not be underestimated. Some characteristics of sleep, including its timing and duration, differ between men and women[6] and change throughout the life span:[7,8] older people wake up earlier, and younger people sleep longer. Age-related changes in sleep duration persist when all social constraints are removed.[9] Individuals differ in their diurnal preferences for the timing of sleep and waking activities, including cognitive activities. This traitlike characteristic, which differs between men and women and shifts towards morning preference with aging,[10] has a heritability of around 50%.[11]

The magnitude of the differences in sleep timing across the life span and across the spectrum of diurnal preference is considerable, varying by as much as 2 to 3 hours between young adults and older people[10] and by 2 to 3 hours between "larks" and "owls."[12,13] Despite these differences in the timing of the sleep/wake cycle, most healthy people (with the noticeable exception of infants and young children) experience consolidated wake and sleep episodes, during which cognitive performance is upheld throughout the wake episode. The following sections first describe the endogenous oscillatory processes through which this consolidation of sleep and wakefulness is achieved and then presents the endogenous biologic factors contributing to individual differences in the timing of sleep and wakefulness.

Consolidation of Sleep/Wake Cycles Through Opposing Circadian and Homeostatic Sleep Propensity Rhythms

Research during the past 40 to 50 years has established that the consolidation and timing of the daily sleep/wake cycle is generated by the interaction of two oscillatory processes, the deep or stable circadian pacemaker, located in the suprachiasmatic nuclei (SCN) in the hypothalamus, and the labile oscillator or sleep homeostat, the locus of which is not known and may be diffuse. How the two processes interact has been elucidated through laboratory experiments in which the labile sleep–wake oscillator was scheduled to a periodicity well outside the circadian range.[14–17] Because the deep circadian oscillator has a robust endogenous period of nearly 24 hours, living on these noncircadian days leads to sleep and wake episodes that occur at all circadian phases, thereby allowing an analysis of the contribution of these two oscillators to sleep–wake regulation (Fig. 1). Following initial reports, multiple experiments have confirmed that the circadian process generates a rhythm of sleep–wake propensity that has a phase relationship with the sleep/wake cycle that, although paradoxical at first sight, is highly functional: a circadian wake-promoting signal becomes progressively stronger during the course of the biological day, reaching a maximum shortly before habitual bedtime at a phase that has become known as the "wake-maintenance zone," or forbidden zone for sleep. This wake-promoting signal dissipates rapidly after the onset of nocturnal melatonin secretion. Circadian sleep propensity increases as the night progresses to reach a maximum at approximately 7 to 8 AM in healthy young individuals and 6 to 7 AM in older people, which is very close to habitual wake time.[18] The circadian sleep–wake propensity rhythm oscillates in anti-phase with the homeostatic sleep–wake propensity rhythm: homeostatic sleep propensity is at its minimum at the end of the sleep episode and then increases progressively throughout the waking episode, to reach a maximum just before the habitual sleep episode, which is initiated when the circadian drive for wakefulness subsides. Homeostatic sleep propensity then can dissipate throughout the sleep episode. The hypothesis that consolidation of the sleep/wake cycle is achieved through these opposing homeostatic and circadian sleep–wake propensity rhythms is supported by the observation that after lesions of the SCN, which is the hypothalamic locus of the deep circadian oscillator, the sleep/wake cycle becomes fragmented. Detailed analyses of sleep in intact and

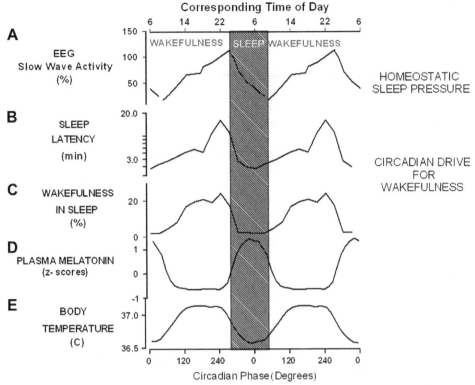

Fig. 1. Circadian and homeostatic regulation of sleep and wakefulness in humans. (*A*) Increase of homeostatic sleep pressure during wakefulness and its dissipation during sleep as reflected in EEG slow-wave activity during daytime naps and nocturnal sleep. (*Data from* Dijk DJ, Beersma DGM, Daan S. EEG power density during nap sleep: reflection of an hourglass measuring the duration of prior wakefulness. J Biol Rhythms 1987;2:207–19.) (*B–E*) Circadian variation in wake/sleep propensity as reflected in (*B*) the latency to sleep onset after 18 hours, 40 minutes of wakefulness, (*C*) wakefulness in sleep opportunities, measured during forced desynchrony of the sleep/wake cycle, (*D*) endogenous circadian rhythms of melatonin, and (*E*) core body temperature. (*Data from* Dijk DJ, Duffy JF, Riel E, et al. Ageing and the circadian and homeostatic regulation of human sleep during forced desynchrony of rest, melatonin and temperature rhythms. J Physiol (Lond) 1999;516.2:611–27.)

SCN-lesioned squirrel monkeys suggest that the SCN primarily generates a strong alerting signal.[19] Other analyses suggest that the SCN also generates a sleep-inducing signal.[20] The importance of an adequate phase relationship between circadian rhythmicity and sleep homeostasis also is underscored by the observation that disruption of the phase relationship between these two oscillators, as occurs during shift work and jetlag, leads to disruption of sleep and waking performance.

These two oscillatory processes profoundly influence sleep physiology as well as sleep–wake timing and sleep propensity. Sleep physiology includes the basic characteristics of sleep, such as the duration of rapid eye movement (REM) sleep, the density of rapid eye movements during REM sleep, alpha (8–12 Hz) electroencephalographic (EEG) activity during REM sleep, the incidence, amplitude, and frequency of sleep spindles (ie, 12- to 14-Hz spindle-like EEG

oscillations) during nonREM sleep, high-frequency EEG activity during nonREM sleep, and slow-wave activity (SWA, 0.75–4.5 Hz) in nonREM sleep.[21–24] The latter variable is unique in that it is determined primarily by the homeostatic oscillator and only minimally by the circadian oscillator. In fact, SWA is considered a primary marker of the sleep homeostat during sleep, because sleep deprivation leads to predictable increases in this variable.

The impact of the sleep homeostat and circadian oscillator on the EEG is not limited to nonREM and REM sleep. An EEG recorded under controlled behavioral conditions during wakefulness also is influenced profoundly by these two oscillators.

For example, alpha activity during wakefulness exhibits a very distinct circadian rhythm with a maximum at approximately 4 PM and a minimum at 6 AM but also is influenced by the time awake, diminishing as time awake increases. By contrast, SWA and theta activity (4.5–8 Hz), although also displaying their circadian maxima during the biological day, increase as time awake increases.[25] The latter two variables also have been considered markers of the sleep homeostat during wakefulness, because sleep deprivation leads to a further increase in these EEG activities. Recent analyses of topographic differences in the circadian and sleep–wake–dependent modulation of EEG activity, especially low-frequency components of the EEG during sleep[26] and wakefulness[25] and EEG spindle activity during sleep,[27] have suggested that frontal areas are more affected by the sleep homeostat than the occipital areas.

Thus, brain activity, as monitored through polysomnography and the analysis of the EEG during both wakefulness and sleep, is modulated dynamically by the circadian and homeostatic oscillator. The changes in low-frequency EEG activity associated with the duration of wakefulness have been hypothesized to represent use-dependent changes in neural networks.[28,29] Such changes may be more prominent in areas that have been used more intensively, and evidence for local changes in SWA in response to local stimulation has been accumulating.[30,31] Currently, it is thought that wakefulness and the intense sensory stimulation and experience associated with waking behaviors lead to local release of adenosine and growth factors that in turn may lead to local increases in SWA.[32,33]

Consolidation of Cognitive Performance Through Circadian Rhythmicity and Sleep Homeostasis

What humans experience during wakefulness is their ability to perform. Waking performance includes both physical performance (eg, athletic performance) and nonphysical performance (eg, sustained attention). This article discusses only aspects of nonphysical performance, loosely referred to as "cognitive performance" (for a discussion of physical performance, see[34]). Cognitive performance comprises many different domains and elements, including working memory, vigilance, attention, and executive function. A discussion of the brain basis and interrelationships between these domains and elements of cognitive performance is well beyond the scope of this article and the expertise of its authors, who merely summarize experiments in which the separate influences of the two oscillatory processes on cognitive performance have been assessed by the use of multiple performance tasks. Wever and Aschoff[35] reported that performance is influenced by both the circadian and sleep–wake oscillator. Subsequent experiments have shown that many aspects of performance deteriorate with time awake and improve with sleep. These observations are in accordance with the view that sleep serves to allow recovery from the wear and tear of wakefulness that interferes with the ability to perform. These experiments also have shown a circadian influence on cognitive performance so that performance is poor during the circadian night and better during the circadian day. This basic rhythm of performance has been observed for all performance tests analyzed to date, although minor differences in the timing of peak performance may exist between specific performance tasks.[36,37] This finding suggests that both the circadian oscillator and the sleep homeostat modulate general determinants of cognitive performance (eg, arousal) rather than only more specific aspects such as executive function. This view also is consistent with the observation, first reported by Kleitman and more recently re-investigated and confirmed,[38] that variables such as core body temperature that display both circadian and sleep–wake–dependent variation are correlated with variation in the performance of a number of tasks. It should be emphasized, however, that very few experiments have been designed to investigate specifically how, within the context of cognitive psychology, the circadian pacemaker and the sleep homeostat interact to affect performance. Noticeable exceptions are the experiments conducted by Horowitz[39] and Santhi.[40] These experiments indicate that the interaction of high sleep pressure and circadian misalignment leads to decrements in selective attention and reduced accuracy as assessed in the visual search task (eg, a fast but careless search). Harrison and colleagues[41] used a sustained attention-to-response task that is thought to depend heavily on frontal lobe function to investigate the contribution of time awake and the circadian system to errors related to failure of response (errors of omission) and errors in automatic aspects of responding arising from failure of inhibitory responses (errors of commission). They reported that both errors of commission and errors of omission were modulated by time awake but not by circadian phase, although the interaction between these two factors was highly significant for errors of commission.

An analysis of the effects of sleep deprivation and circadian phase misalignment on performance found a statistically reliable deterioration in 11 of 16 performance measures, with no clear differential sensitivity between executive and non-executive tasks.[42]

The influence of circadian rhythmicity and sleep homeostasis on aspects of waking function is not limited to performance. The mood of healthy volunteers, as well as that of patients suffering from seasonal affective disorder, exhibits both sleep–wake–dependent and robust circadian modulation. Mood deteriorates with time awake, recovers during sleep, and, from a circadian perspective, is worst in the early morning and best in the evening hours.[43,44]

The impact of circadian and sleep–wake–dependent processes on performance extends beyond laboratory conditions. Thus, the sleep homeostat and the circadian oscillator have been observed to contribute to alertness and mood in abnormally entrained and free-running blind individuals living in their normal environment.[45] These data from the blind also show that the wake-dependent deterioration of mood and performance is not dependent solely on light exposure but also seems to be associated with wakefulness itself.

All the findings summarized thus far have emphasized the effects of the two oscillatory processes on acute aspects of waking performance. There is a rapidly growing interest in the role of sleep and circadian rhythms in the regulation of longer-lasting aspects of performance (ie, learning, memory, and plasticity). Practice effects (ie, the slow long-term improvements in performance that can be observed in throughput tasks such as the Digit Symbol Substitution and Addition task) are diminished when the phase relationship between the sleep/wake cycle and circadian rhythmicity is disrupted.[46] Whether these differences are related to the sleep disruption or circadian misalignment cannot be determined from the available data. Implementation of an implicit procedural memory task in experiments designed to elucidate the contribution of circadian rhythms and sleep to waking performance has revealed that both circadian rhythmicity and sleep pressure modulate the improvement of the learned aspects of this task. Whether this improvement indeed reflects enhanced consolidation or simply an improvement in observed performance cannot be deduced from the available data. In a separate line of research, evidence is accumulating that SWA and sleep spindles are associated with the consolidation of procedural and declarative tasks.[30,47] In general, these experiments have emphasized the role of sleep rather than the role of circadian rhythmicity in learning, memory, and plasticity, even though many aspects of sleep that are thought to be relevant to its memory-consolidating effects (eg, sleep spindles) are influenced profoundly by sleep homeostasis and circadian rhythmicity.[21,22]

The data summarized in this section demonstrate that under conditions of normal entrainment the phase relationship of the sleep–wake–dependent and circadian changes in performance are such that performance can be maintained throughout the waking episode, because the wake-dependent deterioration is countered by the circadian upswing. When wakefulness is extended into the biological night, performance deteriorates rapidly, because the wake-dependent decline no longer is opposed by the circadian arousal signal. The importance of sleep homeostasis and circadian rhythmicity is not limited to acute performance but extends to mood and to long-term changes in performance associated with learning and memory. The next section discusses the nature of the interaction between the two processes and their putative brain bases and neural correlates.

Interaction of Sleep Homeostasis and Circadian Rhythmicity: Observed Circadian Amplitude Depends on Homeostatic Sleep Pressure

The notion that the sleep homeostat and circadian rhythmicity regulate the consolidation of sleep and waking performance is widely accepted. In general, the two processes are thought to be independent: conceptual and mathematical models have assumed that the two oscillatory processes shape sleep and waking performance in an additive manner.[48] This assumption suggests that sleep propensity and waking performance can be predicted at any given time by addition of the circadian and homeostatic process. This assumption, in turn, leads to the prediction that the observed amplitude of the circadian modulation is independent of homeostatic sleep pressure and suggests that the circadian and homeostatic processes contribute independently to the variable of interest. Now, however, there is a wide range of observations that are at variance with such an additive contribution of the two processes. For example, the amplitude of the circadian rhythm of the propensity to wake up from sleep increases as sleep pressure dissipates. In the initial part of the sleep episode, the circadian amplitude is small (ie, humans can sleep at all circadian phases). By contrast, at the end of the sleep episode, when homeostatic sleep pressure is low, the circadian amplitude of the propensity to wake up is very large: humans still can maintain sleep consolidation at around the temperature nadir, but sleep becomes very disrupted on its rising phase. This change in circadian amplitude has been observed for the duration of wakefulness[21] as well as for both the frequency and duration of awakenings.[49] The amplitude of the circadian rhythm of the propensity to initiate sleep also changes with sleep pressure.[50,51]

One interpretation of this change in observed circadian amplitude is that increased homeostatic sleep pressure inhibits the circadian wake-promoting signal and amplifies the circadian sleep-promoting signal. Such an interaction between the circadian and homeostatic regulation leads to more rapid transitions between the vigilance states. The amplitude of the circadian rhythm of EEG characteristics during sleep, such as sleep spindles and the density of REMs during sleep, also changes with homeostatic sleep pressure, so that its amplitude increases as homeostatic sleep pressure dissipates.[23] Evidence for an interaction extends to the EEG during wakefulness: the observed amplitude increases as sleep pressure increases. This increase has been observed for delta and theta EEG activity but not for alpha activity: the robust circadian amplitude of alpha activity is not affected by homeostatic sleep pressure.[25]

The observed circadian amplitude for several aspects of waking performance also increases with homeostatic sleep pressure, so that the wake-dependent deterioration is minimal during the wake-maintenance zone and is most pronounced just after the core body temperature nadir[36] and a few hours after the melatonin maximum.[37] This interaction has been observed for several measures on the psychomotor vigilance task, namely, an addition task (**Fig. 2**), the digit symbol substitution task, and the occurrence of slow eye movements and unintentional sleep onset during scheduled wake episodes. These interactions, which were not observed for the probed-recall memory task, were statistically reliable in subjects living on a very long day (42.85-hour forced desynchrony with 28.57 hours of wakefulness).[16] The observed circadian amplitude of subjective sleepiness, as assessed by the Karolinska Sleepiness Scale, is very sensitive to changes in homeostatic sleep pressure and is statistically reliable in subjects living on a 20-hour day.[37]

Additional evidence for an interaction between the two oscillators stems from the observed modulation of the circadian period and amplitude of the

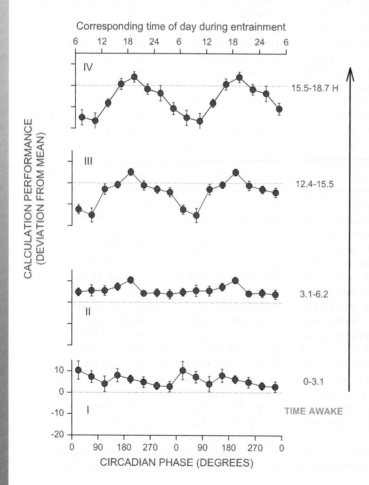

Fig. 2. Increase in the apparent circadian amplitude of calculation performance with increasing homeostatic sleep pressure. The circadian variation in performance was assessed while subjects were scheduled to 28-hour sleep/wake cycles in a forced desynchrony protocol, and data are segmented per quarter of the 18-hour, 40-minute scheduled wake episode. The circadian amplitude is very low during the first quarter of the wake period (0–3.1 hours awake), but it increases progressively so that performance is greatly impaired during the last quarter, particularly at and shortly after the nadir of the core body temperature rhythm (*zero on the x-axis*). (*Data from* Czeisler CA, Dijk DJ, Duffy JF. Entrained phase of the circadian pacemaker serves to stabilize alertness and performance throughout the habitual waking day. In: Ogilvie RD, Harsh JR editors. Sleep onset: normal and abnormal processes. Washington, DC: American Psychological Association, 1994;89–110; and Dijk DJ, Duffy JF, Czeisler CA. Circadian and sleep/wake dependent aspects of subjective alertness and cognitive performance. J Sleep Res 1992;1:112–7.)

melatonin rhythm by the sleep/wake cycle.[52] Thus, even a hormone, the rhythm of which is driven through a multisynaptic neural pathway from the SCN, is modulated by sleep–wake pressure, although these effects are relatively small.[53] These observations suggest that sleep homeostasis and circadian rhythmicity are not independent. The amplitude of any observed circadian rhythm depends on the status of the sleep homeostat.

The question then arises as to where in the central nervous system (CNS) the circadian and homeostatic oscillators meet and interact. Neuroanatomic and functional evidence suggest that output of the SCN reaches target areas such as the ventro-lateral-pre-optic area (VLPO), Tubero mammillary nucleus (TMN), lateral hypothalamus (LH), thalamus, and brain stem nuclei via the dorsal medial hypothalamus (DMH).[54] The diffuse activating systems, serotonin, orexin, noradrenaline, and histamine, all of which are under circadian control, impinge on many areas including thalamic and cortical areas. This very simplified neuroanatomic scheme of the circadian modulation of the CNS already suggests that the interaction with sleep homeostasis could take place at many different levels. In one scenario, for example, the circadian arousal signals a circadian rhythm of noradrenaline released from brainstem locus coeruleus (LC) neurons[55] or serotonin from dorsal raphe nuclei, which impinge on cortical or thalamic networks, to counter wake-dependent changes in these networks. The efficacy of these activating signals may be modified through adenosine, a putative mediator of homeostasis, or may depend on the strength of local connectivity. Alternatively, homeostatic sleep pressure may modify the firing patterns of the LC, dorsal raphe, or other nuclei of the diffuse activating systems. Other areas in which interaction may occur are the VLPO and the neurons synthesizing and releasing orexin. In fact, animal and human studies indicate that orexin is under both circadian and sleep–wake control[56,57] and that SCN lesions indeed abolish the circadian rhythm of orexin.[58,59]

Finally, evidence for feedback of the sleep/wake cycle and associated changes in SWA onto circadian rhythmicity has emerged at the level of multiple unit activity (MUA) of the SCN. This feedback concerns both acute changes in MUA in response to changes in SWA[60] and changes in the circadian amplitude of MUA in response to sleep deprivation.[61] These observations show that the interaction of sleep homeostasis and circadian rhythmicity extends to an output that is very close to the core circadian oscillator. Whether sleep homeostasis indeed can modulate the amplitude of circadian rhythms at the level of clock gene expression and translation, which are thought to constitute the core of the circadian oscillations in humans, remains unknown, although animal studies have provided evidence for such interactions.[62] Thus, there now is abundant evidence for an interaction of circadian rhythmicity at many different levels of description and many different areas in the brain. The discovery that canonical clock genes are expressed not only in the loci of the circadian pacemaker but also in many other brain areas adds another level of complexity with respect to the possible ways in which circadian rhythmicity and sleep homeostasis may interact.

Whatever the exact nature of the locus of the interaction may be, one implication of the interaction is that differences in observed circadian amplitude may be related to differences in homeostatic sleep pressure.

INTERINDIVIDUAL DIFFERENCES IN CIRCADIAN SLEEP PHENOMENOLOGY AND THE ROLE OF CLOCK GENES

Individuals differ in the timing and duration of sleep, their preferred timing for waking activities (including cognitive tasks), and their ability to maintain wakefulness and cognitive performance during sleep loss and circadian misalignment. Many of these characteristics have been shown to be trait-like, and variations in circadian and sleep physiology and genetic makeup associated with these phenotypes are being investigated intensively.

Circadian Correlates: Physiology and Clock Gene Expression

One line of investigation into circadian and sleep phenotypes is inspired by classic circadian entrainment theory, according to which the phase of a circadian pacemaker is determined by its intrinsic period (as well as by light sensitivity and light exposure, which are not discussed in this article). Variation in sleep–wake timing is predicted to be associated with variation in the phase of physiologic markers of the circadian pacemaker, even when assessed in the absence of the sleep/wake cycle (ie, in constant-routine conditions). These differences in phase are, in turn, predicted to be associated with differences in endogenous circadian period. The timing of the melatonin and core body temperature rhythms is earlier in morning types than evening types,[63] and the endogenous period of these variables, as assessed during forced desynchrony, is shorter in the former group.[64] The association between the entrained phase and endogenous period is reliable in young individuals but not in older people. Associations between sleep–wake timing and circadian markers extend to the level of clock gene expression in vivo and in vitro. Many clock genes are expressed rhythmically in peripheral tissues and cells, including peripheral blood cells in humans (**Fig. 3**).[65–67] In young adults, the timing of the rhythm of RNA expression of *PER3* in leukocytes, as assessed under constant-routine conditions, is associated with habitual sleep–wake timing, although this association is much weaker than the association with the melatonin rhythm.[65] This association was not significant for the clock genes *PER2* and *BMAL1*. The period of circadian gene expression, as monitored in vitro in fibroblast cell cultures through a luciferase reporter gene driven by the *Bmal1* promoter, differs between morning and evening types.[68] Morning types had an average period of 24.33 hours compared with 24.74 hours in evening types, and entrained phase correlated with period length, although there was significant spread and overlap between the two sets of data. This overlap suggests that other factors could account for circadian behavioral variation. Differences in the amplitude of clock gene expression could affect phase of entrainment. The study showed that, in individuals who have a normal circadian period, the clock gene expression was low in morning-type subjects and high in the evening types and that this difference correlated with larger phase shifts in the morning types.

The circadian oscillator also has been implicated in interindividual differences in sleep duration. Short sleepers have a shorter biological night, as indexed by the period of melatonin secretion, than long sleepers.[69]

Homeostatic Correlates

In another line of investigations, differences in sleep–wake timing and preference for the timing of waking activities are related to differences in the sleep homeostat. It has long been known that morning types have more slow-wave sleep (SWS) and SWA, in particular in the beginning of the sleep episode, and a more rapid decline of SWA during sleep.[70,71] This finding was confirmed recently in a series of analyses in which morning and evening types were subdivided into those who had an early or late circadian phase and those who had a normal circadian phase despite an extreme diurnal preference.[72,73] These analyses have suggested that people may be morning types either because of an early circadian phase or because of a more rapid build-up of homeostatic sleep pressure and associated changes in neural networks. In fact, it has been reported that, during wakefulness, theta activity in the EEG increases

more rapidly in morning types than in the evening types.[74] Individual differences in SWS and SWA, primary markers of the sleep homeostat, have been linked to polymorphisms in the adenosine-2 receptor and adenosine deaminase,[75] but whether these changes have functional consequences for waking performance remains to be established.

Amplitude Correlates

Analyses of the association between diurnal preference, as assessed by the Horne-Östberg questionnaire,[76] with patterns of clock gene expression in vitro have shown that part of the diurnal preference variation can be explained by differences in circadian period, but an approximately equal portion of the variance can be explained by differences in amplitude of clock gene expression.[68] Young and older people differ in their ability to perform when wakefulness is extended into the biological night. Although young people show a very strong deterioration of performance during the circadian night, the apparent circadian amplitude of this performance decrement is greatly attenuated in older people.[77] It should be noted, however, that SWS and SWA also are very much reduced in older people. Because the observed circadian amplitude is a consequence of the interaction of homeostatic sleep pressure and circadian rhythmicity,[21,36] differences in homeostasis may underlie these age-related changes in circadian amplitude of performance deterioration.

Role of PER3 in the Circadian and Homeostatic Regulation of Sleep and Cognition

The clock gene *PER3* is thought to exert a statistically significant but minor impact on traditional circadian assays such as the free-running period in animals.[78,79] In humans, the role of this clock gene has been investigated by analyzing the association of polymorphisms in the gene with circadian and sleep phenotypes. To date, a number of laboratories have reported polymorphisms in *PER3* to be associated with diurnal preference and delayed sleep phase syndrome.[80–82] The authors and colleagues[83] have reported that a primate-specific, variable-number tandem repeat (VNTR) polymorphism in *PER3*, the allele frequency of which varies with ethnicity,[84] exhibits a statistically significant but weak association with diurnal preference, as assessed with the Horne-Östberg scales. Individuals homozygous for the longer, 5-repeat allele (*PER3^{5/5}*) are more likely to show morning preference than individuals homozygous for the shorter, 4-repeat allele (*PER3^{4/4}*),[80]

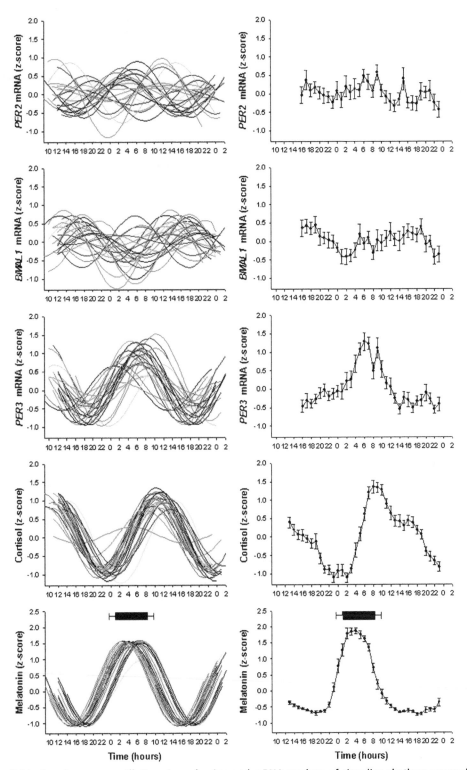

Fig. 3. Individual and average oscillations in endocrine and mRNA markers of circadian rhythms assessed during constant routine conditions. (*Left*) Z-scored normalized rhythms for *PER2*, *BMAL1*, *PER3*, cortisol, and melatonin are plotted relative to clock time. (*Right*) Average z-score curves (± SD). Mean sleep onset and wake times (± SD) are indicated by the black bar above the melatonin profile. (*From* Archer SN, Viola AU, Kyriakopoulou V, et al. Inter-individual differences in habitual sleep timing and entrained phase of endogenous circadian rhythms of *BMAL1*, *PER2* and *PER3* mRNA in human leukocytes. Sleep 2008;31(5):608–17; with permission.)

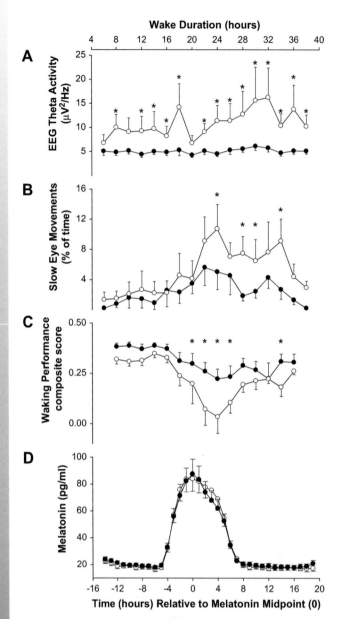

Fig. 4. Faster increase of homeostatic sleep pressure and more rapid deterioration of waking performance in *PER3*[5/5] (*open symbols*) than *PER3*[4/4] (*filled symbols*) during approximately 40 hours of wakefulness. Homeostatic sleep pressure is assessed by the increase in theta EEG activity and slow eye movements during wakefulness. Error bars represent SEMs. Data are plotted relative to the melatonin midpoint. (*From* Viola AU, Archer SN, James LM, et al. *PER3* polymorphism predicts sleep structure and waking performance. Curr Biol 2007;17(7):613–8; with permission.)

although the strength of this association declines with age.[85] As discussed earlier in this article, diurnal preference is a complex phenotype and may be determined by differences in both circadian rhythmicity and sleep homeostasis, among other unidentified factors. To investigate the contribution of the VNTR *PER3* polymorphism to circadian and sleep physiology, the authors and colleagues conducted a prospective study in which individuals were selected only on the basis of their *PER3* VNTR genotype. The investigators next characterized sleep physiology, circadian physiology, and the effects of sleep loss and circadian misalignment on cognitive decline in subjects

homozygous for the longer or shorter allele. No differences between the genotypes were observed with respect to circadian physiologic markers (such as the phase and amplitude of the melatonin and cortisol rhythm in plasma) or in the phase and amplitude of clock gene expression in leukocytes. Traditional markers of sleep homeostasis (ie, SWA during sleep, the increase of theta activity during wakefulness and during sleep deprivation, and the autonomic control of heart rate during sleep)[86] indicated a more rapid increase of homeostatic sleep pressure in *PER3*[5/5], however.[87] The more rapid increase in homeostatic sleep pressure was associated with a more rapid decline in a composite measure of cognitive performance during the biological night; that is, the apparent amplitude of the cognitive performance rhythm was much greater in PER3^{5/5} subjects than in PER3^{4/4} subjects (**Fig. 4**). Detailed analyses of the performance data showed that even though sleep loss and circadian phase misalignment affected many performance measures, the effects of genotype on deterioration of performance in the morning was particularly pronounced for measures of executive function, such as the verbal and spatial n-backs, paced visual serial addition tasks, and the delay in response on a serial addition task when a predictable sequence is replaced by a random sequence.[42] This observation, when replicated, may suggest that clock genes could affect specific aspects of cognition, even though these specific aspects also may be mediated through effects on sleep homeostasis.

Modeling the Effects of PER3 on Sleep Homeostasis, Circadian Rhythmicity, and the Cognitive Decline During Sleep Loss

The authors developed a simple conceptual model to describe the effects of the VNTR polymorphism. In this model, it is assumed that the VNTR exerts its effect through effects on sleep homeostasis. The nature and mechanism of these effects are unknown but could be related to effects on neural metabolisms that lead to more rapid changes in local connectivity in response to wakefulness in PER3^{5/5} or, alternatively, could reflect differences in activating influences on the EEG that may appear as changes in sleep homeostasis. The time course and absolute values of SWA during baseline and recovery sleep are consistent with a more rapid buildup and decline of homeostatic sleep pressure in PER3^{5/5} individuals,[87] and this difference is reflected in the differential time course of process S

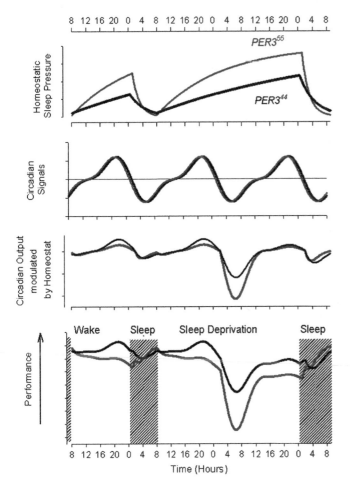

Fig. 5. Conceptual model for the regulation of the sleep/wake cycle and performance in PER3^{5/5} and PER3^{4/4} subjects. (*Top panel*) The homeostatic process S increases during wakefulness and declines during sleep. The time constants of this process are shorter in PER3^{5/5} subjects than in PER3^{4/4} subjects and the amplitude of the homeostatic oscillation during a normal sleep/wake cycle (*left side of panel*) is greater in PER3^{5/5} subjects. During sleep deprivation (*right side of panel*) there is a prolonged increase in process S followed by its return to baseline during recovery sleep. (*Second panel*) A circadian signal promoting wakefulness and sleep does not differ between the genotypes in either phase or amplitude. (*Third panel*) The circadian process modulated by S. At the end of the waking day, the attenuation of the wake-promoting signal by homeostatic sleep pressure is greater in PER3^{5/5} subjects than in PER3^{4/4} subjects. During sleep deprivation, the sleep-promoting signal, which is maximal in the morning hours, is amplified by homeostatic sleep pressure and is amplified to a greater degree in PER3^{5/5} subjects than in PER3^{4/4} subjects. (*Bottom panel*) Performance, which is a simple function of (C modulated by S) and S, is nearly stable during a normal waking day, although a small decline is observed in PER3^{5/5} subjects (as typical for morning types), whereas performance increases in PER3^{4/4} subjects (as typical for evening types). During sleep deprivation, performance is poorest in the early morning hours, particularly in PER3^{5/5} subjects. Note the correspondence between this time course and the time course of performance in **Fig. 4**.

(**Fig. 5**), which is derived from EEG SWA. Thus, during a normal sleep/wake cycle, the amplitude of the homeostatic oscillator, as represented by process S, is greater in $PER3^{5/5}$ subjects than in $PER3^{4/4}$ subjects. The physiologic and molecular circadian data are consistent with an identical amplitude and phase of a core circadian oscillator (C), and the investigators therefore have assumed process C to be identical. Based on data from forced desynchrony protocols, the authors assume that this process C generates a wake-promoting signal and a sleep-promoting signal. The feedback of sleep homeostasis on the process suggests that S modulates the amplitude of the wake- and sleep-promoting signals, inhibiting the wake-promoting signal and amplifying the sleep-promoting signal. As a consequence, the amplitude of the C process modulated by S is greater in $PER3^{5/5}$ subjects than in $PER^{4/4}$ subjects. Performance is represented by the difference of this C*H process and S. Under these assumptions, performance is nearly stable throughout a waking day in both $PER3^{5/5}$ and $PER3^{4/4}$ subjects, although minor differences between the two genotypes do emerge. In $PER3^{5/5}$ subjects, performance reaches its maximum just after awakening in the morning; in $PER3^{4/4}$ subjects this maximum is reached in the evening hours, just before bedtime. When wakefulness is extended into the biological night, the differences between the two genotypes escalate, not because the difference in S becomes much greater between the two genotypes but because of the interaction of S and C. The essence of the model is that a difference in the kinetics of a homeostatic process leads to differences in the negative effects of sleep loss on performance, in particular during the circadian morning. Thus, what is an apparent circadian phenotype derives from differences in sleep homeostasis.

A mutation in $PER2$ has been reported to affect the timing of sleep in members of a family afflicted with familial advanced sleep-phase syndrome.[88] To date, only effects on traditional circadian markers (ie, phase and period)[89] have been reported for this mutation, and the available sleep physiology data are insufficient to warrant any conclusion about effects on sleep homeostasis. Animal experiments, however, have shown that disruption to the clock genes $Cry1$, $Cry2$, $Clock$, $Npas2$, $Bmal1$, and Dbp all lead to effects on sleep physiology or EEG-derived parameters of sleep homeostasis (reviewed in[90]).

SUMMARY

Maintenance of performance throughout consecutive waking episodes requires adequate alignment of a circadian arousal rhythm with the sleep–wake homeostat. The two systems interact dynamically and contribute to many aspects of sleep physiology and waking performance, including learning and memory. How aspects of sleep physiology and their circadian and homeostatic regulation relate to performance remains largely unknown, although a role for SWS often is suggested. The close interaction between circadian rhythmicity and sleep homeostasis is underscored by the interdependence of circadian amplitude and homeostatic sleep pressure for many sleep and performance measures. Such a close interdependence also is consistent with the effects of clock genes on sleep homeostasis and the effects of the VNTR polymorphism in $PER3$ on markers of sleep homeostasis and cognitive decline in the early morning following sleep loss. Understanding the effects of these alterations in clock genes at the cellular level may provide insights into the nature of the sleep homeostat and its interaction with circadian rhythmicity.

ACKNOWLEDGMENTS

The authors thank Wendy May for editorial assistance.

REFERENCES

1. Czeisler CA, Dijk DJ. Human circadian physiology and sleep-wake regulation. In: Takahashi JS, Turek FW, Moore RY, editors. Handbook of behavioral neurobiology: circadian clocks. New York: Kluwer Academic/Plenum Publishing Co.; 2001. p. 531–61.
2. Dijk DJ, Lockley SW. Invited review: integration of human sleep-wake regulation and circadian rhythmicity. J Appl Physiol 2002;92(2):852–62.
3. Dijk DJ, von Schantz M. Timing and consolidation of human sleep, wakefulness, and performance by a symphony of oscillators. J Biol Rhythms 2005; 20(4):279–90.
4. Lockley SW, Skene DJ, Arendt J, et al. Relationship between melatonin rhythms and visual loss in the blind. J Clin Endocrinol Metab 1997;82(11):3763–70.
5. Roenneberg T, Kumar CJ, Merrow M. The human circadian clock entrains to sun time. Curr Biol 2007;17(2):R44–5.
6. Dijk DJ. Sleep of aging women and men: back to basics. Sleep 2006;29(1):12–3.
7. Ohayon MM, Carskadon MA, Guilleminault C, et al. Meta-analysis of quantitative sleep parameters from childhood to old age in healthy individuals: developing normative sleep values across the human lifespan. Sleep 2004;27(7):1255–73.
8. Groeger JA, Zijlstra FR, Dijk DJ. Sleep quantity, sleep difficulties and their perceived consequences

9. Klerman EB, Dijk DJ. Age-related reduction in the maximal capacity for sleep—implications for insomnia. Curr Biol 2008;18(15):1118–23.

10. Roenneberg T, Kuehnle T, Pramstaller PP, et al. A marker for the end of adolescence. Curr Biol 2004;14(24):R1038–9.

11. Koskenvuo M, Hublin C, Partinen M, et al. Heritability of diurnal type: a nationwide study of 8753 adult twin pairs. J Sleep Res 2007;16(2):156–62.

12. Duffy JF, Dijk DJ, Hall EF, et al. Relationship of endogenous circadian melatonin and temperature rhythms to self-reported preference for morning or evening activity in young and older people. J Investig Med 1999;47:141–50.

13. Mongrain V, Lavoie S, Selmaoui B, et al. Phase relationships between sleep-wake cycle and underlying circadian rhythms in morningness-eveningness. J Biol Rhythms 2004;19(3):248–57.

14. Johnson MP, Duffy JF, Dijk DJ, et al. Short-term memory, alertness and performance: a reappraisal of their relationship to body temperature. J Sleep Res 1992;1:24–9.

15. Dijk DJ, Czeislor CA. Paradoxical timing of the circadian rhythm of sleep propensity serves to consolidate sleep and wakefulness in humans. Neurosci Lett 1994;166:63–8.

16. Wyatt JK, Cajochen C, Ritz-De Cecco A, et al. Low dose, repeated caffeine administration for circadian-phase dependent performance degradation during extended wakefulness. Sleep 2004;27(3):374–81.

17. Wyatt JK, Ritz-De Cecco A, Czeisler CA, et al. Circadian temperature and melatonin rhythms, sleep, and neurobehavioral function in humans living on a 20-h day. Am J Physiol 1999;277(4 Pt 2):R1152–63.

18. Dijk DJ, Duffy JF, Riel E, et al. Ageing and the circadian and homeostatic regulation of human sleep during forced desynchrony of rest, melatonin and temperature rhythms. J Physiol (Lond) 1999;516(2):611–27.

19. Edgar DM, Dement WC, Fuller CA. Effect of SCN lesions on sleep in squirrel monkeys: evidence for opponent processes in sleep-wake regulation. J Neurosci 1993;13(3):1065–79.

20. Mistlberger RE. Circadian regulation of sleep in mammals: role of the suprachiasmatic nucleus. Brain Res Brain Res Rev 2005;49(3):429–54.

21. Dijk DJ, Czeisler CA. Contribution of the circadian pacemaker and the sleep homeostat to sleep propensity, sleep structure, electroencephalographic slow waves and sleep spindle activity in humans. J Neurosci 1995;15(5):3526–38.

22. Dijk DJ, Shanahan TL, Duffy JF, et al. Variation of electroencephalographic activity during non-rapid eye movement and rapid eye movement sleep with phase of circadian melatonin rhythm in humans. J Physiol (Lond) 1997;505(3):851–8.

23. Khalsa SBS, Conroy DA, Duffy JF, et al. Sleep- and circadian-dependent modulation of REM density. J Sleep Res 2002;11(1):53–9.

24. Wei HG, Riel E, Czeisler CA, et al. Attenuated amplitude of circadian and sleep-dependent modulation of electroencephalographic sleep spindle characteristics in elderly human subjects. Neurosci Lett 1999;260:29–32.

25. Cajochen C, Wyatt JK, Czeisler CA, et al. Separation of circadian and wake duration-dependent modulation of EEG activation during wakefulness. Neuroscience 2002;114(4):1047–60.

26. Cajochen C, Foy R, Dijk DJ. Frontal predominance of relative increase in sleep delta and theta EEG activity after sleep loss in humans. Sleep Res Online 1999;2(3):65–9.

27. Knoblauch V, Martens WLJ, Wirz-Justice A, et al. Regional differences in the circadian modulation of human sleep spindle characteristics. Eur J Neurosci 2003;18(1):155–63.

28. Krueger JM, Obal F. A neuronal group theory of sleep function. J Sleep Res 1993;2(2):63–9.

29. Tononi G, Cirelli C. Sleep function and synaptic homeostasis. Sleep Med Rev 2006;10(1):49–62.

30. Huber R, Ghilardi MF, Massimini M, et al. Local sleep and learning. Nature 2004;430(6995):78–81.

31. Kattler H, Dijk DJ, Borbély AA. Effect of unilateral somatosensory stimulation prior to sleep on the sleep EEG in humans. J Sleep Res 1994;3:159–64.

32. Basheer R, Porkka-Heiskanen T, Strecker RE, et al. Adenosine as a biological signal mediating sleepiness following prolonged wakefulness. Biol Signals Recept 2000;9(6):319–27.

33. Krueger JM, Obal F Jr. Sleep function. Front Biosci 2003;8:d511–9.

34. Reilly T, Atkinson G, Gregson W, et al. Some chronobiological considerations related to physical exercise. Clin Ter 2006;157(3):249–64.

35. Wever RA. The circadian system of man: results of experiments under temporal isolation. New York: Springer-Verlag; 1979. p. 1–276.

36. Dijk DJ, Duffy JF, Czeisler CA. Circadian and sleep/wake dependent aspects of subjective alertness and cognitive performance. J Sleep Res 1992;1:112–7.

37. Wyatt JK, Ritz-De Cecco A, Czeisler CA, et al. Circadian temperature and melatonin rhythms, sleep, and neurobehavioral function in humans living on a 20-h day. Am J Physiol 1999;277:R1152–63.

38. Wright KP Jr, Hull JT, Czeisler CA. Relationship between alertness, performance, and body temperature in humans. Am J Physiol Regul Integr Comp Physiol 2002;283(6):R1370–7.

39. Horowitz TS, Cade BE, Wolfe JM, et al. Searching night and day: a dissociation of effects of circadian

phase and time awake on visual selective attention and vigilance. Psychol Sci 2003;14(6):549–57.

40. Santhi N, Horowitz TS, Duffy JF, et al. Acute sleep deprivation and circadian misalignment associated with transition onto the first night of work impairs visual selective attention. PLoS ONE 2007;2(11): e1233.

41. Harrison Y, Jones K, Waterhouse J. The influence of time awake and circadian rhythm upon performance on a frontal lobe task. Neuropsychologia 2007;45(8): 1966–72.

42. Groeger JA, Viola AU, Lo JC, et al. Early morning executive functioning during sleep deprivation is compromised by a PERIOD3 polymorphism. Sleep 2008;31(8):1159–67.

43. Boivin DB, Czeisler CA, Dijk DJ, et al. Complex interaction of the sleep-wake cycle and circadian phase modulates mood in healthy subjects. Arch Gen Psychiatry 1997;54:145–52.

44. Koorengevel KM, Beersma DG, Den Boer JA, et al. Mood regulation in seasonal affective disorder patients and healthy controls studied in forced desynchrony. Psychiatry Res 2003;117(1):57–74.

45. Lockley SW, Dijk DJ, Kosti O, et al. Alertness, mood and performance rhythm disturbances associated with circadian sleep disorders in the blind. J Sleep Res 2008;17(2):207–16.

46. Wright KP Jr, Hull JT, Hughes RJ, et al. Sleep and wakefulness out of phase with internal biological time impairs learning in humans. J Cogn Neurosci 2006;18(4):508–21.

47. Schmidt C, Peigneux P, Muto V, et al. Encoding difficulty promotes postlearning changes in sleep spindle activity during napping. J Neurosci 2006; 26(35):8976–82.

48. Achermann P, Borbély AA. Simulation of daytime vigilance by the additive interaction of a homeostatic and a circadian process. Biol Cybern 1994;71:115–21.

49. Dijk DJ, Duffy JF, Czeisler CA. Age-related increase in awakenings: impaired consolidation of nonREM sleep at all circadian phases. Sleep 2001;24(5): 565–77.

50. Carskadon MA, Acebo C. Regulation of sleepiness in adolescents: update, insights, and speculation. Sleep 2002;25(6):606–14.

51. Carskadon MA, Acebo C, Jenni OG. Regulation of adolescent sleep: implications for behavior. Ann N Y Acad Sci 2004;1021:276–91.

52. Cajochen C, Jewett ME, Dijk DJ. Human circadian melatonin rhythm phase delay during a fixed sleep-wake schedule interspersed with nights of sleep deprivation. J Pineal Res 2003;35(3):149–57.

53. Zeitzer JM, Duffy JF, Lockley SW, et al. Plasma melatonin rhythms in young and older humans during sleep, sleep deprivation, and wake. Sleep 2007; 30(11):1437–43.

54. Saper CB, Scammell TE, Lu J. Hypothalamic regulation of sleep and circadian rhythms. Nature 2005; 437(7063):1257–63.

55. Aston-Jones G, Chen S, Zhu Y, et al. A neural circuit for circadian regulation of arousal. Nat Neurosci 2001;4(7):732–8.

56. Zeitzer JM, Buckmaster CL, Lyons DM, et al. Locomotor-dependent and -independent components to hypocretin-1 (orexin A) regulation in sleep-wake consolidating monkeys. J Physiol 2004;557(Pt 3): 1045–53.

57. Zeitzer JM, Buckmaster CL, Parker KJ, et al. Circadian and homeostatic regulation of hypocretin in a primate model: implications for the consolidation of wakefulness. J Neurosci 2003;23(8):3555–60.

58. Deboer T, Overeem S, Visser NA, et al. Convergence of circadian and sleep regulatory mechanisms on hypocretin-1. Neuroscience 2004;129(3):727–32.

59. Zhang S, Zeitzer JM, Yoshida Y, et al. Lesions of the suprachiasmatic nucleus eliminate the daily rhythm of hypocretin-1 release. Sleep 2004;27(4):619–27.

60. Deboer T, VanSteensel MJ, Detari L, et al. Sleep states alter activity of suprachiasmatic nucleus neurons. Nat Neurosci 2003;6(10):1086–90.

61. Deboer T, Detari L, Meijer JH. Long term effects of sleep deprivation on the mammalian circadian pacemaker. Sleep 2007;30(3):257–62.

62. Maret S, Dorsaz S, Gurcel L, et al. Homer1a is a core brain molecular correlate of sleep loss. Proc Natl Acad Sci U S A 2007;104(50):20090–5.

63. Duffy JF, Rimmer DW, Czeisler CA. Association of intrinsic circadian period with morningness-eveningness, usual wake time, and circadian phase. Behav Neurosci 2001;115(4):895–9.

64. Duffy JF, Czeisler CA. Age-related change in the relationship between circadian period, circadian phase, and diurnal preference in humans. Neurosci Lett 2002;318(3):117–20.

65. Archer SN, Viola AU, Kyriakopoulou V, et al. Interindividual differences in habitual sleep timing and entrained phase of endogenous circadian rhythms of BMAL1, PER2 and PER3 mRNA in human leukocytes. Sleep 2008;31(5):608–17.

66. Boivin DB, James FO, Wu A, et al. Circadian clock genes oscillate in human peripheral blood mononuclear cells. Blood 2003;102(12):4143–5.

67. Kusanagi H, Hida A, Satoh K, et al. Expression profiles of 10 circadian clock genes in human peripheral blood mononuclear cells. Neurosci Res 2008;61(2):136–42.

68. Brown SA, Kunz D, Dumas A, et al. Molecular insights into human daily behavior. Proc Natl Acad Sci U S A 2008;105(5):1602–7.

69. Aeschbach D, Sher L, Postolache TT, et al. A longer biological night in long sleepers than in short sleepers. J Clin Endocrinol Metab 2003;88(1):26–30.

70. Kerkhof GA, Lancel M. EEG slow wave activity, REM sleep, and rectal temperature during night and day sleep in morning-type and evening-type subjects. Psychophysiology 1991;28:678–88.

71. Lancel M, Kerkhof GA. Sleep structure and EEG power density in morning types and evening types during a simulated day and night shift. Physiol Behav 1991;49:1195–201.

72. Mongrain V, Carrier J, Dumont M. Difference in sleep regulation between morning and evening circadian types as indexed by antero-posterior analyses of the sleep EEG. Eur J Neurosci 2006;23(2):497–504.

73. Mongrain V, Carrier J, Dumont M. Circadian and homeostatic sleep regulation in morningness-eveningness. J Sleep Res 2006;15(2):162–6.

74. Taillard J, Philip P, Coste O, et al. The circadian and homeostatic modulation of sleep pressure during wakefulness differs between morning and evening chronotypes. J Sleep Res 2003;12(4):275–82.

75. Retey JV, Adam M, Honegger E, et al. A functional genetic variation of adenosine deaminase affects the duration and intensity of deep sleep in humans. Proc Natl Acad Sci U S A 2005;102(43):15676–81.

76. Horne JA, Östberg O. A self-assessment questionnaire to determine morningness-eveningness in human circadian rhythms. Int J Chronobiol 1976;4:97–110.

77. Adam M, Retey JV, Khatami R, et al. Age-related changes in the time course of vigilant attention during 40 hours without sleep in men. Sleep 2006; 29(1):55–7.

78. Bae K, Jin X, Maywood ES, et al. Differential functions of mPer1, mPer2, and mPer3 in the SCN circadian clock. Neuron 2001;30(2):525–36.

79. Shearman LP, Jin X, Lee C, et al. Targeted disruption of the mPer3 gene: subtle effects on circadian clock function. Mol Cell Biol 2000;20(17):6269–75.

80. Archer SN, Robilliard DL, Skene DJ, et al. A length polymorphism in the circadian clock gene Per3 is linked to delayed sleep phase syndrome and extreme diurnal preference. Sleep 2003;26(4):413–5.

81. Ebisawa T, Uchiyama M, Kajimura N, et al. Association of structural polymorphisms in the human period3 gene with delayed sleep phase syndrome. EMBO Rep 2001;2(4):342–6.

82. Pereira DS, Tufik S, Louzada FM, et al. Association of the length polymorphism in the human Per3 gene with the delayed sleep-phase syndrome: does latitude have an influence upon it? Sleep 2005;28(1):29–32.

83. von Schantz M, Jenkins A, Archer SN. Evolutionary history of the vertebrate Period genes. J Mol Evol 2006;62(6):701–7.

84. Nadkarni NA, Weale ME, von Schantz M, et al. Evolution of a length polymorphism in the human PER3 gene, a component of the circadian system. J Biol Rhythms 2005;20(6):490–9.

85. Jones KH, Ellis J, von SM, et al. Age-related change in the association between a polymorphism in the PER3 gene and preferred timing of sleep and waking activities. J Sleep Res 2007;16(1): 12–6.

86. Viola AU, James LM, Archer SN, et al. PER3 polymorphism and cardiac autonomic control: effects of sleep debt and circadian phase. Am J Physiol Heart Circ Physiol 2008;295(5):H2156–63.

87. Viola AU, Archer SN, James LM, et al. PER3 polymorphism predicts sleep structure and waking performance. Curr Biol 2007;17(7):613–8.

88. Toh KL, Jones CR, He Y, et al. An hPer2 phosphorylation site mutation in familial advanced sleep phase syndrome. Science 2001;291(5506):1040–3.

89. Jones CR, Campbell SS, Zone SE, et al. Familial advanced sleep-phase syndrome: a short-period circadian rhythm variant in humans. Nat Med 1999; 5(9):1062–5.

90. Dijk DJ, Franken P. Interaction of sleep homeostasis and circadian rhythmicity: dependent or independent systems. In: Kryger MH, Roth T, Dement WC, editors. Principles and practice of sleep medicine. 4th edition. Philadelphia: Elseviers Saunders; 2005. p. 418–34.

Physiologic and Health Consequences of Circadian Disruption (in Animal Models)

Aaron D. Laposky, PhD[a],*, Fred W. Turek, PhD[b]

KEYWORDS

- Suprachiasmatic nucleus • Circadian rhythms • Sleep
- Energy metabolism • Cardiovascular disease
- Shift work • Animal models

A primary role of the circadian clock is to entrain the organism to environmental cues, such as the light/dark (LD) cycle and food availability (external synchronization). The ability to anticipate changes in the environment, such as dusk and dawn, the presence of nutrients and predators, and temperature fluctuations, allows the organism to prepare its behaviors and physiology for optimal survival potential. Another critical role of the circadian system is to govern internal synchronization between multiple behaviors, physiologic systems, and molecular pathways to ensure that all of these processes, ranging from the sleep/wake cycle, to hormonal rhythms, to gene transcription, are aligned properly. Indeed, the many different diurnal/circadian rhythms throughout the body maintain specific phase relationships to one another. A guiding principal of circadian biology is that disruption of phase relationships between rhythms, whether behaviorally or genetically determined (ie, circadian desynchronization), results in perturbed physiologic functioning and may be a significant factor in a wide range of disease processes.

Advances in the field of circadian biology have resulted in a detailed understanding of the neuroanatomic and molecular components of the core circadian clock system.[1–3] Importantly, a functional transcriptional–translational feedback loop of circadian clock genes has been identified in virtually all organisms and organ systems of the body, suggesting a role for the circadian clock in the physiology and health of all animals, including humans.[4] In recent years, landmark behavioral and genetic discoveries have highlighted the notion that the circadian clock is involved in more than just temporal organization and that it may assert a fundamental role in physiologic homeostasis and be intimately involved in the pathophysiology of diseases.[3,5–9] This article reviews recent advances in circadian biology, with a particular focus on animal models that have elucidated important roles of the circadian system in various aspects of health and disease; references back to relevant human conditions are made when appropriate.

CIRCADIAN SYNCHRONIZATION AS A FACTOR IN HEALTH AND DISEASE

Virtually all behaviors and physiologic processes exhibit a circadian pattern. Some rhythms (ie, the sleep/wake cycle, feeding behavior, cognitive performance, levels of vigilance, body temperature, heart rate, and blood pressure) can be measured conveniently. Other rhythms, such as

This work was supported by Grant Nos. P01 AG011412 and HL075029 from the National Institutes of Health.
[a] National Center on Sleep Disorders Research, National Institutes of Health, National Heart, Lung, and Blood Institute/Division of Lung Diseases, 6701 Rockledge Drive, Suite 10042, Bethesda, MD 20892-7952, USA
[b] Center for Sleep and Circadian Biology, Northwestern University, 2200 Tech Drive/Hogan 2-160, Evanston, IL 60208, USA
* Corresponding author.
E-mail address: laposkya@nhlbi.nih.gov (A.D. Laposky).

hormone and neurotransmitter concentrations, lipid and carbohydrate metabolism, clock-gene expression, and the transcription of clock-controlled genes, are more difficult to measure. An overriding principal of circadian biology is that, under normal conditions, all behavioral, physiologic, and molecular rhythms are organized in a particular phase relationship with one another to confer optimal survival potential and health to the organism. The sleep/wake cycle represents the major circadian output rhythm, because most behavioral and physiologic processes are coordinated across these states of arousal. For example, sleep/wake states are accompanied by behavioral and hormonal changes that affect glucose metabolism.[10] The initial period of nocturnal sleep in humans is characterized by slow-wave sleep, peak growth hormone (GH) concentrations, and elevated blood glucose levels. The coordination of reduced glucose use by tissues throughout the body during slow-wave sleep, the gluconeogenic effects of GH, and decreased insulin release from pancreatic beta cells sustains blood glucose throughout the prolonged fasting state of sleep. In anticipation of morning arousal, cortisol levels begin to increase and contribute to enhanced cardiovascular tone and glucose use, two physiologic processes important for optimal waking behavior. Other hormones and neurotransmitters, such as ghrelin, leptin, hypocretin/orexin, and histamine, which exhibit circadian oscillations, are closely tied to the sleep/wake cycle and have significant roles in appetite regulation and metabolic homeostasis.[11-13] Indeed, disruptions to the sleep/wake cycle resulting from chronic partial sleep restriction and shift work are associated with impaired insulin sensitivity and glucose tolerance.[14,15] The link between sleep and energy metabolism is only one example of circadian-coupled processes. There are many scenarios in which temporal coordination between physiologic systems could affect a wide range of functions, ranging from neurobehavioral performance to the functioning of the immune, respiratory, cardiovascular, renal, gastrointestinal, and sympathetic/parasympathetic systems. Various scenarios will be discussed throughout this article.

than the ability of the circadian system to achieve a complete phase shift, the consequence may be chronic circadian desynchronization. Many adverse physiologic outcomes are linked to shift work, including increased body mass index, severe sleep disturbance, gastrointestinal disorders, cardiovascular disease, diabetes, infertility, and some forms of cancer.[15-19] These epidemiologic findings provide support for the hypothesis that the chronic disruption of circadian organization may lead to or aggravate abnormal functioning in multiple physiologic systems and increase the risk for disease.

Despite these important epidemiologic findings, surprisingly few experimental studies have been conducted to elucidate the precise mechanisms by which circadian desynchronization facilitates or causes physiologic perturbation and disease. Many important questions are open for experimental study. For example, in what situations might circadian disruption be the primary cause of alterations in physiologic functions? Do perturbations in circadian processes provoke the onset or exacerbate conditions to which the individual is genetically predisposed? What factors are responsible for individual differences in the effects of shift work on health? Furthermore, are the effects of circadian disruption based at the molecular and genetic levels in a tissue/organ-specific manner? Importantly, what are the mechanisms by which the circadian clock (ie, clock genes) interface with and co-regulates other molecular pathways? What are the environmental, physiologic, and molecular inputs to the clock that affect its function? The possibility of internal desynchronization as an underlying factor in disease states is particularly attractive in view of the recent and accumulating evidence that many tissues throughout the body contain the molecular circadian clock-gene machinery and may achieve some level of independence from suprachiasmatic nucleus (SCN) regulation.[5,20,21] Therefore, an important advance will be to understand what physiologic and molecular factors are involved in the links between circadian regulation/dysregulation and the function of multiple physiologic systems.

SHIFT WORK: EFFECTS OF CIRCADIAN DESYNCHRONIZATION ON HEALTH

Circadian misalignment may be most pronounced in the context of shift work, when an individual is forced to be awake, to eat, and to perform physical and cognitive tasks at times of day that may not be aligned with internal rhythms. When the demands of entrainment posed by shift work are greater

RESEARCH APPROACHES TO STUDY LINKS BETWEEN CIRCADIAN RHYTHMS, PHYSIOLOGY, AND DISEASE

Valuable behavioral and genetic animal models of circadian function and dysregulation have been developed to identify and understand the mechanisms underlying a wide range of circadian-related processes. Furthermore, the application of biochemical and genetic studies has allowed significant progress in characterizing the circadian system at the molecular level and in defining circadian mechanisms in individual organs/tissues. Most circadian studies have used experimental approaches to

- Elucidate the anatomic and molecular components of the circadian clock. Studies have aimed to identify neuronal pathways in the hypothalamus responsible for the integration of multiple circadian rhythms and to define the role of molecular clock programs in tissues throughout the body. These discoveries demonstrate that a functional molecular clock-gene network exists throughout the body and is positioned to have wide-ranging effects on multiple layers of physiologic regulation.
- Develop animal models of circadian desynchronization. Studies have examined the consequences of behavioral (eg, LD phase reversal and shifting) and genetic perturbations on physiological function (eg, clock-gene mutation, deletion, and overexpression) on physiologic function.
- Examine animal models of disease. Studies have investigated environmental and genetic models of disease (eg, diabetes, cardiovascular disease, gastrointestinal inflammation) to characterize the effects on circadian function.

ANATOMIC ORGANIZATION OF THE CIRCADIAN SYSTEM
The Suprachiasmatic Nucleus: Master Circadian Pacemaker

The SCN is the master circadian pacemaker of the central nervous system and consists of bilaterally paired group of neurons located in the anterior hypothalamus just above the optic chiasm.[22] The notion of the SCN as the central pacemaker arose from rodent models in which SCN lesions eliminated a wide range of rhythms, including the sleep/wake cycle, locomotor activity, corticosterone and leptin levels, glucose tolerance, and feeding and drinking behavior.[23–25] Ralph and colleagues[26] performed classic studies by transplanting the SCN from a host animal into SCN-lesioned wild-type and *tau*-mutant hamsters. The SCN-lesioned hamsters regained rhythms following the transplantation, and their circadian behavior (ie, a circadian free-running period of locomotor activity) reflected rhythms of the donor animal. Further support for a pacemaker function of the SCN was derived from recordings of isolated SCN tissue in which electrical activity and circadian clock-gene expression exhibited nearly 24-hour oscillatory patterns.[27–29] For example, circadian oscillation of *Period1* (*Per1*) gene expression in the SCN, as measured by a bioluminescent reporter transgene (*Per1-luciferase*), is maintained for longer than 1 month in the absence of any input or output signals.[27,30] The significance of these findings is that the SCN contains intrinsic mechanisms sufficient to generate circadian rhythms and to drive circadian output rhythms.

Suprachiasmatic Nucleus: Entrainment To The Light/Dark Cycle

Information about the external LD cycle is transduced into biologic signals primarily by a pathway leading from nonvisual photoreceptive ganglion cells in the retina to the SCN, known as the "retinohypothalamic tract."[31] When LD cues are not present (eg, in constant darkness), the SCN free runs with a period close to, but not exactly, 24 hours. Therefore, the SCN must make small adjustments on a daily basis to maintain the organism on a precise 24-hour cycle, a process termed "entrainment." There are situations in which the capacity and efficiency of the circadian system to entrain is challenged, as with the large phase-shift requirements that occur during shift work or travel across many time zones. Not all behavioral and molecular rhythms entrain at the same rate following a phase shift of the LD cycle. In nocturnal rodents, wheel-running behavior is used commonly as a reliable behavioral assay for entrainment to the LD cycle; rodents exhibit a dramatic increase in activity at dark onset. In response to a phase delay of the LD cycle, the locomotor activity rhythm shifts to the new schedule within 1 to 2 days, whereas following a phase advance, re-entrainment occurs more gradually,[32] as depicted in **Fig. 1**. Reddy and colleagues[32] revealed a dissociation between molecular clock components within the SCN during a 6-hour LD phase advance in mice: *mPer1* expression adjusted quickly to the LD shift, whereas *mCry1* expression shifted more slowly, as did the locomotor activity rhythm.[32] Other studies have identified dissociations between clock-gene expression and electrical activity in the SCN, as well as between central versus peripheral molecular rhythms following phase shifts of the LD cycle.[27,33,34] The studies indicate how the demands of being exposed to phase shifts on a repeated basis may result in a state of chronic circadian desynchronization, whereby the phase relationships of rhythms throughout the body remain uncoupled from one another.

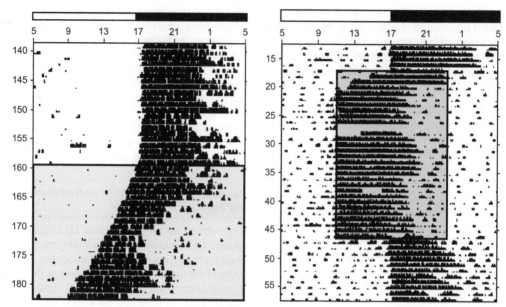

Fig. 1. Locomotor activity recording in a C57BL/6J mouse. (*Left*) A typical recording of mouse wheel-running behavior. There is a sudden onset of wheel running at dark onset (17:00, 5 PM) and minimal wheel running during the light period when animals are entrained to an external 12/12 LD cycle (indicated by the white-and-black bar above the actogram). When the lights are turned off permanently (constant darkness, *shaded box*), there is a clear daily rhythm in wheel-running behavior, but the onset is advanced by about 20 minutes each day (ie, the activity rhythm is free running). The free-running rhythm is taken to indicate the endogenous function of the circadian pacemaker in the absence of LD cues. (*Right*) A recording of mouse locomotor activity detected by counting infrared sensor beam breaks. The mouse was maintained on a 12/12 LD cycle with dark onset at 17:00 (5 PM) for the first 5 days of recording. There is a clear increase in locomotor activity at the beginning of the dark phase and only periodic activity during the light period. Because infrared sensors pick up spontaneous activity, this method detects more movement during the light phase than seen with a running wheel, which is a more specific measure of motivated running behavior. The LD cycle was advanced by 6 hours (lights off at 11:00; *shaded block*) for a period of approximately 32 days. The mouse gradually entrained to the new LD cycle over 5 days. Next, the LD cycle was phase delayed by 6 hours (lights off at 17:00) for the remainder of the recording. The mouse quickly entrained to the phase delay within 1 to 2 days. The principle that adjustments to a phase delay occur more quickly than adjustments to a phase advance is consistent in rodents and humans. In both frames, the y-axis represents consecutive days of recording.

Anatomic Integration of Circadian Regulation

According to the traditional hierarchy of circadian organization, the SCN functions as the primary circadian oscillator entrained to the 24-hour solar day that drives and coordinates all other rhythms of the body. There has been substantial interest in identifying the mechanisms by which the SCN sustains and coordinates output rhythms. In part, the SCN produces diffusible factors (eg, transforming growth factor-α [TGF-α], prokineticin-2 [PK2], cardiotrophin-like cytokine, and vasopressin) that are released in a circadian pattern and that may exert direct effects on behavior, such as locomotor activity. Comprehensive reviews of SCN cellular anatomy and endocrine physiology are available.[22,28,35] (Also see the article by Gillette and Abbot elsewhere in this issue.)

In addition, the SCN is integrated into a network of neuronal projections within the hypothalamus. Based on one anatomic model, a dense projection of fibers leads from the SCN to the ventral and dorsal regions of the subparaventricular zone (SPZ) of the hypothalamus (**Fig. 2**).[2] SPZ fibers project to the dorsomedial nucleus of the hypothalamus (DMH), which is connected to (1) the ventrolateral preoptic area, important in sleep/wake control,[36] (2) the paraventricular nucleus, which contains neurons that synthesize corticotrophin-releasing hormone and neurons that mediate pre-ganglionic outputs of the autonomic nervous system,[35] and (3) the lateral hypothalamic area, where the hunger-stimulating neuropeptides, hypocretin and melanin-concentrating hormone, are produced.[37] Targeted neurotoxic lesions of the SPZ and DMH impair sleep/wake, locomotor activity, body temperature, corticosterone, and

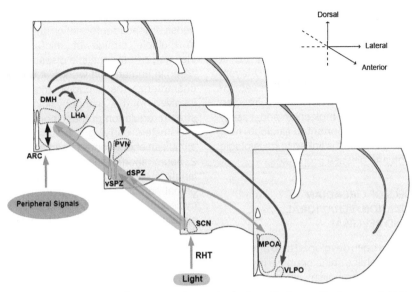

Fig. 2. Suprachiasmatic nuclei input and output pathways in the hypothalamus. Environmental LD cues are transduced to the suprachiasmatic nuclei (SCN) via the retinohypothalamic tract (RHT). The SCN sends a major projection to the ventral and dorsal subparaventricular zone (sPVZ), which then transmits SCN signals to a variety of nuclei involved in sleep/wake, feeding, energy expenditure, and autonomic regulation (details provided in text). ARC, arcuate nucleus; DMH, dorsomedial nucleus of the hypothalamus; LHA, lateral hypothalamic area (including hypocretin and melanin-concentrating hormone–containing neurons); MPOA, medial preoptic area; PVN, paraventricular nucleus; VLPO, ventrolateral preoptic area. In the coronal sections of the anterior and posterior hypothalamic areas, note that the SCN, SPVZ and ACR are located in the mediobasal hypothalamus surrounding the third ventricle. (*From* Laposky AD, Bass J, Kohsaka A, et al. Sleep and circadian rhythms: key components in the regulation of energy metabolism. FEBS Lett 2007;582:147; with permission.)

metabolic rhythms, indicating that these areas are important relay sites where the SCN integrates multiple physiologic processes.[38] Kalsbeek and colleagues[35] have performed detailed anatomic studies identifying the paraventricular nucleus as an integrative site for SCN and autonomic communication. An important hypothesis resulting from these studies is that alteration in the temporal control of sympathetic/parasympathetic output can have a major effect on glucose homeostasis and liver function and ultimately on the pathophysiology of diabetes and cardiometabolic disease.[39]

The DMH has been considered a possible neural locus of the food-entrainable oscillator (FEO).[40] In nocturnal rodents, when food availability is restricted to a block of time during the normal fasting period (ie, light phase), rhythms such as sleep/wake, locomotor activity (ie, food-anticipatory activity), corticosterone, body temperature, and gene expression in the liver shift to anticipate feeding time by a few hours.[38,41,42] Surprisingly, data from circadian gene-expression and SCN-lesion studies indicate that the FEO operates independently from the light-entrainable oscillator.[41,43–45] In one rat study, neurotoxic lesions targeted to the DMH eliminated food-anticipatory behavior, particularly in

general cage activity, sleep/wake, and body temperature rhythms.[38] In contrast, a separate study in rats that measured food bin approaches rather than locomotor activity reported intact food entrainment following large electrolytic DMH lesions.[46] Molecular-based studies have identified that c-fos activation in the DMH shifts to correspond with meal timing and that the expression of *Period2* (*Per2*), a core circadian clock gene, in the DMH entrains to feeding time.[47] The DMH receives input from the arcuate nucleus, an area of the mediobasal hypothalamus that has been well characterized with respect to the regulation of food intake and energy expenditure, as well as for the ability to monitor peripheral energy status, particularly through leptin receptor signaling.[2,48] Despite the discrepant findings between lesion studies[38,46] and disagreements about the interpretation of data involving the DMH and synchronization to feeding cycles,[49,50] the DMH remains a potentially important integrative region of the hypothalamus for food entrainment as well as for the coordination of multiple physiologic signals under normal and phase-shifted conditions.

In summary, although light is the major input signal to entrain the SCN, other oscillators have been identified that are responsive to food availability and to methamphetamine administration, independently of the SCN.[41,51,52] These important discoveries reveal that circadian alignment results from multiple input signals and from many layers of physiologic and molecular integration. As investigations continue to operationalize "circadian desynchronization" at the molecular and tissue-specific levels, it will be important to elucidate how chronic circadian disruption is linked to physiologic systems function and disease processes.

ANIMAL MODELS OF CIRCADIAN DESYNCHRONIZATION: BEHAVIORAL PHASE SHIFT AND REVERSAL

Animal models have been developed to examine the effects of persistent phase shifts or phase reversals on life span, energy metabolism, and cardiovascular function. Nearly a decade ago, Penev and colleagues[53] discovered that continuous reversal of the LD cycle each week in cardiomyopathic hamsters reduced median life span by 11% compared with nonshifted cardiomyopathic control animals. Repeated 6-hour phase advances or delays of the LD cycle increase mortality in very old mice (27–31 months of age) when compared with nonshifted age-matched control animals.[54] A recent study shows that repeated LD phase reversals dramatically exacerbate weight loss and increase mortality in mice with chemically induced (ie, dextran sodium sulfate) colitis versus nonshifted animals receiving the same chemical.[55] These studies show that circadian desynchronization, when combined with risk factors or underlying disease processes (eg, cardiovascular disease, advanced age, or gastrointestinal insult), can worsen the respective disease conditions and/or produce synergistically detrimental effects.

Increases in body weight occur in young healthy rats following 3 months of LD phase reversal (biweekly) compared with nonshifted rats.[56,57] Using a different phase-shifting paradigm, Salgado-Delgado and colleagues[58] held the LD cycle constant but phase shifted the sleep/wake cycle in rats by placing them in slowly rotating wheels during either the light or dark phase on alternating weeks. This phase shifting led to an increase in weight gain compared with control animals.[58] In contrast, phase shifting the LD cycle in healthy CD1F2 female or C57BL6 J mice has no effect on body weight.[55,59] Because few studies have been performed, there is insufficient evidence on how the effects of circadian desynchronization are influenced by species, by the methodology used to disrupt the rhythms, or by genetic background. Differences in genetic background may

be particularly important because of the comprehensive genetic information that now is available in multiple strains of mice. Considering the elevated risk for multiple disease conditions implicated in human shift work,[17] it will be important to characterize the circadian mechanisms that are involved in the pathophysiology and/or downstream regulation of these conditions.

Hamsters carrying a mutation in the *tau* gene exhibit an endogenous circadian period of 22 hours, 2 hours shorter than the external 24-hour day length.[60] Heterozygous *tau* mutants develop cardiorenal pathology when maintained on a 12/12 LD cycle, but the condition is improved when they are entrained to an 11/11 LD cycle that is closer to their endogenous circadian period.[61] Furthermore, the adverse cardiovascular effects of experimentally induced cardiac hypertrophy (ie, transverse aortic constriction) are more pronounced in mice maintained on a 10/10 LD regimen than in those on a 12/12 LD cycle.[62] The homozygous *Clock*-mutant mouse has an extremely long free-funning period, close to 28 hours.[63] These mice are hyperphagic and obese and exhibit other symptoms reflective of the metabolic syndrome when housed in a 12/12 LD environment.[9] The effect of placing *Clock*-mutant mice on a 28-hour day (eg, 14/14 LD) to alleviate their cardiometabolic symptoms has not been examined, however.

Drosophila is a fundamental organism in circadian research, particularly in the discovery of genes and molecular pathways. Interestingly, flies maintained on a non–24-hour LD cycle (eg, a 21- or 27-hour cycle) or in constant light have shorter life spans than flies kept on a 12/12 LD cycle.[64] Furthermore, flies harboring mutations in a core circadian clock gene, *cycle*, suffer higher mortality in response to sleep deprivation than wild-type flies.[65] In combination, these findings are provocative, pointing to the importance of circadian alignment between the lengths of external and endogenous periods in cardiovascular, metabolic, and renal function and undoubtedly also in as-yet-undiscovered processes. These studies also highlight the opportunity to use a range of experimental paradigms (eg, LD phase reversal, LD phase shifting, and environmental-endogenous period mismatch) to examine the effects of circadian desynchronization on specific physiologic systems and health outcomes.

THE MOLECULAR BASIS OF CIRCADIAN RHYTHMS: CIRCADIAN CLOCK GENES
The Core Circadian Clock Machinery

The discovery of the molecular basis of circadian rhythms represents a seminal advance in circadian biology and has profound implications for the understanding of physiology and disease. The first clock genes were discovered using forward genetics approaches in flies, and *Drosophila* models have remained instrumental in circadian gene discovery and in elucidating the complexity of circadian genetics.[66,67] Importantly, the molecular circadian clock is highly conserved from at least flies to mice to humans and exists in organisms as diverse as bacteria, *Neurospora*, *Drosophila*, mammals, and even plants.[4] The retention of a circadian clock across diverse organisms and millions of years of evolution suggests that circadian machinery is an integral component of life. The molecular basis for circadian rhythm generation involves an integrated circuit of circadian clock genes that exists in individual cells and functions in a cell-autonomous manner. This molecular program involves transcriptional–translational feedback loops with positive- and negative-acting components that cycle naturally with a nearly 24-hour periodicity.[68] The first mammalian circadian clock gene, named *Clock* (c̲ircadian l̲ocomotor o̲utput c̲ycles k̲aput), was discovered using a mutagenesis and locomotor activity–screening approach in mice.[63,69] When placed in constant darkness, homozygous *Clock* mutant mice exhibit a strikingly long (approximately 28-hour) free-running period in locomotor activity, often followed in a few weeks by a complete loss of rhythmicity.[63] After the discovery of *Clock*, rapid progress was made in identifying other molecular components of the mammalian circadian transcriptional–translational feedback loop as well as various posttranslational mechanisms that contribute to the fine-tuned kinetics of this circuitry.[3] Interestingly, circadian phenotypes vary by specific clock-gene mutations or deletions, indicating that individual clock genes have a unique role in the output function of the circadian clock. **Fig. 3** depicts the core circadian clock genes; comprehensive reviews are available that describe this genetic system in great detail and provide a comparative analysis between species.[3,4,70] In brief, mammalian *Clock* and *Bmal1* (B̲rain and m̲uscle Arnt-like 1, also called "*Mop3*") encode transcription factors CLOCK and BMAL1, which contain the basic helix-loop-helix PAS (P̲eriod-A̲rnt-S̲ingle-minded) domain. CLOCK:BMAL1, which forms the positive limb of

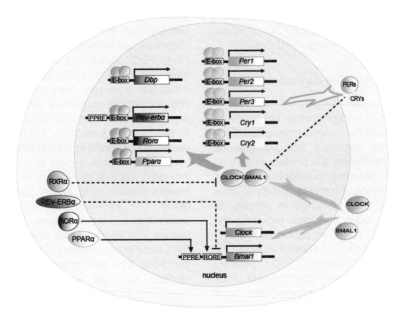

Fig. 3. Transcriptional–translational feedback loop of core circadian clock genes. This diagram depicts the positive (CLOCK:BMAL1) and negative (PER:CRY) limbs of the circadian clock-gene feedback loop that is present in virtually all cells throughout the body. REV-ERBα and RORα represent components of a secondary feedback loop that either activate (*solid line*) or inhibit (*dashed line*) *Bmal1* activity. The CLOCK:BMAL1 transcription complex has the ability to directly mediate the activity of genes (clock-controlled genes) critically involved in energy metabolism, including *Dbp* and *Pparα*. In turn, PPARα can bind directly to *Bmal1* and influence activation of the positive limb of the feedback loop. BMAL1, brain muscle Arnt-like factor; CLOCK, circadian locomotor output cycles kaput; CRY, cryptochrome; DBP, albumin D-element binding protein; PER, period; PPARα, peroxisome proliferators-activated factor α; REV-ERBα, reverse erythroblastosis virus α; RORα, retinoic acid receptor-related orphan receptor α. (*From* Laposky AD, Bass J, Kohsaka A, et al. Sleep and circadian rhythms: key components in the regulation of energy metabolism. FEBS Lett 2007;582:148; with permission.)

the feedback loop, binds to E-box *cis*-regulatory enhancer elements in the promoter region of *Period* (*Per1*, *Per2*, and *Per3*) and *Cryptochrome* (*Cry1* and *Cry2*) genes and drives the expression of these transcripts. Cytoplasmic PER:CRY translocates to the nucleus to inhibit *Per* and *Cry* transcription further by repressing activation of CLOCK:BMAL1, thus forming the negative limb of the circuitry. The kinetics of the feedback loop can be modified significantly by posttranslational mechanisms, such as casein kinase 1ε, which modulates the phosphorylation of cytoplasmic PER:CRY and subsequent translocation into the nucleus. The identification of posttranslational mechanisms and additional elements of the feedback loop continues to be an active area of circadian biology research.[70] Recent findings that some proteins oscillate, even when their respective mRNA sequences do not, has highlighted the importance of understanding circadian regulation at the posttranslational and proteomic levels.[5] As discussed later, the circadian circuitry is integrated directly at the level of DNA binding with other metabolic pathways, such as those regulating energy metabolism and cardiovascular physiology. Therefore, alteration in clock-gene function not only has the potential to alter temporal organization but also may impact homeostatic regulation in multiple physiologic systems.

Peripheral Clocks and Cell-Autonomous Oscillators

A paradigm shift in understanding the range of possible functions of the molecular circadian clock occurred with the discovery that autonomous circadian clock oscillators are present in tissues outside the SCN, including multiple brain regions and peripheral organs. Rhythmic activity in core clock genes has been detected in virtually all tissues that have been analyzed, including the heart,[71,72] liver,[41,71] lung[27,73] pancreas,[74] gut,[75] vascular smooth muscle,[72,76] skeletal muscle,[27,77] adipose tissue,[78,79] kidney,[30,73,80] pituitary gland,[73] and bone marrow.[81] Not only are clock genes present in peripheral tissues, the clock circuitry maintains an architecture (ie, phase relationships) similar to that of the central pacemaker (eg, *Bmal1* and *Period* transcripts cycle in antiphase to one another). A common ex vivo approach to detect patterns in clock-gene expression is to collect tissue samples at multiple time points across the LD cycle or in constant darkness (ie, usually every 2–4 hours) and to quantify mRNA expression levels. This approach yields a profile of peak and nadir mRNA levels; the precision of the profile depends on how frequently the tissue samples are collected. Examination of mRNA expression also provides a way to examine whether the oscillators in different tissues are cycling in alignment or are out of phase with each other.

An important aspect of circadian function that cannot be ascertained using ex vivo tissue analysis is whether the circadian clock is operating in an independent and self-sustaining manner in peripheral tissues: it is possible that the clock gene rhythms detected in tissue isolated at specific time points are simply passive reflections of central clock output signals. This scenario would be consistent with a traditional hierarchical model of circadian organization. As previously discussed, however, the ability of locomotor activity, corticosterone, and clock genes in the liver to entrain to food restriction (ie, FEO) provides important clues that particular behavioral, physiologic, and molecular rhythms can be regulated independently of SCN output.[41] A completely dominant hierarchical model also does not explain adequately why, after a phase shift of the LD cycle, SCN and peripheral rhythms entrain with different time courses or, in some instances, never achieve complete phase readjustment.

Balsalobre and colleagues[82] performed classic experiments to show that, after serum shock, immortalized rat-1 fibroblasts exhibit repetitive circadian oscillations in core clock genes (eg, *Per1*, *Per2*, *Rev-Erbα*) and in clock-controlled genes (eg, *Dbp*). Inventive studies using the bioluminescent transgene *Per1-luciferase* allowed the first opportunity to monitor clock-gene (ie, *Per1*) rhythms in real time over prolonged periods of time in culture. Amazingly, *Per1*-driven *luciferase* expression exhibits spontaneous circadian rhythmicity for multiple cycles in peripheral tissues, including extra-SCN regions of the brain, liver, skeletal muscle, lung, kidney, cornea, and pineal gland.[27,41,83] *Per1-luciferase* read-outs also reveal unique features of circadian regulation in individual tissues. For example, the free-running period of *Per1* and *Per2-luciferase* cycling is tissue specific, indicating that the molecular clock program is similar, but not identical, throughout the body.[27,73] In peripheral tissues extracted from SCN-lesioned animals, *Per2-luciferase* expression continues to oscillate in a circadian manner, but the phase relationships between the individual tissues are altered, suggesting some autonomy in clock function between different tissues.[73] In response to 6-hour phase advances or delays in the LD cycle, *Per1-luciferase* expression shifts almost immediately in the SCN but takes several days to entrain or shows incomplete entrainment in skeletal muscle, liver, and the lung.[27] Furthermore, the period length of *Per1-luciferase* expression is altered in aged rats as compared with young animals in some tissues (eg, paraventricular nucleus of the hypothalamus, pineal gland, and kidney), but not in others (eg, SCN, arcuate nucleus, pituitary, cornea, liver, and lung).[30] Yoo and colleagues[73] found *Per2-luciferase* circadian oscillations in the periphery, with some tissues exhibiting persistent rhythms for more than 20 days in undisturbed culture. In combination, these studies provide definitive evidence that peripheral circadian clocks are cell autonomous and generate self-sustained oscillations yielding unique phenotypes in different tissues/organ systems. These results also highlight the potential heterogeneity in the physiologic and molecular functions that the clock may serve, depending on the respective tissue/organ system or cell type. The fundamental question remains, however, as to what local functions self-sustained clock programs serve in individual tissue/organ systems.

Because clock genes function as transcription factors, they have the potential to drive oscillations in many other genes, referred to as "clock-controlled genes." Microarray techniques allow the expression of hundreds to thousands of genes to be measured simultaneously using rigorous statistical analyses. The most comprehensive microarray studies in SCN, liver, heart, and adipose tissue indicate that a notable proportion of the transcriptome (ie, 5%–20%) is under circadian regulation.[71,78,84,85] Importantly, these studies show there is little overlap in the genes that cycle between different tissues, and the same clock gene can exhibit different expression profiles in different tissues. Many clock-controlled genes represent key components (eg, rate-limiting steps) in molecular pathways related to intermediary metabolism, cell division, and xenobiotic detoxification. This diversity in gene expression indicates that the downstream targets of the core clock are largely tissue specific, so that particular tissues and cells are able to carry out unique functions. Through its effects on distinct clock-controlled pathways, the core circadian clock can diversify its role in physiologic and molecular regulation. The anatomic and molecular architecture of the clock is designed in a way that allows circadian rhythms to affect a wide range of behavioral, physiologic, and molecular systems.

CIRCADIAN REGULATION OF SLEEP/WAKE HOMEOSTASIS

Genetic models of circadian clock disruption have pointed toward unique roles of the molecular clock in sleep/wake regulation. For example, homozygous *Clock* mutant mice have large increases in wake time (approximately 2 hours/day), in addition to increased sleep fragmentation, impaired recovery from sleep deprivation, and a trend for reduced electroencephalographic non–rapid eye movement delta power compared with wild-type controls.[86] This study was the first mammalian study to show that clock genes affect aspects of sleep homeostasis, not just the temporal organization of sleep/wake states. Interestingly, *Bmal1* deficient (*Bmal1*$^{-/-}$) mice have large increases in sleep time (approximately 1.5 hours/day) and elevated electroencephalographic non–rapid eye movement delta power, in sharp contrast to *Clock* mutants.[86,87] Despite elevated sleep time, *Bmal1*$^{-/-}$ mice have fragmented sleep across the LD cycle, with increased arousals and sleep bouts of short duration. Sleep patterns between *Bmal1*$^{-/-}$ and *Cryptochrome 1,2*-deficient (*Cry1,2*$^{-/-}$) mice are similar, except that *Cry1,2*$^{-/-}$ mice have enhanced sleep consolidation.[88] Data from other animals with altered function of core clock genes (eg, *Period* mutants and *Npas2* [*Neuronal PAS domain protein 2*]-deficient mice) and clock-controlled genes (eg, *Dbp*, *PK2*, and *TGF-α* knockouts) also show distinct alterations in sleep/wake regulation.[89–92] Although a comprehensive comparison of sleep/wake patterns between genetic models is beyond the scope of this article, it is important to note that each circadian model exhibits a unique sleep/wake phenotype. These results demonstrate that the circadian clock does not have a ubiquitous role in sleep/wake regulation, but the interplay between sleep phenotype and circadian genetics is specific and certainly complex.

It is interesting that in female mice, wake time is significantly increased and consolidated at the beginning of the active (ie, dark) period compared with male mice and that this sex difference is eliminated following gonadectomy.[93] It is tempting to hypothesize that the circadian drive for wakefulness may be greater in female mice than in male mice, but this conjecture remains to be determined experimentally. In future studies, it will be important to determine exactly how genetic circadian perturbations interface with sleep regulatory mechanisms. For example, is sleep mediated purely by circadian processes in the SCN, or are extra-SCN and peripheral clocks involved? The authors' laboratory has found that SCN-lesioned *Clock* mutant mice still exhibit a high-wake phenotype (F.W. Turek, unpublished observations, 2000), suggesting that the *Clock* mutation affects sleep through extra-SCN mechanisms. Furthermore, *Npas2* is a paralogue of *Clock* but is not expressed in the SCN of mice. *Npas2*$^{-/-}$ animals show a high-wake phenotype, indicative of extra-SCN–mediated sleep/wake effects.[89,90] Advanced genetic techniques, such as knocking out or overexpressing clock genes in a tissue-specific manner, will provide substantial opportunities to understand clock–sleep interactions in greater detail.[94,95] Ultimately, circadian molecular investigations may lead the way for the discovery of novel drug targets and perhaps for developing nonpharmacologic approaches to treat sleep/wake problems.

CIRCADIAN REGULATION AND ENERGY METABOLISM

Major organs involved in carbohydrate and lipid metabolism, including the liver, pancreas, and adipose tissue, contain cell-autonomous clock-gene programs.[27,74,79] Microarray studies have identified circadian expression of many clock-controlled genes that are components of intermediary metabolic pathways.[71,78,85] Of particular interest is the direct interaction between CLOCK:BMAL1 and the nuclear orphan receptors, including reverse erythroblastosis virus-alpha (Rev-Erbα) and retinoic acid receptor-related orphan receptor-alpha (RORα), which form a secondary circadian clock feedback loop,[25] as depicted in **Fig. 3**. CLOCK:BMAL1 drives the transcription of *Rev-Erbα* and *Rorα* through binding to *ROR* response elements in the promoter region of these genes. In response, REV-ERBα and RORα inhibit and activate *Bmal1* transcription, respectively, to fine tune the kinetics of the clock-gene circuitry. Studies have implicated both *Rev-Erbα* and *Bmal1* in the process of adipocyte differentiation and lipogenesis.[5,96,97] The direct links between clock genes and nuclear orphan receptors point to distinct co-regulation between the circadian clock and gluconeogenic and lipogenic pathways. Other examples of interlinked circadian and metabolic pathways include direct transcriptional regulation between core circadian clock genes and *Pparα* (*peroxisome proliferator-activator receptor alpha*), a fatty acid–responsive nuclear receptor involved in lipid and glucose metabolism, *Gsk3* (*glycogen synthase kinase 3*), a key modulator of carbohydrate metabolism, and *Srebp-1* (*sterol regulatory element binding protein 1*), a transcriptional regulator of lipogenesis.[5,25] In fact, a large number of nuclear orphan receptors display circadian expression patterns, although the extent to which each of these transcripts is driven directly or indirectly by the circadian clock has not been determined.[98] A critical aspect of these circadian–metabolic molecular interactions is the extent to which they are important for normal physiologic functioning and/or contribute to disease processes. For example, it

will be important to determine whether obesity, diabetes, cardiovascular disease, and other disease conditions are accompanied by alterations in circadian regulation that could have a causative and/or exacerbating role in these disease processes and interfere with the effectiveness of therapies. The following paragraphs present an overview some of the progress made in developing animal models to examine the circadian–metabolism interplay.

An analysis of homozygous *Clock* mutant mice (C57BL/6 J background) revealed a surprising metabolic phenotype consisting of obesity and other symptoms of the metabolic syndrome: hyperleptinemia, hyperlipidemia, hepatic steatosis, and hyperglycemia with impaired insulin production.[9] These mice have attenuated diurnal rhythms in locomotor activity and metabolic rate and consume a high proportion of daily calories (47% versus 25% in wild-type mice) during the light phase, the normal fasting period for nocturnal mice. Furthermore, mRNA levels of *Per2* and appetite-regulating neuropeptides in the mediobasal hypothalamus (ie, hypocretin, ghrelin, and cocaine-amphetamine–related transcript) are significantly attenuated.[9] *Clock* mutants have alterations in gluconeogenesis following insulin administration, impaired insulin responsiveness following glucose infusion, and modifications in glucose homeostasis in response to a chronic high-fat (HF) content diet.[99] In the context of a different genetic background (Jcl:ICR), however, the *Clock* mutation protects animals from excessive weight gain and elevations in triglyceride and free-fatty acid levels in response to an HF diet, possibly because of impaired fat absorption.[100] Overall, the importance of these findings is that genetic perturbation of a core clock gene can result in dramatic alterations in metabolic homeostatic regulation, results that have led to intensive biochemical research using animal models to investigate the role of circadian mechanisms in cardiometabolic health and other important disease conditions. The role of clock genes in metabolic and other physiologic functions may depend on the genetic background of the strain under investigation, and it is important to consider this factor when comparing and contrasting data from different studies. In the genetic models discussed previously, the *Clock* mutation is expressed throughout the body, and it is not possible to pinpoint whether the metabolic phenotypes are caused by tissue-specific effects of altered *Clock* function. Recent transgenic models, including tissue-specific gene deletion and overexpression of clock genes, will provide the opportunity to gain deeper insights into the role of the *Clock* gene and other clock molecular components in metabolic regulation.[94,95,101]

Although the circadian clock is designed to integrate inputs and generate outputs to orchestrate physiologic systems precisely, it allows some degree of flexibility for sudden changes in behavior or physiology that may be required for adaptation to unexpected or acute environmental or physiologic demands. For example, the circadian system is responsive to changes in the LD cycle, the availability of food, and possibly to other situations, such as changes in caloric intake, stress, and sleep deprivation.[45,102–104] A number of signals, including factors related to energy balance, can affect the circadian clock, directly either in vivo or in cultured cell/tissue preparations. In vitro, clock gene oscillations are initiated by glucocorticoids, components of cAMP and protein kinase C pathways, $Ca2^+$ signaling, glucose, and insulin.[21] Leptin and ghrelin, two appetite-regulating neuropeptides with signaling properties in the mediobasal hypothalamus, have the ability to stimulate clock gene oscillations in vitro.[105,106] A variety of diurnal and circadian rhythm alterations occur in genetic models of leptin deficiency (ob/ob mice and Zucker obese rats) and leptin resistance (db/db mice), as well as in pharmacologic models of impaired glucose signaling and diabetes.[107–115] Rutter and colleagues[116] made the important discovery that the metabolic cell environment (ie, re-dox state) affects the transcriptional activity of NPAS2, a paralogue of CLOCK. Therefore, alterations in metabolic homeostasis may present a significant challenge to the circadian system to function normally and in an adaptive manner.

Diet-induced obesity in mice is associated with significant changes in behavioral and molecular circadian rhythms.[117] Within 1 week of receiving an HF content diet, mice show a significant lengthening in their free-running period of locomotor activity and a severe attenuation in the diurnal rhythm of food intake (ie, they consume a high proportion of calories during the light phase), compared with animals fed regular chow. These alterations in behavioral rhythm occur before notable weight gain appears.[117] HF feeding dampens the diurnal rhythms of *Clock*, *Bmal1*, and *Per2* mRNA expression in peripheral tissues (ie, white adipose tissue and liver) but not in the mediobasal hypothalamus, which contains the SCN. Furthermore, the diurnal patterns of a broad range of metabolism-related transcripts are altered in fat and liver in a time- and tissue-dependent manner following HF administration. Consistent with the study just described,[117] a HF diet interferes with the ability of mice to phase advance, but not to phase delay, locomotor

activity and SCN rhythms in response to shifts in the LD cycle and to light pulses in constant darkness.[118] Surprisingly, calorie restriction, whether applied using a single timed meal or evenly spaced meals across the LD cycle, leads to changes in the locomotor activity rhythm and clock-gene expression in the SCN, suggesting that metabolic status can be a driving force for central pacemaker regulation.[102,119,120] Even a timed palatable meal in otherwise ad lib–fed mice may influence SCN activity and clock protein levels, raising the possibility that reward or arousal systems affect circadian regulation.[121] In combination, a variety of experimental paradigms have been used to demonstrate complex interactions between circadian clock regulation, meal timing, and nutrient status. Although particular experimental designs, such as restricting food for animals using regular chow, have effects predominantly on the peripheral clock system, other situations, including restricting caloric intake and the availability of palatable food, have clear effects on the central pacemaker. These data raise the interesting hypothesis that the combination of meal time and dietary content may have profound effects on the synchronization of the central pacemaker and cell-autonomous oscillators in the periphery, directly affecting the ability to control body weight and other aspects of energy metabolism.

There are various indications that the temporal organization of caloric intake may be a contributing and modifiable factor in weight control. As previously noted, nocturnal rodents eat almost exclusively during the active (ie, dark) phase of the diurnal cycle. In rodent models of obesity, a large proportion of daily caloric intake is consumed during the light period.[9,13,114,117,122] In experiments where nocturnal rodents are given access to food only during the light phase but are not calorie restricted, weight gain is more rapid than if the same amount of calories is provided only during the dark phase (F.W. Turek, unpublished observations, 2008). Therefore, simply eating at the "wrong" time of day presents a challenge to weight control. Although the mechanisms underlying this relationship are unknown, it is reasonable to hypothesize that when food is consumed at times when the body is not primed to metabolize nutrients, the mismatch between food intake and nutrient metabolism leads to impaired energy homeostasis. In humans, excess caloric intake in the evening has been reported in obese individuals and in an intriguing sleep disorder, night-eating syndrome.[123,124] Because food intake is a potentially modifiable behavior, developing circadian-based strategies for controlling the time of feeding may represent a viable approach for weight loss.

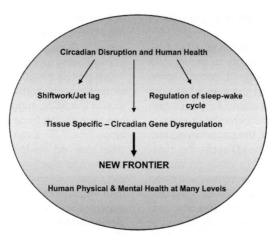

Fig. 4. Role of the circadian rhythms and the molecular circadian clock in health and disease. Recent discoveries in the field of circadian biology have demonstrated the importance of the circadian clock in virtually all aspects of behavior, physiology, and molecular function. The use of animal models has played a critical role in developing a blueprint of circadian clock function, which now is being translated to understanding circadian-based mechanisms of health and disease. The intersections between circadian regulation and health are complex and undoubtedly result from a combination of direct and indirect interactions between the organism's external and internal environments. It is becoming clear that new methods to measure and modify circadian function may provide the opportunity to integrate circadian biology into the practice of clinical medicine to prevent, diagnose, and treat diseases that affect millions of people. Indeed, circadian biology represents a new frontier in the understanding of human physical and mental health.

PERSPECTIVE AND SUMMARY

In the wild, unpredictable changes in weather conditions or food availability may present acute challenges to an animal's behavioral routine. Industrialized society presents many opportunities to ignore the circadian clock and to eat, work, and relax at any time of day. Therefore, the circadian system must allow some degree of flexibility; however, optimal function may not be maintained in conditions of chronic challenge. Short-term adjustments in physiology that serve an initial adaptive purpose can lead to system overload and maladaptive responses if forced to continue over long periods of time.[125,126] It will be important to continue to examine the role of repeated circadian desynchronization as a risk/causative factor in the development and/or exacerbation of multiple disease processes.

Although this article has focused primarily on the role of circadian biology in energy metabolism, important advances have been made in understanding the interplay between the circadian clock and cardiovascular function[72,76,97] as well as in more recent areas of investigation, including tumor formation/regulation of the cell cycle,[127,128] respiration,[129,130] mood disorders,[131,132] reproduction, neurologic diseases,[6] and pharmacotherapy.[133] Animal models will continue to be valuable in developing translational-level research to discover and elucidate how the circadian clock is interlinked with critical aspects of health and disease. Based on the tremendous advances that have been made in basic circadian biology research, the circadian field now is positioned to forge ahead and make a major impact in the biomedical sciences (**Fig. 4**). It is reasonable to predict that behavioral, pharmacologic, and genetic-based therapies involving the circadian clock will be developed to treat and prevent major disorders, such as psychiatric illness, cardiometabolic disease, and cancer. A blueprint for the place of circadian biology in medicine exists. Now, research must continue to build on this framework and seek new directions to treat disease and to optimize human health.

ACKNOWLEDGMENTS

The authors thank Dr. Joe Bass, Dr. Ravi Allada, and members of their laboratories for thought-provoking discussions regarding the topics presented in this article.

REFERENCES

1. Ko CH, Takahashi JS. Molecular components of the mammalian circadian clock. Hum Mol Genet 2006; 15(Spec no 2):R271–7.
2. Saper CB. Staying awake for dinner: hypothalamic integration of sleep, feeding, and circadian rhythms. Prog Brain Res 2006;153:243–52.

3. Takahashi JS, Hong HK, Ko CH, et al. The genetics of mammalian circadian order and disorder: implications for physiology and disease. Nat Rev Genet 2008;9:764–75.

4. Wijnen H, Young MW. Interplay of circadian clocks and metabolic rhythms. Annu Rev Genet 2006;40:409–48.

5. Green CB, Takahashi JS, Bass J. The meter of metabolism. Cell 2008;134:728–42.

6. Maywood ES, O'Neill J, Wong GK, et al. Circadian timing in health and disease. Prog Brain Res 2006;153:253–69.

7. Curtis AM, Fitzgerald GA. Central and peripheral clocks in cardiovascular and metabolic function. Annu Mediaev 2006;38:552–9.

8. Ishida N. Circadian clock, cancer and lipid metabolism. Neurosci Res 2007;57:483–90.

9. Turek FW, Joshu C, Kohsaka A, et al. Obesity and metabolic syndrome in circadian clock mutant mice. Science 2005;308:1043–5.

10. Van Cauter E, Polonsky KS, Scheen AJ. Roles of circadian rhythmicity and sleep in human glucose regulation. Endocr Rev 1997;18:716–38.

11. Wisor JP, Kilduff TS. Molecular genetic advances in sleep research and their relevance to sleep medicine. Sleep 2005;28:357–67.

12. Bodosi B, Gardi J, Hajdu I, et al. Rhythms of ghrelin, leptin, and sleep in rats: effects of the normal diurnal cycle, restricted feeding, and sleep deprivation. Am J Physiol Regul Integr Comp Physiol 2004;287:R1071–9.

13. Masaki T, Yoshimatsu H. The hypothalamic H1 receptor: a novel therapeutic target for disrupting diurnal feeding rhythm and obesity. Trends Pharmacol Sci 2006;27:279–84.

14. Spiegel K, Leproult R, Van Cauter E. Impact of sleep debt on metabolic and endocrine function. Lancet 1999;354:1435–9.

15. Haus E, Smolensky M. Biological clocks and shift work: circadian dysregulation and potential long-term effects. Cancer Causes Control 2006;17:489–500.

16. Karlsson B, Knutsson A, Lindahl B. Is there an association between shift work and having a metabolic syndrome? Results from a population based study of 27,485 people. Occup Environ Med 2001;58:747–52.

17. Knutsson A. Health disorders of shift workers. Occup Med (Lond) 2003;53:103–8.

18. Costa G. Shift work and occupational medicine: an overview. Occup Med (Lond) 2003;53:83–8.

19. Driscoll TR, Grunstein RR, Rogers NL. A systematic review of the neurobehavioural and physiological effects of shiftwork systems. Sleep Med Rev 2007;11:179–94.

20. Hastings M, O'Neill JS, Maywood ES. Circadian clocks: regulators of endocrine and metabolic rhythms. J Endocrinol 2007;195:187–98.

21. Nagoshi E, Brown SA, Dibner C, et al. Circadian gene expression in cultured cells. Meth Enzymol 2005;393:543–57.

22. Antle MC, Silver R. Orchestrating time: arrangements of the brain circadian clock. Trends Neurosci 2005;28:145–51.

23. Stephan FK, Zucker I. Circadian rhythms in drinking behavior and locomotor activity of rats are eliminated by hypothalamic lesions. Proc Natl Acad Sci U S A 1972;69:1583–6.

24. Moore RY, Eichler VB. Loss of a circadian adrenal corticosterone rhythm following suprachiasmatic lesions in the rat. Brain Res 1972;42:201–6.

25. Kohsaka A, Bass J. A sense of time: how molecular clocks organize metabolism. Trends Endocrinol Metab 2007;18:4–11.

26. Ralph MR, Foster RG, Davis FC, et al. Transplanted suprachiasmatic nucleus determines circadian period. Science 1990;247:975–8.

27. Yamazaki S, et al. Resetting central and peripheral circadian oscillators in transgenic rats. Science 2000;288:682–5.

28. Kriegsfeld LJ, Silver R. The regulation of neuroendocrine function: timing is everything. Horm Behav 2006;49:557–74.

29. Gillette MU, Mitchell JW. Signaling in the suprachiasmatic nucleus: selectively responsive and integrative. Cell Tissue Res 2002;309:99–107.

30. Yamazaki S, Straume M, Tei H, et al. Effects of aging on central and peripheral mammalian clocks. Proc Natl Acad Sci U S A 2002;99:10801–6.

31. Lockley SW, Gooley JJ. Circadian photoreception: spotlight on the brain. Curr Biol 2006;16:R795–7.

32. Reddy AB, Field MD, Maywood ES, et al. Differential resynchronisation of circadian clock gene expression within the suprachiasmatic nuclei of mice subjected to experimental jet lag. J Neurosci 2002;22:7326–30.

33. Vansteensel MJ, Yamazaki S, Albus H, et al. Dissociation between circadian Per1 and neuronal and behavioral rhythms following a shifted environmental cycle. Curr Biol 2003;13:1538–42.

34. Nagano M, Adachi A, Nakahama K, et al. An abrupt shift in the day/night cycle causes desynchrony in the mammalian circadian center. J Neurosci 2003;23:6141–51.

35. Kalsbeek A, Palm IF, La Fleur SE, et al. SCN outputs and the hypothalamic balance of life. J Biol Rhythms 2006;21:458–69.

36. Lu J, Greco MA, Shiromani P, et al. Effect of lesions of the ventrolateral preoptic nucleus on NREM and REM sleep. J Neurosci 2000;20:3830–42.

37. Horvath TL, Diano S. The floating blueprint of hypothalamic feeding circuits. Nat Rev Neurosci 2004;5:662–7.

38. Gooley JJ, Schomer A, Saper CB. The dorsomedial hypothalamic nucleus is critical for the expression

of food-entrainable circadian rhythms. Nat Neurosci 2006;9:398–407.

39. Kreier F, Kalsbeek A, Sauerwein HP, et al. "Diabetes of the elderly" and type 2 diabetes in younger patients: possible role of the biological clock. Exp Gerontol 2007;42:22–7.

40. Davidson AJ. Search for the feeding-entrainable circadian oscillator: a complex proposition. Am J Physiol Regul Integr Comp Physiol 2006;290: R1524–6.

41. Stokkan KA, Yamazaki S, Tei H, et al. Entrainment of the circadian clock in the liver by feeding. Science 2001;291:490–3.

42. Stephan FK. The "other" circadian system: food as a zeitgeber. J Biol Rhythms 2002;17:284–92.

43. Damiola F, Le Minh N, Preitner N, et al. Restricted feeding uncouples circadian oscillators in peripheral tissues from the central pacemaker in the suprachiasmatic nucleus. Genes Dev 2000;14:2950–61.

44. Hara R, Wan K, Wakamatsu H, et al. Restricted feeding entrains liver clock without participation of the suprachiasmatic nucleus. Genes Cells 2001;6: 269–78.

45. Saper CB, Fuller PM. Inducible clocks: living in an unpredictable world. Cold Spring Harb Symp Quant Biol 2007;72:543–50.

46. Landry GJ, Simon MM, Webb IC, et al. Persistence of a behavioral food-anticipatory circadian rhythm following dorsomedial hypothalamic ablation in rats. Am J Physiol Regul Integr Comp Physiol 2006;290:R1527–34.

47. Mieda M, Williams SC, Richardson JA, et al. The dorsomedial hypothalamic nucleus as a putative food-entrainable circadian pacemaker. Proc Natl Acad Sci U S A 2006;103:12150–5.

48. Nogueiras R, Tschop MH, Zigman JM. Central nervous system regulation of energy metabolism: ghrelin versus leptin. Ann N Y Acad Sci 2008; 1126:14–9.

49. Mistlberger RE, Yamazaki S, Pendergast JS, et al. Comment on "Differential rescue of light- and food-entrainable circadian rhythms". Science 2008;322:675 author reply 675.

50. Fuller PM, Lu J, Saper CB. Differential rescue of light- and food-entrainable circadian rhythms. Science 2008;320:1074–7.

51. Honma K, Honma S, Hiroshige T. Activity rhythms in the circadian domain appear in suprachiasmatic nuclei lesioned rats given methamphetamine. Physiol Behav 1987;40:767–74.

52. Davidson AJ, Tataroglu O, Menaker M. Circadian effects of timed meals (and other rewards). Methods Enzymol 2005;393:509–23.

53. Penev PD, Kolker DE, Zee PC, et al. Chronic circadian desynchronization decreases the survival of animals with cardiomyopathic heart disease. Am J Physiol 1998;275:H2334–7.

54. Davidson AJ, Sellix MT, Daniel J, et al. Chronic jet-lag increases mortality in aged mice. Curr Biol 2006;16:R914–6.

55. Preuss F, Tang Y, Laposky AD, et al. Adverse effects of chronic circadian desynchronization in animals in a "challenging" environment. Am J Physiol Regul Integr Comp Physiol 2008;295(6):R2034–40.

56. Tsai LL, Tsai YC, Hwang K, et al. Repeated light-dark shifts speed up body weight gain in male F344 rats. Am J Physiol Endocrinol Metab 2005; 289:E212–7.

57. Tsai LL, Tsai YC. The effect of scheduled forced wheel activity on body weight in male F344 rats undergoing chronic circadian desynchronization. Int J Obes (Lond) 2007;31:1368–77.

58. Salgado-Delgado R, Angeles-Castellanos M, Buijs MR, et al. Internal desynchronization in a model of night-work by forced activity in rats. Neuroscience 2008;154:922–31.

59. Nelson W, Halberg F. Schedule-shifts, circadian rhythms and lifespan of freely-feeding and meal-fed mice. Physiol Behav 1986;38:781–8.

60. Ralph MR, Menaker M. A mutation of the circadian system in golden hamsters. Science 1988;241: 1225–7.

61. Martino TA, Oudit GY, Herzenberg AM, et al. Circadian rhythm disorganization produces profound cardiovascular and renal disease in hamsters. Am J Physiol Regul Integr Comp Physiol 2008;294: R1675–83.

62. Martino TA, Tata N, Belsham DD, et al. Disturbed diurnal rhythm alters gene expression and exacerbates cardiovascular disease with rescue by resynchronization. Hypertension 2007;49:1104–13.

63. Vitaterna MH, King DP, Chang AM, et al. Mutagenesis and mapping of a mouse gene, clock, essential for circadian behavior. Science 1994;264:719–25.

64. Pittendrigh CS, Minis DH. Circadian systems: longevity as a function of circadian resonance in Drosophila melanogaster. Proc Natl Acad Sci U S A 1972;69:1537–9.

65. Shaw PJ, Tononi G, Greenspan RJ, et al. Stress response genes protect against lethal effects of sleep deprivation in Drosophila. Nature 2002;417:287–91.

66. Zheng X, Sehgal A. Probing the relative importance of molecular oscillations in the circadian clock. Genetics 2008;178:1147–55.

67. Konopka RJ, Benzer S. Clock mutants of Drosophila melanogaster. Proc Natl Acad Sci U S A 1971;68:2112–6.

68. Lowrey PL, Takahashi JS. Mammalian circadian biology: elucidating genome-wide levels of temporal organization. Annu Rev Genomics Hum Genet 2004;5:407–41.

69. King DP, Zhao Y, Sangoram AM, et al. Positional cloning of the mouse circadian clock gene. Cell 1997;89:641–53.

70. Reppert SM, Weaver DR. Coordination of circadian timing in mammals. Nature 2002;418:935–41.

71. Storch KF, Lipan O, Leykin I, et al. Extensive and divergent circadian gene expression in liver and heart. Nature 2002;417:78–83.

72. Young ME, Bray MS. Potential role for peripheral circadian clock dyssynchrony in the pathogenesis of cardiovascular dysfunction. Sleep Med 2007; 8(6):656–67.

73. Yoo SH, Yamazaki S, Lowrey PL, et al. PERIOD2: LUCIFERASE real-time reporting of circadian dynamics reveals persistent circadian oscillations in mouse peripheral tissues. Proc Natl Acad Sci U S A 2004;101:5339–46.

74. Muhlbauer E, Wolgast S, Finckh U, et al. Indication of circadian oscillations in the rat pancreas. FEBS Lett 2004;564:91–6.

75. Hoogerwerf WA. Biologic clocks and the gut. Curr Gastroenterol Rep 2006;8:353–9.

76. Maemura K, Takeda N, Nagai R. Circadian rhythms in the CNS and peripheral clock disorders: role of the biological clock in cardiovascular diseases. J Pharm Sci 2007;103:134–8.

77. McCarthy JJ, Andrews JL, McDearmon EL, et al. Identification of the circadian transcriptome in adult mouse skeletal muscle. Physiol Genomics 2007;31: 86–95.

78. Zvonic S, Ptitsyn AA, Conrad SA, et al. Characterization of peripheral circadian clocks in adipose tissues. Diabetes 2006;55:962–70.

79. Ando H, Yanagihara H, Hayashi Y, et al. Rhythmic messenger ribonucleic acid expression of clock genes and adipocytokines in mouse visceral adipose tissue. Endocrinology 2005; 146:5631–6.

80. Oishi K, Kasamatsu M, Ishida N. Gene- and tissue-specific alterations of circadian clock gene expression in streptozotocin-induced diabetic mice under restricted feeding. Biochem Biophys Res Commun 2004;317:330–4.

81. Tsinkalovsky O, Smaaland R, Rosenlund B, et al. Circadian variations in clock gene expression of human bone marrow CD34+ cells. J Biol Rhythms 2007;22:140–50.

82. Balsalobre A, Damiola F, Schibler U. A serum shock induces circadian gene expression in mammalian tissue culture cells. Cell 1998;93:929–37.

83. Abe M, Herzog ED, Yamazaki S, et al. Circadian rhythms in isolated brain regions. J Neurosci 2002;22:350–6.

84. Panda S, Antoch MP, Miller BH, et al. Coordinated transcription of key pathways in the mouse by the circadian clock. Cell 2002;109:307–20.

85. Oishi K, Miyazaki K, Kadota K, et al. Genome-wide expression analysis of mouse liver reveals CLOCK-regulated circadian output genes. J Biol Chem 2003;278:41519–27.

86. Naylor E, Bergmann BM, Krauski K, et al. The circadian clock mutation alters sleep homeostasis in the mouse. J Neurosci 2000;20:8138–43.

87. Laposky A, Easton A, Dugovic C, et al. Deletion of the mammalian circadian clock gene BMAL1/Mop3 alters baseline sleep architecture and the response to sleep deprivation. Sleep 2005;28:395–409.

88. Wisor JP, O'Hara BF, Terao A, et al. A role for cryptochromes in sleep regulation. BMC Neurosci 2002; 3:20.

89. Franken P, Dudley CA, Estill SJ, et al. NPAS2 as a transcriptional regulator of non-rapid eye movement sleep: genotype and sex interactions. Proc Natl Acad Sci U S A 2006;103:7118–23.

90. Dudley CA, Erbel-Sieler C, Estill SJ, et al. Altered patterns of sleep and behavioral adaptability in NPAS2-deficient mice. Science 2003;301:379–83.

91. Kopp C, Albrecht U, Zheng B, et al. Homeostatic sleep regulation is preserved in mPer1 and mPer2 mutant mice. Eur J Neurosci 2002;16:1099–106.

92. Shiromani PJ, Xu M, Winston EM, et al. Sleep rhythmicity and homeostasis in mice with targeted disruption of mPeriod genes. Am J Physiol Regul Integr Comp Physiol 2004;287:R47–57.

93. Paul KN, Dugovic C, Turek FW, et al. Diurnal sex differences in the sleep wake cycle of mice are dependent on gonadal function. Sleep 2006;29: 1211–23.

94. Hong HK, Chong JL, Song W, et al. Inducible and reversible clock gene expression in brain using the tTA system for the study of circadian behavior. PLoS Genet 2007;3:e33.

95. McDearmon EL, Patel KN, Ko CH, et al. Dissecting the functions of the mammalian clock protein BMAL1 by tissue-specific rescue in mice. Science 2006;314:1304–8.

96. Shimba S, Ishii N, Ohta Y, et al. Brain and muscle Arnt-like protein-1 (BMAL1), a component of the molecular clock, regulates adipogenesis. Proc Natl Acad Sci U S A 2005;102:12071–6.

97. Fontaine C, Staels B. The orphan nuclear receptor Rev-erbalpha: a transcriptional link between circadian rhythmicity and cardiometabolic disease. Curr Opin Lipidol 2007;18:141–6.

98. Yang X, Downes M, Yu RT, et al. Nuclear receptor expression links the circadian clock to metabolism. Cell 2006;126:801–10.

99. Rudic RD, McNamara P, Curtis AM, et al. BMAL1 and CLOCK, two essential components of the circadian clock, are involved in glucose homeostasis. PLoS Biol 2004;2:e377.

100. Oishi K, Atsumi G, Sugiyama S, et al. Disrupted fat absorption attenuates obesity induced by a high-fat diet in clock mutant mice. FEBS Lett 2006;580: 127–30.

101. Kornmann B, Schaad O, Bujard H, et al. System-driven and oscillator-dependent circadian

transcription in mice with a conditionally active liver clock. PLoS Biol 2007;5:e34.

102. Mendoza J. Circadian clocks: setting time by food. J Neuroendocrinol 2007;19:127–37.

103. Deboer T, Detari L, Meijer JH. Long term effects of sleep deprivation on the mammalian circadian pacemaker. Sleep 2007;30:257–62.

104. Colwell CS, Michel S. Sleep and circadian rhythms: do sleep centers talk back to the clock? Nat Neurosci 2003;6:1005–6.

105. Yannielli PC, Molyneux PC, Harrington ME, et al. Ghrelin effects on the circadian system of mice. J Neurosci 2007;27:2890–5.

106. Prosser RA, Bergeron HE. Leptin phase-advances the rat suprachiasmatic circadian clock in vitro. Neurosci Lett 2003;336:139–42.

107. Mistlberger RE, Marchant EG. Enhanced food-anticipatory circadian rhythms in the genetically obese Zucker rat. Physiol Behav 1999;66:329–35.

108. Mistlberger RE, Lukman H, Nadeau BG. Circadian rhythms in the Zucker obese rat: assessment and intervention. Appetite 1998;30:255–67.

109. Young ME, Wilson CR, Razeghi P, et al. Alterations of the circadian clock in the heart by streptozotocin-induced diabetes. J Mol Cell Cardiol 2002;34:223–31.

110. Laposky AD, Shelton J, Bass J, et al. Altered sleep regulation in leptin-deficient mice. Am J Physiol Regul Integr Comp Physiol 2006;290:R894–903.

111. Challet E, Losee-Olson S, Turek FW. Reduced glucose availability attenuates circadian responses to light in mice. Am J Physiol 1999;276:R1063–70.

112. Challet E, van Reeth O, Turek FW. Altered circadian responses to light in streptozotocin-induced diabetic mice. Am J Physiol 1999;277:E232–7.

113. Ando H, Oshima Y, Yanagihara H, et al. Profile of rhythmic gene expression in the livers of obese diabetic KK-A(y) mice. Biochem Biophys Res Commun 2006;346:1297–302.

114. Kudo T, Akiyama M, Kuriyama K, et al. Night-time restricted feeding normalises clock genes and Pai-1 gene expression in the db/db mouse liver. Diabetologia 2004;47:1425–36.

115. Davidson AJ, Stokkan KA, Yamazaki S, et al. Food-anticipatory activity and liver per1-luc activity in diabetic transgenic rats. Physiol Behav 2002;76:21–6.

116. Rutter J, Reick M, Wu LC, et al. Regulation of clock and NPAS2 DNA binding by the redox state of NAD cofactors. Science 2001;293:510–4.

117. Kohsaka A, Laposky AD, Ramsey KM, et al. High-fat diet disrupts behavioral and molecular circadian rhythms in mice. Cell Metab 2007;6:414–21.

118. Mendoza J, Pevet P, Challet E. High-fat feeding alters the clock synchronization to light. J Physiol 2008;586:5901–10.

119. Mendoza J, Graff C, Dardente H, et al. Feeding cues alter clock gene oscillations and photic responses in the suprachiasmatic nuclei of mice exposed to a light/dark cycle. J Neurosci 2005;25:1514–22.

120. Mendoza J, Drevet K, Pevet P, et al. Daily meal timing is not necessary for resetting the main circadian clock by calorie restriction. J Neuroendocrinol 2008;20:251–60.

121. Mendoza J, Angeles-Castellanos M, Escobar C. A daily palatable meal without food deprivation entrains the suprachiasmatic nucleus of rats. Eur J Neurosci 2005;22:2855–62.

122. Parmentier R, Ohtsu H, Djebbara-Hannas Z, et al. Anatomical, physiological, and pharmacological characteristics of histidine decarboxylase knock-out mice: evidence for the role of brain histamine in behavioral and sleep-wake control. J Neurosci 2002;22:7695–711.

123. Howell MJ, Schenck CH, Crow SJ. A review of nighttime eating disorders. Sleep Med Rev 2008;13:23–34.

124. Stunkard AJ, Allison KC. Two forms of disordered eating in obesity: binge eating and night eating. Int J Obes Relat Metab Disord 2003;27:1–12.

125. McEwen BS, Wingfield JC. The concept of allostasis in biology and biomedicine. Horm Behav 2003;43:2–15.

126. Kim Y, Laposky AD, Bergmann BM, et al. Repeated sleep restriction in rats leads to homeostatic and allostatic responses during recovery sleep. Proc Natl Acad Sci U S A 2007;104:10697–702.

127. Canaple L, Kakizawa T, Laudet V. The days and nights of cancer cells. Cancer Res 2003;63:7545–52.

128. Filipski E, Delaunay F, King VM, et al. Effects of chronic jet lag on tumor progression in mice. Cancer Res 2004;64:7879–85.

129. Stephenson R. Circadian rhythms and sleep-related breathing disorders. Sleep Med 2007;8:681–7.

130. Burioka N, Fukuoka Y, Takata M, et al. Circadian rhythms in the CNS and peripheral clock disorders: function of clock genes: influence of medication for bronchial asthma on circadian gene. J Pharm Sci 2007;103:144–9.

131. Turek FW. From circadian rhythms to clock genes in depression. Int Clin Psychopharmacol 2007;22(Suppl 2):S1–8.

132. Roybal K, Theobold D, Graham A, et al. Mania-like behavior induced by disruption of CLOCK. Proc Natl Acad Sci U S A 2007;104:6406–11.

133. Bruguerolle B, Boulamery A, Simon N. Biological rhythms: a neglected factor of variability in pharmacokinetic studies. J Pharm Sci 2008;97:1099–108.

Influence of the Circadian System on Disease Severity

Mikhail Litinski, MD[a], Frank A.J.L. Scheer, PhD[b],
Steven A. Shea, PhD[b],*

KEYWORDS

- Sleep • Circadian • Asthma
- Cardiovascular • Epilepsy • Chronotherapy

The severity of many diseases varies by time of day. For example, myocardial infarction occurs most frequently in the morning a few hours after waking up, epileptic seizures of the brain's temporal lobe usually occur in the late afternoon or early evening, and asthma is generally worse at night (**Fig. 1**). There are also differences across the 24-hour period in cancer development and on chemotherapeutic effectiveness. In addition, shift work is generally associated with chronic misalignment between the endogenous circadian timing system and the behavioral cycles, including sleep/wake and fasting/feeding cycles, and this misalignment could be a cause of the increased risk of diabetes, obesity, cardiovascular disease, and certain cancers in shift workers. This article describes the existence and magnitude of such daily changes in disease severity. This article also explores the mechanisms underlying these time-variant changes in disease severity, in particular in terms of whether or not these changes are caused by the endogenous circadian system or are due to behaviors that occur on a regular daily basis, including the sleep/wake cycle. Understanding the biologic basis of these changes across the day and night can lead to better therapy. This means, for example, giving medications at more appropriate times to target specific phases of the body clock or to coincide with specific behaviors that cause vulnerability, while withholding higher doses at other times when deleterious side effects could outweigh the benefits. Thus, current and future chronotherapeutic practices and targets are presented where appropriate.

CARDIOVASCULAR DISEASE
Day/night Rhythm in Adverse Cardiovascular Events, Arrhythmias, and Blood Pressure

Cardiovascular disease is the leading cause of death in the United States. Myocardial ischemia (insufficient supply of oxygenated blood relative to the demand of the cardiac muscle) can be caused by hypoxia, by coronary vasospasm, or by rupture of an atherosclerotic plaque and subsequent thrombosis affecting the coronary circulation. In extreme cases "sudden cardiac death" can result from an ischemic event in association with severe myocardial infarction or ventricular tachycardia/fibrillation. Robust epidemiologic evidence indicates that the peak incidence of cardiac ischemic events, including angina, acute myocardial infarction, and sudden cardiac death occurs between 6 AM and noon.[1–6] The reasons for this day/night pattern are not yet known,

This work was supported by grant K24 HL76446 from the National Institutes of Health to SA Shea, by grant R21 AT002713 from the National Institutes of Health to FAJL Scheer, and by grant 43-PA-08 from the American Sleep Medicine Foundation (a foundation of the American Academy of Sleep Medicine) to M Litinski.
[a] Division of Sleep Medicine, Department of Medicine, Brigham & Women's Hospital, teaching affiliate of Harvard Medical School, 221 Longwood Avenue, Boston, MA 02115, USA
[b] Harvard Medical School and Division of Sleep Medicine, Brigham & Women's Hospital, 221 Longwood Avenue, Boston, MA 02115, USA
* Corresponding author.
E-mail address: sshea@hms.harvard.edu (S.A. Shea).

Sleep Med Clin 4 (2009) 143–163
doi:10.1016/j.jsmc.2009.02.005

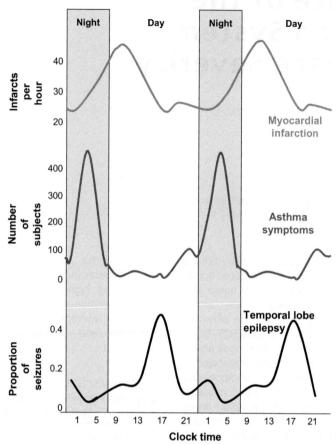

Fig. 1. The day/night patterns of disease severity. Results of three epidemiologic studies demonstrating robust day/night patterns of disease severity for myocardial infarction (*top panel*), asthma (*middle panel*), and temporal lobe seizures (*bottom panel*). The disease severity for myocardial infarction broadly peaks around 10 AM. The disease severity for asthma sharply peaks around 4 AM. The disease severity for temporal lobe seizures peaks around 5 PM. Data are double plotted to emphasize rhythmicity. (*Data from* Muller JE. Circadian variation and triggering of acute coronary events. Am Heart J 1999;137(4 Pt 2):S1–8; Dethlefsen U, Repgas R. [Ein neues therapieprinzip bei nachtlichen asthma]. Clin Med 1985;80:44; and Pavlova MK, Shea SA, Bromfield EB. Day/night patterns of focal seizures. Epilepsy Behav 2004;5(1):44–9.)

although triggering behaviors occurring at specific times of day have been suggested as a cause. It is equally possible that endogenous circadian rhythms in an array of hemodynamic, hemostatic, endothelial, and autonomic variables could cause a day/night pattern in adverse events.[6]

Ventricular tachyarrhythmias are the most common cause of sudden cardiac death. Studies of patients undergoing 24-hour electrocardiographic monitoring have revealed a robust and prominent peak in ventricular tachyarrhythmias during the morning and a trough at night.[7–16] For example, Mallavarapu and colleagues[13] analyzed the electrocardiograms from 390 implantable cardioverter–defibrillator recipients who sustained a total of 2692 episodes of ventricular tachycardia or ventricular fibrillation. The peak incidence of the arrhythmias occurred between 10 and 11 AM, with

a nadir between 2 and 3 AM. This day/night pattern persisted regardless of age, gender, ejection fraction, or ventricular tachycardia cycle length. Further evidence of the morning increase in susceptibility to serious arrhythmias comes from defibrillation thresholds in patients with implantable cardioverter–defibrillators: Venditti and colleagues[17] found that (1) the defibrillation threshold was higher when implantation occurred in the morning than when implanted at other times of day (thus greater energy is required for termination of morning tachyarrhythmias) and (2) first shocks in ambulant patients applied in the morning were more likely to fail than those applied at other times.

Arterial blood pressure generally falls during sleep and rises during activity, contributing to a day/night pattern in blood pressure in most normotensive people as well as in most of those with uncomplicated essential hypertension. However, a "nondipping" hypertensive phenotype exists without much of a decline during sleep, which presents an independent predictor of cardiovascular morbidity and mortality.[18] Mechanisms for this phenotype could include enhanced sodium sensitivity;[19–22] underlying circadian rhythmicity; the presence of sleep disorders, such as insomnia and obstructive sleep apnea; and more sleep during the daytime, which would blunt the day/night pattern.

Circadian Rhythm Versus Behavioral Influences on Cardiovascular Risk Markers

Sympathetic nervous activity is modulated in most circumstances as a protective homeostatic response. However, in some individuals with underlying pathophysiology or susceptibility, sympathetic activation can provoke adverse cardiovascular events. For instance, sympathetic activation can increase blood pressure and arterial wall sheer forces, which can potentially rupture vulnerable atherosclerotic plaques in coronary arteries. Thus, a day/night pattern in the activity of the sympathetic nervous system might underlie the day/night pattern of adverse events in vulnerable individuals. The day/night pattern could occur simply from a day/night pattern of behaviors, such as a surge of sympathetic activity upon standing up and becoming active in the morning or during rapid eye movement sleep.[23–28] Indeed, Deedwania and colleagues[29] found that the morning increase in heart rate and blood pressure may cause a 40% increase in cardiac oxygen demand. Andrews and colleagues[30] found that about 80% of ambulatory ischemic events are accompanied by tachycardia. Tachycardia, while normally promoting blood supply to peripheral tissues, actually decreases blood supply to the myocardium. This decrease is due to a relative reduction in diastole (when coronary arterioles receive most flow) versus systole. In addition, platelets are a cornerstone of the hemostatic system and facilitate thrombus formation, which could impede coronary blood flow. Several in vivo and in vitro studies have found day/night variation in a number of functional platelet factors, with peaks in both activation and adhesiveness between 6 and 9 AM.[31–35] The increased morning platelet activation possibly could be caused by increased circulating catecholamines[36,37] or decreasing plasma melatonin.[38]

Most of the evidence demonstrating the existence of a 24-hour pattern in adverse cardiovascular events is epidemiologic, which cannot attribute the underlying behavioral or circadian causes. Laboratory studies clearly show marked systematic changes in most hemodynamic and hemostatic variables with changes in behavior, such as exercise. Usually people sleep at the same phase of the circadian cycle so the relative contribution of behavioral and circadian influences on cardiovascular vulnerability cannot be determined. Such separation can be examined when keeping people awake and in the same conditions across at least 24 hours or by shifting the time-relationship between the endogenous circadian clock and the behaviors (as occurs with shift work and during jet lag) and examining the changes in relevant variables. A few laboratory studies have examined endogenous circadian influences on cardiovascular variables, principally by employing a "constant routine" protocol in which subjects remain in the same posture and awake for over 24 hours in dim light and with regular small snacks rather than larger irregular meals.[39–41] For example, Burgess and colleagues[40] studied 16 subjects during a 26-hour constant routine protocol (to reveal underlying circadian rhythmicity) and in a similar study in which sleep was permitted (to assess the additional effect of sleep beyond underlying circadian rhythmicity). They found that sympathetic activity was reduced during sleep (estimated from cardiac isovolumetric contraction time), whereas parasympathetic nervous system activity (estimated from heart rate variability) increased during the circadian "night" with little additional effect of sleep itself. Kerkhof and colleagues[41] were unable to find a circadian fluctuation in blood pressure in 12 healthy normotensive adults, but found significant circadian variation in heart rate (7-beats-per-minute range, peak around 11 AM). Hu and colleagues[42] found in healthy humans that the scale invariance of heart rate fluctuations changes toward an "unhealthy" state at a circadian phase corresponding to the peak in adverse events in other studies and populations. Experiments on rats discovered that circadian fluctuations in heart rate as well as the scale invariance of heart rate fluctuations were abolished upon lesioning of the suprachiasmatic nucleus (SCN).[43,44] To quantify both circadian and behavioral effects as well as any interactions, Scheer and colleagues[45] performed a forced desynchrony protocol that scheduled all behaviors evenly across all phases of the circadian cycle. They found robust circadian-related increases in heart rate and plasma epinephrine and norepinephrine throughout the circadian "morning," with maxima occurring later than the time when cardiovascular risk is highest (~9 AM), raising the untested hypothesis that the rate of change of some sympathetic markers may be more relevant than the absolute level for the timing of adverse cardiovascular events. These same investigators found that certain behavioral stressors (mental stress, postural tilt, or exercise) resulted in similar autonomic, hemostatic, or hemodynamic effects when these stressors were presented at different phases of the circadian cycle. This result suggests that there is little functional interaction between the behavioral stressors and the circadian system, suggesting that these factors are additive in terms of affecting vulnerability to an adverse cardiovascular event.[46]

Chronotherapy for Cardiovascular Disorders

Although clinical pharmacology for cardiovascular disorders is a rapidly evolving field, the current standard of care often involves the use of a number of medications, depending on each individual's disease or diseases (eg, coronary artery disease, congestive heart failure, arrhythmias, hypertension, or a combination of these), disease severity, and presence of comorbidities (eg, diabetes mellitus, renal insufficiency). The main classes of cardiovascular medications include (1) beta-adrenoreceptor antagonists (beta-blockers), which block the effects of endogenous catecholamines to decrease cardiac output and heart rate, and prolong diastole leading to improved myocardial blood supply; (2) nitrates, which increase coronary artery diameter and blood flow to alleviate angina; (3) calcium channel blockers, which are strong arterial vasodilators and may have negative inotropic effects (decreasing the force of myocardial contractions) and negative chronotropic effects (decreasing heart rate); (4) antiplatelet drugs such as aspirin, which reduces platelet aggregation and thrombus formation; (5) angiotensin-converting enzyme inhibitors and angiotensin receptor blockers, used primarily for reducing blood pressure; (6) cholesterol-lowering medications (eg, statins) to reduce circulating low-density lipoprotein and inflammatory markers and thereby reduce the risk of atheroma formation on arterial walls; and (7) experimental treatments, such as use of melatonin in hypertension.

Chronotherapy refers to the appropriately timed medication to achieve the most efficacious therapeutic levels in the body at the most needed times, while avoiding higher doses at other times when side effects could outweigh the benefits. For instance, rather than perpetually giving patients the maximum tolerated dose of beta-blocker, it may be better to time the beta-blockade to coincide with the periods of greatest sympatho-excitation. This strategy may improve exercise tolerance in those with chronotropic incompetence (inadequate heart rate response) by allowing periods of reduced beta-blockade during lower-risk periods. Similarly, antiplatelet agents in cardiovascular disease could specifically target the periods of greatest platelet aggregability to reduce thrombotic complications, while minimizing hemorrhagic complications during periods of reduced platelet aggregation. Furthermore, by determining if certain behaviors alter disease severity (eg, exercise-induced angina), timed medication can be planned to coincide with those behaviors, or such triggering behaviors could be scheduled outside periods of greater vulnerability.

Calcium channel blockers

Calcium channel blockers are commonly used in hypertension, Prinz-Metal angina, supraventricular tachyarrhythmias (eg, atrial fibrillation), and "non–Q wave" myocardial infarction. For example, verapamil has potent negative inotropic and negative chronotropic effects and has a relatively weak arterial vasodilatory effect compared with nifedipine. Chronotherapy with calcium channel blockers, marketed in the United States since 1996, has been designed to achieve the highest plasma concentration during the most vulnerable time period while maintaining an adequate therapeutic dose throughout the remainder of the 24-hour period. A variety of calcium channel blocker delivery formulations (eg, with controlled-onset, extended release, or both) have been approved by the Food and Drug Administration,[47–49] and may be beneficially prescribed to lower blood pressure, heart rate, and rate-pressure product between 6 AM and noon, depending on the time of administration.[50–52] One study has demonstrated an improvement in the duration of exercise with evening doses of a preparation of diltiazem, a calcium channel blocker, versus morning dosing.[53]

Beta-adrenoreceptor antagonists

Beta-adrenoreceptor blockers are associated with an overall decrease in adverse cardiovascular events as well as the abolition of the day/night pattern of adverse coronary events.[54–56] Andrews and colleagues[30] also found that beta-blockers decrease the incidence of coronary events associated with tachycardia, but not with a normal heart rate, suggesting that this effect of beta-blockers is mediated via decreased myocardial demand (reduced tachycardia), or improved myocardial blood supply (prolonged diastole), or both. An evening dose of propranolol extended release results in peak levels sustained throughout the most vulnerable time for ischemic events. Such propranolol chronotherapy was approved by the Food and Drug Administration in 2003 for treating systemic hypertension. Propranolol chronotherapy also seems to possess optimal pharmacokinetic properties for treating ischemic heart disease.[57] A potential setback for beta-blocker chronotherapy is that it can suppress nighttime melatonin production and could disrupt normal circadian rhythms.[58]

Nitrates

Short-acting nitrates control angina most effectively when administered in the morning.[59] In contrast, long-acting nitrates are designed for once-per-day dosing and should normally be administered at bedtime to maintain a therapeutic concentration in the plasma throughout the night and the subsequent vulnerable morning hours.[60]

Aspirin

Aspirin inhibits cyclooxygenase in platelets, which normally induces tromboxane A2 to promote platelet aggregation and thrombus formation. Aspirin has reduced the incidence of myocardial infarction in males by 59% during morning hours and only 34% during the rest of the 24-hour cycle.[61] However, low-dose aspirin in females decreased risk for ischemic stroke but not myocardial infarction,[62] and the mechanisms for this gender difference are currently unknown. Although the effect of aspirin on platelets is irreversible (lasting throughout the thrombocyte's lifespan, ~12 days), some data show that the effect of aspirin has marked diurnal variation with a peak during morning,[63] possibly due to day/night variation in pharmacodynamics, bioavailability, and rate of elimination.[63–65]

Angiotensin-converting enzyme inhibitors and cholesterol-lowering medication

No solid evidence has been found showing any benefit of chronotherapy with angiotensin-converting enzyme inhibitors in patients with hypertension or coronary artery disease.[66–68] For example, Kohno and colleagues[67] found no significant difference in blood pressure decrease between morning and evening doses of imidaprol in either "dipping" and "nondipping" hypertensive patients. Similarly, to the best of our knowledge, no evidence shows any benefit from chronotherapy with cholesterol-lowering medication.

Melatonin and hypertension

Generally used therapeutic strategies for suboptimally controlled arterial hypertension include increasing the dose of current medications, adding another medication, or switching to a medication with a different mechanism of action. A recent review[69] indicates that most hypertensive patients take their medications once a day in the morning, which would likely prove sufficient for patients with a normal nighttime fall in blood pressure. However, this strategy may be inadequate for the "nondipper" phenotype as effective medication levels are still needed across the night. Thus, sustained-release preparations or twice-a-day dosing may be better suited for "nondipping" hypertensive patients who are at higher risk for cardiovascular complications.[70] One paper found that "nondippers" have impaired nocturnal melatonin secretion.[71] Moreover, a randomized placebo-controlled crossover trial in men with uncontrolled essential hypertension found that melatonin administration for 3 weeks (2.5 mg orally 1 hour before sleep) decreased nighttime systolic and diastolic blood pressure by 6 and 4 mm Hg, respectively.[72] These results have recently been extended to females, in whom 3 weeks of melatonin significantly decreased nocturnal systolic and diastolic blood pressure.[73] Thus, the approach of supplementing the traditional management of hypertension with melatonin therapy appears promising, but requires more investigation into both the mechanism and the clinical use.

ASTHMA
Day/Night Rhythm in Asthma Severity

Bronchial asthma can be quite unstable especially when untreated. Asthmatic events occur most frequently during the night.[74] More severe asthma is associated with more nocturnal symptoms.[75] Patients with nocturnal asthma demonstrate increased morbidity and mortality relative to patients without noticeable worsening of asthma at night.[76] Asthma has three defining components: chronic inflammation, airway hyperresponsiveness, and reversible airway obstruction.[77] Each of these parameters exhibit 24-hour fluctuations with worsening around 4 AM compared with 4 PM.[78–84] Such changes could be caused by the physiologic consequences of sleep (eg, increased vagal tone, decreased sympathetic activity, decreased temperature), the supine posture (causing reduced functional residual capacity of the lungs, affecting the lower airway caliber), the environment (eg, allergies to dust mites in the bedding), or factors related to the endogenous circadian system (eg, increased pulmonary vagal bronchoconstrictive tone during the biologic night). The relative contributions of these varied factors are not firmly established and these potentially change from patient to patient and even within a patient from one day to the next, although some general findings may be applicable. For example, Hetzel and colleagues[81] studied airway obstruction as indicated by peak expiratory flow (PEF) in 221 healthy and asthmatic subjects and found that, even though the timing of the 24-hour rhythm in PEF was similar between these two groups, the amplitude of the fluctuation was 51% larger in asthma patients, who experienced more obstruction during the night. In patients with nocturnal worsening of asthma, airway-provoking agents (eg, histamine, methacholine, house dust) had a greater effect on indices of airway obstruction during the night than during the day. For instance, Bonnet and colleagues[82] found 24-hour oscillations in the pulmonary sensitivity to histamine and methacholine, with at least doubling concentrations required for the same effect at certain times of day. There is day/night variability in sympathetic activity, related to sleep or circadian rhythms.[26,85–88] The lowest plasma epinephrine concentration generally occurs at about 4 AM, corresponding to the nadir of PEF, suggesting that these may be linked.[86,89] Patients with symptoms and signs of "nocturnal asthma" (ie, disturbed sleep, nocturnal wheeze, and overnight decreases in pulmonary function) exhibit significantly higher concentrations of inflammatory markers in the distal airways (e.g. leukocyte, neutrophil, and eosinophil counts) at 4 AM compared with 4 PM.[79] The increase in neutrophils and eosinophils correlates with the overnight change in PEF.[79,90] There is some evidence suggesting that patients with nocturnal asthma have abnormal functioning of the hypothalamo-pituitary-adrenal axis or impaired cortisol binding and steroid responsiveness.[91,92]

Circadian Rhythm Versus Behavioral Influences on Pulmonary Function and Asthma Severity

Many studies of nocturnal asthma have relied on assessments made at 4 PM, when the subject is awake, and then at 4 AM, when the subject must be awakened. Such approaches have obvious limitations. For example, measurements at two time points likely underestimate the underlying peaks and troughs in a rhythmic signal. Also, arousal provoked by waking someone to make measurements can presumably affect pulmonary function. Furthermore, there may be a carry-over effect from the differences in posture, state, and environmental conditions preceding the measurements at 4 AM versus 4 PM on the subsequent assessments of pulmonary function. The separate contributions of behavioral and circadian influences on asthma severity can be examined by

keeping people awake and in the same conditions for at least 24 hours or by shifting the time-relationship between the endogenous circadian clock and the behaviors, as occurs in a relatively uncontrolled way with shift work. While such designs are well suited to assess the separate circadian influence on pulmonary function and asthma severity assessed during wakefulness, assessments of asthma during sleep within these protocols are difficult because most indices of asthma severity (eg, from forced spirometry or bronchoalveolar lavage) can only be performed when awake. To specifically assess the contribution of the endogenous circadian system to the day/night pattern of pulmonary function, Spengler and colleagues[93] studied 10 healthy subjects during continuous wakefulness throughout a "constant routine" protocol performed in the same posture for 40 hours in dim light, with small, evenly distributed meals, and with pulmonary function measured every 2 hours. There was a significant circadian variation in forced expired volume in 1 second (FEV_1), with a trough during the biologic night at the time when sleep would normally occur. To further explore this in patients with asthma, Shea and colleagues[94] examined endogenous circadian variations in pulmonary function throughout a "forced desynchrony" protocol conducted over 10 days in the laboratory, during which the behavioral sleep/wake cycles were adjusted systematically to occur across all phases of the endogenous circadian cycle, enabling analytical separation of the circadian and behavioral cycle effects on pulmonary function. PEF and airway resistance exhibited circadian rhythms, with worsening asthma during the biologic night, and an additional worsening caused by sleep itself (independent of the phase of the circadian cycle). The same investigators found an endogenous circadian rhythm in rescue inhaler use in asthma, peaking during the biologic night.[95] Although most people usually sleep at night, many people—such as those experiencing jet lag, those with sleep disorders, and those performing shift work—occasionally or even systematically stay awake throughout the biologic night. So it is important to determine the extent to which the severity of asthma is affected by being awake and active through the night (as well as the effect on asthma of sleep during the day). Assuming that the behavioral and circadian cycle effects summate, these data suggest that when sleep occurs at night, asthma severity will be highest in some individuals because of the combined effects of sleep and the circadian system. Moreover, sleep can mask the severity of bronchoconstriction across the night because the sleeping subject may not awaken during bronchoconstriction, may experience reduced sensations due to "sleep inertia" upon awakening, or may have reduced ventilatory demands at night.

Chronotherapy for Asthma

Despite substantial advances in our knowledge of the pathogenesis of bronchial asthma, as well as in the development of therapeutic measures, morbidity and mortality related to asthma remains high.[96] Asthma is usually classified based on severity of symptoms and pulmonary function.[96] Thus, mild intermittent asthma (daytime symptoms less than once a week and nocturnal symptoms less than twice a month) does not require daily medication, and short-acting beta-2 agonist inhalers are used as sporadic "rescue" medication. Mild persistent asthma (daytime symptoms on 1–6 d/wk, with more than two nocturnal symptoms per month) is commonly treated with low-dose inhaled corticosteroids. Before the wide availability of inhaled corticosteroids, oral theophylline was a mainstream therapy for moderate asthma. Nowadays, treatment of moderate persistent asthma requires higher doses of inhaled corticosteroids (compared with lower doses used in mild persistent asthma) with or without sporadic "rescue"-use inhaled beta-2 adrenoreceptor agonists. In severe asthma (daily and frequent nocturnal symptoms) and for asthma exacerbations, systemic corticosteroids might be indicated. To counter the daily variation in asthma severity, chronotherapy has been attempted. Theophylline was prescribed as a chronotherapy for asthma as early as 1980.[97] The recommended daily pattern of dosing is either a single evening dose, or one third of the daily dose in the morning and two thirds in the evening. Several studies have shown that the bioavailability of theophylline is greater if administered in the evening than in the morning, and that such chronotherapy is more effective in preventing the nighttime dip in FEV_1 than the conventional theophylline administration (equally divided daily dose between morning and evening administration),[98–100] although this effect may be concentration-dependent.[101] Kraft and colleagues[102] have also shown that administration of theophylline to subjects with asthma in the evening improved the inflammatory profile of the distal airways, and this was correlated with improved nocturnal FEV_1.

A series of investigations has revealed that (1) administration of corticosteroids in the midafternoon (3 PM) is the most effective in preventing a nocturnal drop of FEV_1 and improving the respiratory inflammatory profile in patients with nocturnal asthma;[103,104] (2) glucocorticoids given in the morning or late at night did not prevent the drop of FEV_1 during the nighttime;[104,105] and (3) systemic glucocorticoids in healthy subjects during the daytime (8 AM–3 PM) minimized suppression of the hypothalamo-pituitary-adrenal axis activity.[103,106] Thus, by administering systemic corticosteroids around 3 PM, one might achieve the best therapeutic effect across the night while avoiding hypothalamo-pituitary-adrenal suppression. Similar results were obtained for inhaled corticosteroids.[107–109] For example, Pincus and colleagues[108] studied the effects on asthma of inhaled triamcinolone given four times per 24 hours (QID), or once at 8 AM, or once at 5 PM. There were clear improvements in FEV_1, PEF, use of beta-2–agonist rescue medication, nocturnal awakenings, and quality-of-life score in the QID group and in the 5 PM group, but not in the 8 AM group.

Several studies have investigated the benefits of chronotherapy with beta-2–agonist medication in the management of nocturnal asthma. Gaultier and colleagues[110] measured total lung resistance in six children with asthma at 7:30 AM, 11:30 AM, 4:30 PM, and 10:30 PM, each before and 10 minutes after 2-mg orciprenaline (beta-adrenoreceptor agonist) aerosol. Inhaled orciprenaline was mainly effective around 7:30 AM and to a lesser extent around 10:30 AM, whereas there was no detectable effect at the other times. The effect of time of 20-mg oral bambuterol (a long-acting beta-adrenoreceptor agonist) was assessed in a double-blind crossover design study in 30 adult patients with asthma, and a trend toward higher FEV_1 throughout the 24-hour period was found when bambuterol was administered in the evening compared with the morning.[111] In a double-blind randomized crossover designed study, salmeterol aerosol 100 mg inhaled at night was as effective as 50 mg inhaled twice a day in improving PEF and FEV_1.[112] Montelukast-leukotriene inhibitors, which are widely used as add-on therapy for treating asthma, particularly in patients with a prominent allergic component to asthma and comorbid allergic rhinitis, improve FEV_1 more effectively when dosed in the evening compared with the morning.[113,114] These studies demonstrate that varied modes of chronotherapy remain potentially useful in some patients with nocturnal worsening of asthma. While the role of theophylline has decreased over the last few decades, it still is an add-on therapy or used for patients who are unable to tolerate inhaled corticosteroids. Some data suggest positive effects of theophylline on diaphragmatic function as well as mucociliary clearance,[115,116] which may be of particular importance in asthma patients suffering from respiratory muscle fatigue and excessive bronchial mucus secretion. The emergence of a new generation of inhaled corticosteroids was recently heralded by the appearance of ciclesonide (approved by the Food and Drug Administration in 2008 for maintenance treatment and prophylactic therapy of bronchial asthma in adults). The most remarkable feature of ciclesonide is that it becomes activated by intracellular esterases located in the lower airways. Therefore the side effects in the upper airways (such as oropharyngeal candidiasis and hoarseness) may potentially be less prominent compared with those associated with other inhaled corticosteroids. Anticholinergic agents represent another class of agents that theoretically may be useful in the management of nocturnal asthma, as these cause bronchodilation by opposing the effects of the parasympathetic nervous system, and such vagal effects are greatest at night (including during sleep).

CANCER

Existing epidemiologic data indicate a link between various physiologic parameters having well-established day/night rhythms and carcinogenesis. For example, Rafnsson and colleagues[117] found a higher rate of breast cancer in female flight attendants and female shift workers than in other women. Severely disrupted rest/activity cycles in patients with metastatic colorectal cancer is accompanied by decreased survival compared with patients with a well-preserved rest/activity pattern.[118] A number of biomolecular and genetic factors might be responsible for the relationship between the circadian system and carcinogenesis. First, by influencing the expression of numerous genes, circadian clock proteins play an important role in regulating cell apoptosis, proliferation and differentiation; DNA repair; and the cell cycle. For example, c-Myc is a proto-oncogene that regulates cell differentiation and proliferation, has a day/night rhythm,[119] and is overexpressed in cells of many human cancers. Compared with their wild-type counterparts, mPER2 and clock knock-out mice have overexpressed c-Myc, are cancer prone, and more susceptible to gamma radiation with reduced survival.[120,121] PER2 has a tumor suppressor effect, depletion of PER2 protein was observed in varied types of cancer cells in humans,[122,123] and induction of PER2 expression in cancer cells inhibits growth, arrests the cell cycle, and reduces apoptosis (at least partially through inhibiting c-Myc gene transcription). Such effects of PER2 induction do not occur in normal human cell lines.[124] Some data suggest that cytidine-cytidine-adenosine-adenosine-thymedine (CCAAT)/enhancer binding protein (C/EBP) alfa, a transcription factor that is ubiquitous in human tissues and plays a role in regulation of cell growth and differentiation, mediates part of its influence through up-regulation of PER2 protein expression.[122] Gery and colleagues[125] induced expression of C/EBP alfa in chronic myeloid leukemia, Burkitt lymphoma, and murine fibroblast cell lines. Using microarray analysis, these investigators showed that induction of the C/EBP alfa gene increased expression of the PER2 gene, which may explain C/EBP's inhibitory effect on c-Myc expression in cancer cells. Circadian clock proteins, such as PER1, also participate in cell apoptosis via modulation of the "checkpoint" proteins: ataxia telangiectasia mutated kinase-1 and kinase-2.[123] Clock proteins modulate the cell cycle by affecting the expression of cell-cycle–related genes cyclin B1 and cyclin D1, and transcription of WEE1.[126] The c-Myc oncogene participates in G0/G1 cell phase transition in normal and tumor cells,[127,128] such that circadian clock proteins may influence the cell cycle through expression of the c-Myc gene as well. Thus, circadian clock genes affect each aspect of a cell's life cycle, including proliferation, differentiation, cell cycle phase shifting, and apoptosis, providing the theoretical basis for cancer chronotherapy. Chemotherapy for different types of malignancy at specific points of the molecular clock cycle and cell cycle can minimize adverse effects, increase tolerable doses, and help achieve better therapeutic responses and survival.[129] In addition, gene therapy is now being used in some fields, including oncology.[130] Thus, in the future, modulating the expression of certain clock genes could be a therapeutic target in treating or preventing certain types of cancer[131,132] both in the general population as well as populations at risk, such as night-shift workers. Finally, there is need for future studies on the potential therapeutic value of melatonin as anti-oncogenic therapy.[133]

EPILEPSY

Epilepsy is another disorder that often exhibits a day/night variation in clinical presentation. Pavlova and colleagues[134] found that temporal lobe epileptic seizures occur more frequently between 3 and 7 PM, whereas the peak incidence for extra–temporal lobe epileptic seizures occurs between 7 and 11 PM. Among those seizures that occurred during sleep, the majority originated in the temporal lobe.[134] Similarly, analysis of 131 adults with localized epilepsy revealed that the day/night distribution of epileptiform activity depended on the specific brain area involved: Most frontal and parietal seizures occurred between 4 and 7 AM, whereas temporal lobe seizures had two peaks (4–7 PM and 7–10 AM). Seizures of occipital origin occurred mostly between 4 and 7 PM.[135] Whether these patterns are caused by the behavioral sleep/wake cycle, by a circadian rhythm in vulnerability, or a combination of both is unknown. Some preliminary data indicate an endogenous circadian rhythm in epileptiform interictal discharges while awake in some subjects with generalized epilepsy, with a peak in the beginning of habitual sleep period (11 PM–3 AM).[136] However considering all interictal discharges—regardless of sleep/wake state—the distribution appeared random.[136] Sleep is well known to activate some seizures, including benign Rolandic epilepsy of childhood and autosomal dominant nocturnal frontal lobe epilepsy, but the mechanism of interaction between sleep physiology and cryptogenic- and localization-related epilepsy is yet to be clarified.[137]

Yegnaranayan and colleagues[138] randomized 103 epileptic subjects who were receiving subtherapeutic plasma levels of antiepileptic medications (phenytoin/carbamazepin) to two treatment groups: One was allowed to increase the dose but not the timing of medication; the second group maintained the same dose but potentially altered the time of administration to 8 PM (regardless of when it was previously scheduled). This latter "chronotherapy" was better as it achieved more therapeutic levels of plasma medication and improved clinical outcomes (no seizures within 1 year), whereas symptoms of toxicity were more often observed in the conventional dose-scheduling group ($P < .05$). Thus, while data on chronotherapy for epilepsy are quite limited, there may be clinical utility in investigating this more.

GASTROESOPHAGEAL REFLUX DISEASE

Gastroesophageal reflux disease that occurs during wakefulness is usually postprandial and rapidly cleared. Nocturnal gastroesophageal reflux events occur less frequently than those occurring during the daytime but are associated with longer acid-clearance time[139] due to sleep or circadian-related decreases in swallowing,[140] saliva production (saliva contains mucous and bicarbonates that neutralize acid from the stomach),[141] peristalsis[142] and reduced symptoms of heartburn such that protective mechanisms are not as quickly initiated.[143] These all may potentially be paired with decreased gastric emptying during non–rapid eye movement sleep. While sleep and the supine posture can promote some of these deleterious effects, no study has determined whether the endogenous circadian system also contributes to any of these effects, and no consistent data have been gathered on chronotherapy for gastroesophageal reflux disease.

ALZHEIMER'S DISEASE

Alzheimer's disease affects about 15 million people worldwide and is most commonly seen after the age of 50, with progressive cognitive decline, and circadian rhythm and sleep disturbances, including insomnia. It is tragic for the patient, causes major physical and emotional burden for primary caregivers, and represents a large economic burden for society. The most common reason for institutionalizing patients with Alzheimer's disease is need for care during the night, stemming from altered sleep/wake regulation because of increased locomotor activity.[144] One feature of Alzheimer's disease is "sundowning," which is characterized by a late afternoon/evening predominance of activity.[145] Some investigators attribute sundowning to insufficient melatonin production.[146] A pathoanathomical sign of Alzheimer's disease is the deposition of beta-amyloid in certain areas of the brain, including the SCN.[147] Beta-amyloid is a potent generator of free radicals, which may cause neuronal damage and cell loss in the SCN and other brain structures, mediating circadian rhythm disruption[148] and cognitive deficits in Alzheimer's disease.[149] Within the SCN of patients with Alzheimer's disease is a significant decrease in neurons that express vasoactive intestinal peptide (VIP).[150,151] VIP plays an important role in the synchronization of clock gene expression across the SCN.[152] Lack of VIP or its receptors eliminates diurnal fluctuations of corticosteroids secretion in rats.[153] Disruption of the SCN neuronal output or the lack of a 24-hour fluctuation in beta-1 adrenoreceptor expression in the pineal gland[154,155] are thought to underlie the observed decrease in melatonin secretion in Alzheimer's disease. Moreover, melatonin deficiency might also be implicated in the pathogenesis of Alzheimer's disease because melatonin is a potent antioxidant that may protect neural tissue from the effects of reactive oxygen species.[156] A series of studies also support the notion that melatonin may decrease beta-amyloid–related neurotoxicity.[157–159] The peak of melatonin serum concentration at night is decreased with age, which may be, in part, due to comorbidities and medication use.[58,160]

Some data suggest that exogenous melatonin administration may improve sleep, decrease sundowning, and slow the progression of cognitive deficit in Alzheimer's disease patients.[161,162] The anti-inflammatory effect of melatonin,[163,164] as well as its protective effect on the cholinergic system demonstrated in rats,[165,166] may have a therapeutic effect on some aspects of Alzheimer's disease pathogenesis in humans. In a recent, double-blind, placebo-controlled trial on the effects of light and melatonin in 189 elderly subjects, it was shown that increased daytime environmental light exposure resulted in decreased cognitive deterioration, improved depressive symptoms, and attenuated the increase in functional limitations.[167] In this same study, melatonin supplementation shortened sleep-onset latency and increased total sleep time. However, melatonin also decreased affect ratings and increased withdrawn behavior, which was counteracted by light. Combined treatment reduced aggressive behavior, increased sleep efficiency, and improved nocturnal restlessness.

EFFECT OF CIRCADIAN MISALIGNMENT ON HEALTH

About 10% of the United States labor force works rotating, irregular, or permanent night shifts. Shift work is generally associated with chronic misalignment between the endogenous circadian timing system and the behavioral cycles, including sleep/wake and fasting/feeding cycles. Thus, such people may be attempting to sleep during the daytime at a circadian phase better for activity and, conversely, attempting to remain awake during the night at a circadian phase better for sleep and fasting. The effect of jet lag is similar. Resulting from rapid travel across a number of time zones, jet lag is characterized by insomnia or hypersomnolence, fatigue, behavioral symptoms, headaches, and gastrointestinal disturbances. Symptoms of jet lag syndrome usually last not more than a week. With shift work, however, there can be chronic circadian misalignment together with increased risk of diabetes, obesity, cardiovascular disease, gastrointestinal disorders, and certain cancers. These adverse consequences of working night shifts could be mediated by (1) direct effects of the misalignment between the endogenous circadian cycle and behavioral cycles (ie, sleep/wake, feed/fast, and rest/activity schedule), or (2) secondary effects of such misalignment, including altered family and social schedules, leading to generalized stress and (3) the potential development of mood disorders, such as depression

and anxiety, as well as (4) chronic partial sleep deprivation, which can cause a number of adverse cardiovascular, endocrine, and neurocognitive outcomes.[168–170] For instance, some surveys suggest that night-shift workers sleep 10 fewer hours per week than those who work day shifts.[171] Gander and colleagues[172] found that crew members on long-haul flights were sleep-deprived with only 6.5 hours of sleep over a 24-hour period. Mittler and colleagues[173] found that truck drivers had on average 3.8 hours of sleep over a 24-hour period. Similar data have emerged for other professions that require night shifts, including police officers and medical residents. The direct effects of misalignment are presented below.

Night-Shift Work and Cardiovascular Disorders

From a study of 79,109 female nurses, the relative risk for development of coronary heart disease in women working night shifts more than 6 years was 1.51 (95% CI 1.12–2.03) compared with those who had never worked night shifts.[174] The risk persisted after adjustment for smoking, alcohol intake, history of hypertension, diabetes mellitus, hypercholesterolemia, postmenopausal status, hormone replacement therapy, aspirin use, and family history of myocardial infarction. From a study of 2354 shift workers and 3088 day workers, shift workers demonstrated increased mortality from coronary heart disease after adjusting for age, lifestyle, blood pressure, and lipid profile (odds ratio 1.83 [95% CI 1.01–3.32]).[175] However, Boggild and colleagues[176] found no increased risk for ischemic heart disease with night shifts in a prospective study with a 22-year follow-up period (relative risk 1.0 [95% CI 0.9–1.2]; n = 5249 Danish males), whether or not adjusting for age and social class. The investigators discuss the potential of "healthy worker effect" and "survival bias" leading to a relatively healthy population among these middle-aged shift workers as a potential explanation for the lack of an effect. Several cross-sectional and longitudinal prospective studies confirm the higher prevalence of cardiovascular disorders in people working rotating or night shifts.[177–180] A number of autonomic consequences of circadian misalignment could be implicated in the adverse cardiovascular effects, such as increased cortisol, increased catecholamine output, increased cardiac sympathetic predominance, and reduced parasympathetic activity.[181] For instance, there is less of a drop in blood pressure during the sleep periods of shift workers.[182,183]

Night-Shift Work and Metabolic Disorders

A cross-sectional study found that among 6676 workers, night-shift work was associated with a higher body mass index and higher waist-to-hip ratio.[184] A longitudinal study found that weight gains that exceeded 7 kg were more frequent among nurses on night work than among nurses at work during the day.[185] In a study of 27,485 individuals, obesity was more prevalent in shift workers than in day workers even after adjustment for age and socioeconomic status (odds ratio 1.41 [95% CI 1.25–1.59]).[186] Obesity is a risk factor for insulin resistance and diabetes mellitus, and it was found that markers associated with insulin resistance, including hyperglycemia, increased triglyceride concentrations, low high-density lipoprotein cholesterol, and hypertension, were more prevalent among night-shift workers than among day workers.[187] In the study of female nurses noted above, the risk of developing diabetes also rose with increasing duration of night-shift work.[174] In a study by Mikuni and colleagues,[188] the prevalence of diabetes in rotating shift workers was 2.1% versus 0.9% in day-shift workers. Night-shift work increases the likelihood of developing insulin resistance.[189]

These adverse metabolic effects of night-shift work could be mediated via deleterious effects on glucose regulation or indirectly via increased appetite, leading to weight gain and obesity, a major risk factor for insulin resistance and type 2 diabetes.[190] Leptin is secreted by adipocytes and inhibits appetite and food intake to produce energy balance in normal-weight individuals. Low leptin levels have been associated with chronic short habitual sleep duration in epidemiologic studies,[191,192] following acute sleep deprivation in laboratory studies (eg, 2 nights of 4 hours of sleep per night),[193] and following reduced sleep for 1 week.[194] Reduced leptin signals a negative energy balance, leading to increased appetite. Leptin resistance eventually appears in obesity and has been implicated in sympathetic activation[195] and insulin resistance.[196,197] There is a significant circadian rhythm in leptin secretion, and circadian misalignment was predicted to alter the day/night range in circulating leptin, which could increase appetite.[198] Other hormones that are secreted by adipose tissue and exhibit day/night patterns that could be affected by shift work include adiponectin, which is positively correlated with insulin sensitivity (adiponectin concentrations are high during the day and low at night),[199] and resistin, which causes insulin resistance in rodents[200] (concentrations are high during the dark/feeding phase in nocturnal rodents). Furthermore, ghrelin, an appetite-stimulating hormone primarily secreted from the gastric fundic mucosa,[201] is associated with type 2 diabetes,[202] may have a direct effect on the SCN,[203] and is increased by sleep loss.[192] Complementary epidemiologic evidence links short sleep with reduced leptin and increased ghrelin levels with increased body mass index.[204] Since these hormones are affected by time of day, food intake or fasting, and, in some cases, circadian rhythms, misalignment of these factors due to shift work may cause prominent metabolic effects. Indeed, circadian misalignment leads to a suppression of leptin levels and an increase in postprandial glucose and insulin levels, indicating decreased insulin sensitivity, which may play a role in explaining the increased risk for obesity and diabetes in shift workers.[205]

Night-Shift Work and Cancer

An early study by Taylor and Pocock[206] found higher cancer-attributed mortality in night-shift workers than in day workers. More recent investigations have confirmed and extended these findings, showing a higher risk for breast cancer in females whose job involves shift or night work, such as flight attendants,[117] nurses,[207] radio operators, and telegraph operators.[208] In a study of 7565 women with breast cancer, past employment requiring work at night for more than 6 months was associated with higher risk of development of breast cancer compared with a daytime working schedule (odds ratio 1.5 [95% CI 1.3–1.7]), after adjusting for age, social class, age at birth of last child, and number of children.[209] In a prospective, 10-year longitudinal study of 78,586 women working at least 3 nights per month for more than 15 years, women who worked rotating night shifts had increased risk of developing colon cancer compared with those who never worked rotating night shifts (relative risk 1.35 [95% CI 1.03–1.77]).[210] A higher risk for prostate cancer was reported among those whose profession requires working rotating night shifts at least occasionally, including police officers, firefighters, physicians, and pilots.[211,212] The International Agency for Research of Cancer, a unit of the World Health Organization, recently announced that night-shift work is probably carcinogenic. The underlying pathologic mechanism could include exposure to light during the biologic night, which causes the pineal gland to secrete less melatonin. This loss of melatonin may affect cancer rates because melatonin has growth-inhibitory and oncostatic properties. Melatonin has been shown to (1) inhibit the proliferation of breast cancer cells in vitro by 60% to 78%,[213] (2) inhibit invasive and metastatic properties of breast cancer cells in vitro by decreasing attachment to basal membrane and counteracting the stimulatory effect of estradiol on cell adhesiveness,[214] (3) enhance apoptosis of breast cancer cells,[215] (4) increase expression of p53 and p21WAF1 genes (tumor suppression genes) in breast cell culture,[216] (5) reverse the mammary tumor promoting effects of pinealectomy in rats,[217] and (6) have an antitumor effect on prostate cancer in vitro.[218] Interestingly, Zhu and colleagues[219] found that a polymorphism in *PER3* might be linked to breast cancer. Several animal experiments demonstrate the modulating effect of light exposure on PER2 gene expression in the SCN,[220,221] which may affect its neurohumoral output, leading to alteration in clock gene expression in peripheral tissues. Finally, alteration in *PER2* affects the DNA damage response and tumor suppression in mice and may play a role in apoptosis of cancerous cells.[120] Thus, it is plausible that light exposure during night-shift work may affect clock gene expression and alter the regulatory effects of clock genes on cell proliferation, differentiation, apoptosis, and DNA damage responses.

Night Shifts and Gastrointestinal and Reproductive Disorders

A study of 11,657 employees found significant increases in both gastric and duodenal ulcers in shift workers compared with stable day workers.[222] Many gastrointestinal variables exhibit robust day/night fluctuations that may be affected by shift work. For example, in rats there are day/night fluctuations in gastrin receptor expression,[223] acid production, bicarbonate secretion, gastric mucus efflux volumes, gastric mucosa blood flow during fasting;[224,225] and in prostacyclin activity in gastric tissue during fasting.[226] Meanwhile, in humans, there are day/night rhythms in gastric mucosa vulnerability for aspirin- and ethanol-related injury;[227,228] in gastric emptying (longer at 8 PM versus 8 AM);[229] in gastrointestinal motor propagation speed (slower during the night);[230] and in basal gastric secretion (highest from 9 PM until midnight).[231] Studies on rats indicated that the peak of gastric acid secretion in rats is out of phase with that of bicarbonate secretion by about 7 hours,[232] creating a period of gastric mucosa vulnerability to injury. Thus, it is reasonable to speculate that an imbalance between acid secretion and protective factors, as well as alterations in the inflammatory profile and activation of stress responses due to circadian and rest/activity and fasting/feeding rhythm

misalignment, might cause gastrointestinal morbidity in night-shift workers compared with day workers.

Furthermore, a number of reports have noted increased reproductive function abnormalities in those who work night or rotating shifts, including irregular menstruation, increased risk of miscarriage, premature birth, and low birth weight.[233,234]

SUMMARY AND FUTURE DIRECTIONS

We have reviewed (1) how interactions between the circadian and behavioral systems affect disease severity, notably the day/night pattern of adverse cardiovascular events, seizures, and asthma exacerbations; (2) how a disease can affect circadian rhythmicity, notably the circadian disruption of Alzheimer's disease; and (3) the adverse health consequences of circadian misalignment, typical of chronic shift work. In each case, chronotherapeutic considerations are presented. With a few notable exceptions described above, chronotherapy is probably underused in most fields of medicine considering the very prominent day/night variation in disease severity. This reticence may be due to a need for improved physician education, availability of suitable medications with appropriate pharmacodynamics, and greater understanding of whether the vulnerable periods are produced by specific behaviors, by the circadian phase, or by both. This last point is important when determining the therapeutic target, which becomes particularly relevant to consider when circadian rhythms and behaviors become differently aligned, as with sleep deprivation, shift work, jet lag, and certain sleep disorders. While there are numerous options to improve neurocognitive function and sleep in conditions of circadian misalignment, less is known about the therapeutic countermeasures to the many physiologic changes that accompany circadian misalignment that might underlie the increased hypertension, cardiovascular disease, diabetes, obesity, cancer, and gastroesophageal and reproductive problems in shift workers. However, there is growing recognition of these problems. In addition, researchers are now beginning to study how functional circadian clocks exist in many peripheral tissues (eg, heart, liver, lung, circulating blood), which potentially can become desynchronized from the central circadian pacemaker in the SCN. The consequences of peripheral-central desynchronization are not well understood, but may have implications for physiologic function, metabolism, sleep, neurocognitive function, and health. The molecular and genetic underpinnings of this rhythmicity are being studied in numerous animal models, laying the groundwork for future translational research to the bedside. The practical implementation of chronotherapy for many disorders warrants further exploration. Finally, determination of useful biomarkers or genetic analyses that can be reliably used to identify individuals at particular risk for adverse circadian disease-related effects, or adverse consequences of circadian misalignment, would have numerous far-reaching consequences.

REFERENCES

1. Cohen MC, Rohtla KM, Lavery CE, et al. Meta-analysis of the morning excess of acute myocardial infarction and sudden cardiac death. Am J Cardiol 1997;79(11):1512–6.
2. Ogawa H, Yasue H, Oshima S, et al. Circadian variation of plasma fibrinopeptide a level in patients with variant angina. Circulation 1989;80(6):1617–26.
3. Deedwania PC. Circadian rhythms of cardiovascular disorders. Armonk (NY): Futura Publishing Company, Inc; 1997.
4. Rocco MB, Barry J, Campbell S, et al. Circadian variation of transient myocardial ischemia in patients with coronary artery disease. Circulation 1987;75(2):395–400.
5. Arntz HR, Willich SN, Oeff M, et al. Circadian variation of sudden cardiac death reflects age-related variability in ventricular fibrillation. Circulation 1993;88(5 Pt 1):2284–9.
6. Shea SA, Hilton MF, Muller JE. Day/night patterns of myocardial infarction and sudden cardiac death: interacting roles of the endogenous circadian system and behavioral triggers. In: White WB, editor. Blood pressure monitoring in cardiovascular medicine and therapeutics. 2nd ed. Totowa (NJ): Humana Press Inc.; 2007. p. 251–89.
7. Canada WB, Woodward W, Lee G, et al. Circadian rhythm of hourly ventricular arrhythmia frequency in man. Angiology 1983;34(4):274–82.
8. Twidale N, Taylor S, Heddle WF, et al. Morning increase in the time of onset of sustained ventricular tachycardia. Am J Cardiol 1989;64(18):1204–6.
9. Valkama JO, Huikuri HV, Linnaluoto MK, et al. Circadian variation of ventricular tachycardia in patients with coronary arterial disease. Int J Cardiol 1992; 34(2):173–8.
10. Rebuzzi AG, Lucente M, Lanza GA, et al. Circadian rhythm of ventricular tachycardia. Prog Clin Biol Res 1987;227B:153–8.
11. d'Avila A, Wellens F, Andries E, et al. At what time are implantable defibrillator shocks delivered? Evidence for individual circadian variance in sudden cardiac death. Eur Heart J 1995;16(9): 1231–3.
12. Behrens S, Galecka M, Bruggemann T, et al. Circadian variation of sustained ventricular tachyarrhythmias terminated by appropriate shocks in patients with an implantable cardioverter defibrillator. Am Heart J 1995;130(1):79–84.
13. Mallavarapu C, Pancholy S, Schwartzman D, et al. Circadian variation of ventricular arrhythmia recurrences after cardioverter-defibrillator implantation in patients with healed myocardial infarcts. Am J Cardiol 1995;75(16):1140–4.
14. Fries R, Heisel A, Huwer H, et al. Incidence and clinical significance of short-term recurrent ventricular tachyarrhythmias in patients with implantable cardioverter-defibrillator. Int J Cardiol 1997;59(3): 281–4.
15. Tofler GH, Gebara OC, Mittleman MA, et al. Morning peak in ventricular tachyarrhythmias detected by time of implantable cardioverter/defibrillator therapy. The CPI Investigators. Circulation 1995;92(5):1203–8.
16. Nanthakumar K, Newman D, Paquette M, et al. Circadian variation of sustained ventricular tachycardia in patients subject to standard adrenergic blockade. Am Heart J 1997;134(4):752–7.
17. Venditti FJ Jr, John RM, Hull M, et al. Circadian variation in defibrillation energy requirements. Circulation 1996;94(7):1607–12.
18. Staessen JA, Thijs L, Fagard R, et al. Predicting cardiovascular risk using conventional vs ambulatory blood pressure in older patients with systolic hypertension. Systolic Hypertension in Europe Trial Investigators. JAMA 1999;282(6):539–46.
19. Uzu T, Fujii T, Nishimura M, et al. Determinants of circadian blood pressure rhythm in essential hypertension. Am J Hypertens 1999;12(1 Pt 1):35–9.
20. Uzu T, Ishikawa K, Fujii T, et al. Sodium restriction shifts circadian rhythm of blood pressure from non-dipper to dipper in essential hypertension. Circulation 1997;96:1859–62.
21. Kimura G, Uzu T, Nakamura S, et al. High sodium sensitivity and glomerular hypertension/hyperfiltration in primary aldosteronism. J Hypertens 1996; 14(12):1463–8.
22. Kario K, Motai K, Mitsuhashi T, et al. Autonomic nervous system dysfunction in elderly hypertensive patients with abnormal diurnal blood pressure variation—relation to silent cerebrovascular disease. Hypertension 1997;30(6):1504–10.
23. Millar-Craig MW, Bishop CN, Raftery EB. Circadian variation of blood-pressure. Lancet 1978;1(8068):795–7.
24. Floras JS, Jones JV, Johnston JA, et al. Arousal and the circadian rhythm of blood pressure. Clin Sci Mol Med Suppl 1978;4:395s–7s.
25. Mancia G, Ferrari A, Gregorini L, et al. Blood pressure and heart rate variabilities in normotensive

and hypertensive human beings. Circ Res 1983; 53(1):96–104.

26. Somers VK, Phil D, Dyken ME, et al. Sympathetic-nerve activity during sleep in normal subjects. N Eng J Med 1993;328:303–7.

27. Kirby DA, Verrier RL. Differential effects of sleep stage on coronary hemodynamic function during stenosis. Physiol Behav 1989;45(5):1017–20.

28. Turton MB, Deegan T. Circadian variations of plasma catecholamine, cortisol and immunoreactive insulin concentrations in supine subjects. Clin Chim Acta 1974;55(3):389–97.

29. Deedwania PC, Nelson JR. Pathophysiology of silent myocardial ischemia during daily life. Hemodynamic evaluation by simultaneous electrocardiographic and blood pressure monitoring. Circulation 1990;82(4):1296–304.

30. Andrews TC, Fenton T, Toyosaki N, et al. Subsets of ambulatory myocardial ischemia based on heart rate activity. Circadian distribution and response to anti-ischemic medication. The Angina and Silent Ischemia Study Group (ASIS). Circulation 1993; 88(1):92–100.

31. Undar L, Turkay C, Korkmaz L. Circadian variation in circulating platelet aggregates. Ann Med 1989; 21(6):429–33.

32. Undar L, Ertugrul C, Altunbas H, et al. Circadian variations in natural coagulation inhibitors protein C, protein S and antithrombin in healthy men: a possible association with interleukin-6. Thromb Haemost 1999;81(4):571–5.

33. Haus E, Cusulos M, Sackett-Lundeen L, et al. Circadian variations in blood coagulation parameters, alpha-antitrypsin antigen and platelet aggregation and retention in clinically healthy subjects. Chronobiol Int 1990;7(3):203–16.

34. Jovicic A, Ivanisevic V, Nikolajevic R. Circadian variations of platelet aggregability and fibrinolytic activity in patients with ischemic stroke. Thromb Res 1991;64(4):487–91.

35. Tofler GH, Stone PH, Maclure M, et al. Analysis of possible triggers of acute myocardial infarction (the MILIS study). Am J Cardiol 1990;66(1):22–7.

36. Andrews NP, Goldstein DS, Quyyumi AA. Effect of systemic alpha-2 adrenergic blockade on the morning increase in platelet aggregation in normal subjects. Am J Cardiol 1999;84(3):316–20.

37. Willich SN, Tofler GH, Brezinski DA, et al. Platelet alpha 2 adrenoceptor characteristics during the morning increase in platelet aggregability. Eur Heart J 1992;13(4):550–5.

38. Del Zar MM, Martinuzzo M, Falcon C, et al. Inhibition of human platelet aggregation and thromboxane-B2 production by melatonin: evidence for a diurnal variation. J Clin Endocrinol Metab 1990; 70(1):246–51.

39. Krauchi K, Wirz-Justice A. Circadian rhythm of heat production, heart rate, and skin and core temperature under unmasking conditions in men. Am J Physiol 1994;267(3 Pt 2):R819–29.

40. Burgess HJ, Trinder J, Kim Y, et al. Sleep and circadian influences on cardiac autonomic nervous system activity. Am J Physiol 1997;273(4 Pt 2): H1761–8.

41. Kerkhof GA, Dongen HPAv, Bobbert AC. Absence of endogenous circadian rhythmicity in blood pressure? Am J Hypertens 1998;11(3):373–7.

42. Hu K, Ivanov P, Hilton MF, et al. Endogenous circadian rhythm in an index of cardiac vulnerability independent of changes in behavior. Proc Natl Acad Sci U S A 2004;101(52):18223–7.

43. Scheer FAJL, Ter Horst GJ, Van der Vliet J, et al. Physiological and anatomic evidence for regulation of the heart by suprachiasmatic nucleus in rats. Am J Physiol 2001;280(3):H1391–9.

44. Hu K, Scheer FA, Buijs RM, et al. The endogenous circadian pacemaker imparts a scale-invariant pattern of heart rate fluctuations across time scales spanning minutes to 24 hours. J Biol Rhythms 2008;23(3):265–73.

45. Scheer FA, Hu Kun, Evoniuk Heather, et al. Additive influences of the endogenous circadian system and mental stress on cardiovascular risk factors. Sleep 2008;31(Suppl):S51.

46. Scheer FA, Hu Kun, Evoniuk Heather, et al. Influence of endogenous circadian system, physical exercise and their interaction on cardiovascular risk factors. Sleep 2008;31(suppl):S46.

47. Cutler NR, Anders RJ, Jhee SS, et al. Placebo-controlled evaluation of three doses of a controlled-onset, extended-release formulation of verapamil in the treatment of stable angina pectoris. Am J Cardiol 1995;75(16):1102–6.

48. Frishman WH, Glasser S, Stone P, et al. Comparison of controlled-onset, extended-release verapamil with amlodipine and amlodipine plus atenolol on exercise performance and ambulatory ischemia in patients with chronic stable angina pectoris. Am J Cardiol 1999;83(4):507–14.

49. Prisant LM, Devane JG, Butler J. A steady-state evaluation of the bioavailability of chronotherapeutic oral drug absorption system verapamil PM after nighttime dosing versus immediate-acting verapamil dosed every eight hours. Am J Ther 2000; 7(6):345–51.

50. Smith DH, Neutel JM, Weber MA. A new chronotherapeutic oral drug absorption system for verapamil optimizes blood pressure control in the morning. Am J Hypertens 2001;14(1):14–9.

51. Prisant Lm WH, Black. Role of circadian rhtyhm in cardiovascular function-efficacy of a chronotherapeutic approach to controlling hypertensionwith

Verelan PM (verapamil HCL). Todays Ther Trends 2003;21:201–13.

52. Glasser SP, Neutel JM, Gana TJ, et al. Efficacy and safety of a once daily graded-release diltiazem formulation in essential hypertension. Am J Hypertens 2003;16(1):51–8.

53. Glasser SP, Gana TJ, Pascual LG, et al. Efficacy and safety of a once-daily graded-release diltiazem formulation dosed at bedtime compared to placebo and to morning dosing in chronic stable angina pectoris. Am Heart J 2005;149(2):e1–9.

54. Spengler CM, Czeisler CA, Shea SA. An endogenous circadian rhythm of respiratory control in humans. J Physiol 2000;526(3):683–94.

55. Muller JE, Stone PH, Turi ZG, et al. Circadian variation in the frequency of onset of acute myocardial infarction. N Engl J Med 1985;313(21):1315–22.

56. Cohn PF, Lawson WE. Effects of long-acting propranolol on A.M. and P.M. peaks in silent myocardial ischemia. Am J Cardiol 1989;63(12):872–3.

57. Sica D, Frishman WH, Manowitz N. Pharmacokinetics of propranolol after single and multiple dosing with sustained release propranolol or propranolol CR (innopran XL), a new chronotherapeutic formulation. Heart Dis 2003;5(3):176–81.

58. Scheer FAJL, Cajochen C, Turek FW, et al. Melatonin in the regulation of sleep and circadian rhythms. In: Kryger MH, Roth T, Dement WC, editors. Principles and practice of sleep medicine. 4th edition. Philadelphia: W.B. Saunders; 2005. p. 395–404.

59. Yasue H, Omote S, Takizawa A, et al. Circadian variation of exercise capacity in patients with Prinzmetal's variant angina: role of exercise-induced coronary arterial spasm. Circulation 1979;59(5): 938–48.

60. Wortman AB. Chronotherapy in coronary heart disease: comparison of two nitrate treatments. Chronobiol Int 1991;8:399–408.

61. Ridker PM, Manson JE, Buring JE, et al. Circadian variation of acute myocardial infarction and the effect of low-dose aspirin in a randomized trial of physicians. Circulation 1990;82(3):897–902.

62. Ridker PM, Cook NR, Lee IM, et al. A randomized trial of low-dose aspirin in the primary prevention of cardiovascular disease in women. N Engl J Med 2005;352(13):1293–304.

63. Cornelissen G, Halberg F, Prikryl P, et al. Prophylactic aspirin treatment: the merits of timing. International Womb-to-Tomb Chronome Study Group. JAMA 1991;266(22):3128–9.

64. Reinberg A, Zagula-Mally ZW, Ghata J, et al. Circadian rhythm in duration of salicylate excretion referred to phase of excretory rhythms and routine. Proc Soc Exp Biol Med 1967;124(3):826–32.

65. Markiewicz A, Semenowicz K. Time dependent changes in the pharmacokinetics of aspirin. Int J Clin Pharmacol Biopharm 1979;17(10):409–11.

66. Shibasaki T, Obara T, Ohkubo T, et al. Time-dependent effects of imidapril administration in patients with morning hypertension measured as home blood pressure. Clin Exp Hypertens 2008;30(3): 243–54.

67. Kohno I, Ijiri H, Takusagawa M, et al. Effect of imidapril in dipper and nondipper hypertensive patients: comparison between morning and evening administration. Chronobiol Int 2000;17(2): 209–19.

68. Dagenais GR, Pogue J, Teo KK, et al. Impact of ramipril on the circadian periodicity of acute myocardial infarction. Am J Cardiol 2006;98(6): 758–60.

69. Hermida RC, Calvo C, Ayala DE, et al. Relationship between physical activity and blood pressure in dipper and non-dipper hypertensive patients. J Hypertens 2002;20(6):1097–104.

70. Ohkubo T, Imai Y, Tsuji I, et al. Relation between nocturnal decline in blood pressure and mortality. The Ohasama Study. Am J Hypertens 1997; 10(11):1201–7.

71. Jonas M, Garfinkel D, Zisapel N, et al. Impaired nocturnal melatonin secretion in non-dipper hypertensive patients. Blood Press 2003;12(1):19–24.

72. Scheer FAJL, van Montfrans GA, Van Someren EJW, et al. Daily nighttime melatonin reduces blood pressure in male patients with essential hypertension. Hypertension 2004;43(2):192–7.

73. Cagnacci A, Cannoletta M, Renzi A, et al. Prolonged melatonin administration decreases nocturnal blood pressure in women. Am J Hypertens 2005.

74. Bohadana AB, Hannhart B, Teculescu DB. Nocturnal worsening of asthma and sleep-disordered breathing. J Asthma 2002;39(2):85–100.

75. Global Initiative for asthma (GINA). Global strategy for asthma management and prevention. NHLBI/WHO Workshop report. Bethesda MNH: Lung and Blood Institute; 1995. Available at: http://www.ginasthma.com/ReportItem.asp?l1=2&l2=2&intld=96. [updated March, 2002]. Accessed September 1, 2008.

76. Hetzel MR, Clark TJ, Branthwaite MA. Asthma: analysis of sudden deaths and ventilatory arrests in hospital. Br Med J 1977;1(6064):808–11.

77. Masoli M, Fabian D, Holt S, et al. The global burden of asthma: executive summary of the GINA Dissemination Committee report. Allergy 2004;59(5):469–78.

78. Martin RJ, Cicutto LC, Smith HR, et al. Airways inflammation in nocturnal asthma. Am Rev Respir Dis 1991;143(2):351–7.

79. Kraft M, Djukanovic R, Wilson S, et al. Alveolar tissue inflammation in asthma. Am J Respir Crit Care Med 1996;154(5):1505–10.

80. Smolensky MH, Barnes PJ, Reinberg A, et al. Chronobiology and asthma. I. Day-night differences in bronchial patency and dyspnea and circadian

rhythm dependencies. J Asthma 1986;23(6): 321–43.

81. Hetzel MR, Clark TJ. Comparison of normal and asthmatic circadian rhythms in peak expiratory flow rate. Thorax 1980;35(10):732–8.

82. Bonnet R, Jorres R, Heitmann U, et al. Circadian rhythm in airway responsiveness and airway tone in patients with mild asthma. J Appl Physiol 1991; 71(4):1598–605.

83. Gervais P, Reinberg A, Gervais C, et al. Twenty-four-hour rhythm in the bronchial hyperreactivity to house dust in asthmatics. J Allergy Clin Immunol 1977;59(3):207–13.

84. Jarjour NN. Circadian variation in allergen and nonspecific bronchial responsiveness in asthma. Chronobiol Int 1999;16(5):631–9.

85. Morrison JF, Pearson SB, Dean HG. Parasympathetic nervous system in nocturnal asthma. Br Med J (Clin Res Ed) 1988;296(6634):1427–9.

86. Barnes P, FitzGerald G, Brown M, et al. Nocturnal asthma and changes in circulating epinephrine, histamine, and cortisol. N Engl J Med 1980; 303(5):263–7.

87. Khatri IM, Freis ED. Hemodynamic changes during sleep. J Appl Physiol 1967;22(5):867–73.

88. Hornyak M, Cejnar M, Elam M, et al. Sympathetic muscle nerve activity during sleep in man. Brain 1991;114(3):1281–95.

89. Soutar CA, Costello J, Ijaduola O, et al. Nocturnal and morning asthma. Relationship to plasma corticosteroids and response to cortisol infusion. Thorax 1975;30(4):436–40.

90. Kraft M, Martin RJ, Wilson S, et al. Lymphocyte and eosinophil influx into alveolar tissue in nocturnal asthma. Am J Respir Crit Care Med 1999;159(1): 228–34.

91. Kraft M, Vianna E, Martin RJ, et al. Nocturnal asthma is associated with reduced glucocorticoid receptor binding affinity and decreased steroid responsiveness at night. J Allergy Clin Immunol 1999;103(1 Pt 1):66–71.

92. Kraft M, Hamid Q, Chrousos GP, et al. Decreased steroid responsiveness at night in nocturnal asthma. Is the macrophage responsible? Am J Respir Crit Care Med 2001;163(5):1219–25.

93. Spengler CM, Shea SA. Endogenous circadian rhythm of pulmonary function in healthy humans. Am J Respir Crit Care Med 2000;162(3 Pt 1):1038–46.

94. Shea SA, Scheer FA, Hilton MF. Predicting the daily pattern of asthma severity based on relative contributions of the circadian timing system, the sleep-wake cycle and the environment. Sleep 2007; 30(suppl):S65.

95. Shea Sa HM, Scheer FAJL, Ayers RT, et al. An endogenous circadian rhythm in bronchodilators rescue medication use in asthma. Sleep 2004; 27(suppl):S81.

96. National Asthma Education and Prevention Program (NAEPP). Guidelines for the diagnosis and management of asthma: expert panel report 2. Bethesda MNH: Lung, and Blood Institute; 1997.

97. Darow PSV. Therapeutic advantage of unequal dosing of theophylline in patients with nocturnal asthma. Chronobiol Int 1987;4:349–57.

98. Smolensky MH, Scott PH, Harrist RB, et al. Administration-time-dependency of the pharmacokinetic behavior and therapeutic effect of a once-a-day theophylline in asthmatic children. Chronobiol Int 1987;4(3):435–47.

99. D'Alonzo GE, Smolensky MH, Feldman S, et al. Twenty-four hour lung function in adult patients with asthma. Chronoptimized theophylline therapy once-daily dosing in the evening versus conventional twice-daily dosing. Am Rev Respir Dis 1990;142(1):84–90.

100. Neuenkirchen H, Wilkens JH, Oellerich M, et al. Nocturnal asthma: effect of a once per evening dose of sustained release theophylline. Eur J Respir Dis 1985;66(3):196–204.

101. Reinberg A, Pauchet F, Ruff F, et al. Comparison of once-daily evening versus morning sustained-release theophylline dosing for nocturnal asthma. Chronobiol Int 1987;4(3):409–19.

102. Kraft M, Torvik JA, Trudeau JB, et al. Theophylline: potential antiinflammatory effects in nocturnal asthma. J Allergy Clin Immunol 1996;97(6):1242–6.

103. Reinberg A, Guillet P, Gervais P, et al. One month chronocorticotherapy (Dutimelan 8 15 mite). Control of the asthmatic condition without adrenal suppression and circadian rhythm alteration. Chronobiologia 1977;4(4):295–312.

104. Beam WR, Weiner DE, Martin RJ. Timing of prednisone and alterations of airways inflammation in nocturnal asthma. Am Rev Respir Dis 1992; 146(6):1524–30.

105. Reinberg A, Gervais P, Chaussade M, et al. Circadian changes in effectiveness of corticosteroids in eight patients with allergic asthma. J Allergy Clin Immunol 1983;71(4):425–33.

106. Ceresa F, Angeli A, Boccuzzi G, et al. Once-a-day neurally stimulated and basal ACTH secretion phases in man and their response to corticoid inhibition. J Clin Endocrinol Metab 1969;29(8): 1074–82.

107. Toogood JH, Baskerville JC, Jennings B, et al. Influence of dosing frequency and schedule on the response of chronic asthmatics to the aerosol steroid, budesonide. J Allergy Clin Immunol 1982; 70(4):288–98.

108. Pincus DJ, Humeston TR, Martin RJ. Further studies on the chronotherapy of asthma with inhaled steroids: the effect of dosage timing on drug efficacy. J Allergy Clin Immunol 1997;100(6): 771–4.

109. Kemp JP, Berkowitz RB, Miller SD, et al. Mometasone furoate administered once daily is as effective as twice-daily administration for treatment of mild-to-moderate persistent asthma. J Allergy Clin Immunol 2000;106(3):485–92.

110. Gaultier C, Reinberg A, Motohashi Y. Circadian rhythm in total pulmonary resistance of asthmatic children. Effects of a beta-agonist agent. Chronobiol Int 1988;5(3):285–90.

111. D'Alonzo GE, Smolensky MH, Feldman S, et al. Bambuterol in the treatment of asthma. A placebo-controlled comparison of once-daily morning vs evening administration. Chest 1995;107(2):406–12.

112. Faurschou P, Engel AM, Haanaes OC. Salmeterol in two different doses in the treatment of nocturnal bronchial asthma poorly controlled by other therapies. Allergy 1994;49(10):827–32.

113. Noonan MJ, Chervinsky P, Brandon M, et al. Montelukast, a potent leukotriene receptor antagonist, causes dose-related improvements in chronic asthma. Montelukast Asthma Study Group. Eur Respir J 1998;11(6):1232–9.

114. Altman LC, Munk Z, Seltzer J, et al. A placebo-controlled, dose-ranging study of montelukast, a cysteinyl leukotriene-receptor antagonist. Montelukast Asthma Study Group. J Allergy Clin Immunol 1998;102(1):50–6.

115. Iravani JM. Theophylline and mucocilliary function. Chest 1987;92(Suppl):38–43.

116. Murciano D, Aubier M, Lecocguic Y, et al. Effects of theophylline on diaphragmatic strength and fatigue in patients with chronic obstructive pulmonary disease. N Engl J Med 1984;311(6):349–53.

117. Rafnsson V, Tulinius H, Jonasson JG, et al. Risk of breast cancer in female flight attendants: a population-based study (Iceland). Cancer Causes Control 2001;12(2):95–101.

118. Mormont MC, Waterhouse J, Bleuzen P, et al. Marked 24-h rest/activity rhythms are associated with better quality of life, better response, and longer survival in patients with metastatic colorectal cancer and good performance status. Clin Cancer Res 2000;6(8):3038–45.

119. Nakamura KD, Duffy PH, Lu MH, et al. The effect of dietary restriction on myc protooncogene expression in mice: a preliminary study. Mech Ageing Dev 1989;48(2):199–205.

120. Fu L, Pelicano H, Liu J, et al. The circadian gene period2 plays an important role in tumor suppression and DNA damage response in vivo. Cell 2002;111(1):41–50.

121. Miller BH, McDearmon EL, Panda S, et al. Circadian and CLOCK-controlled regulation of the mouse transcriptome and cell proliferation. Proc Natl Acad Sci U S A 2007;104(9):3342–7.

122. Gery S, Gombart AF, Yi WS, et al. Transcription profiling of C/EBP targets identifies Per2 as a gene implicated in myeloid leukemia. Blood 2005;106(8):2827–36.

123. Gery S, Komatsu N, Baldjyan L, et al. The circadian gene per1 plays an important role in cell growth and DNA damage control in human cancer cells. Mol Cell 2006;22(3):375–82.

124. Hua H, Wang Y, Wan C, et al. Circadian gene mPer2 overexpression induces cancer cell apoptosis. Cancer Sci 2006;97(7):589–96.

125. Johansen LM, Iwama A, Lodie TA, et al. c-Myc is a critical target for c/EBPalpha in granulopoiesis. Mol Cell Biol 2001;21(11):3789–806.

126. Matsuo T, Yamaguchi S, Mitsui S, et al. Control mechanism of the circadian clock for timing of cell division in vivo. Science 2003;302(5643):255–9.

127. Wang H MS, Grachtchouk V, Zhuang D, et al. c-myc depletion inhibits proliferation of human cells at various stages of the cell cycle. Oncogene 2008;27:1905–15.

128. Prathapam T, Tegen S, Oskarsson T, et al. Activated Src abrogates the Myc requirement for the G0/G1 transition but not for the G1/S transition. Proc Natl Acad Sci U S A 2006;103(8):2695–700.

129. Levi F, Focan C, Karaboue A, et al. Implications of circadian clocks for the rhythmic delivery of cancer therapeutics. Adv Drug Deliv Rev 2007;59(9-10):1015–35.

130. Dang CV, Gerson SL, Litwak M, et al. Gene therapy and translational cancer research. Clin Cancer Res 1999;5(2):471–4.

131. Lissoni P, Brivio F, Fumagalli L, et al. Neuroimmunomodulation in medical oncology: application of psychoneuroimmunology with subcutaneous low-dose IL-2 and the pineal hormone melatonin in patients with untreatable metastatic solid tumors. Anticancer Res 2008;28(2B):1377–81.

132. Lissoni P, Chilelli M, Villa S, et al. Five years survival in metastatic non–small cell lung cancer patients treated with chemotherapy alone or chemotherapy and melatonin: a randomized trial. J Pineal Res 2003;35(1):12–5.

133. Blask DE, Brainard GC, Dauchy RT, et al. Melatonin-depleted blood from premenopausal women exposed to light at night stimulates growth of human breast cancer xenografts in nude rats. Cancer Res 2005;65(23):11174–84.

134. Pavlova MK, Shea SA, Bromfield EB. Day/night patterns of focal seizures. Epilepsy Behav 2004;5(1):44–9.

135. Durazzo TS, Spencer SS, Duckrow RB, et al. Temporal distributions of seizure occurrence from various epileptogenic regions. Neurology 2008;70(15):1265–71.

136. Pavlova Mk BE, Evoniuk H, Shea SA. Endogenous circadian variation of epileptiform abnormalities in

idiopathic generalized epilepsy. Sleep 2005; 28(Suppl):S71.

137. Herman ST, Walczak TS, Bazil CW. Distribution of partial seizures during the sleep–wake cycle: differences by seizure onset site. Neurology 2001; 56(11):1453–9.

138. Yegnanarayan R, Mahesh SD, Sangle S. Chronotherapeutic dose schedule of phenytoin and carbamazepine in epileptic patients. Chronobiol Int 2006;23(5):1035–46.

139. Orr WC, Allen ML, Robinson M. The pattern of nocturnal and diurnal esophageal acid exposure in the pathogenesis of erosive mucosal damage. Am J Gastroenterol 1994;89(4):509–12.

140. Lear CS, Flanagan JB Jr, Moorrees CF. The frequency of deglutition in man. Arch Oral Biol 1965;10:83–100.

141. Schneyer LH, Pigman W, Hanahan L, et al. Rate of flow of human parotid, sublingual, and submaxillary secretions during sleep. J Dent Res 1956; 35(1):109–14.

142. Elsenbruch S, Orr WC, Harnish MJ, et al. Disruption of normal gastric myoelectric functioning by sleep. Sleep 1999;22(4):453–8.

143. Orr WC, Johnson LF, Robinson MG. Effect of sleep on swallowing, esophageal peristalsis, and acid clearance. Gastroenterology 1984;86(5):814–9.

144. Satlin A, Volicer L, Stopa EG, et al. Circadian locomotor activity and core-body temperature rhythms in Alzheimer's disease. Neurobiol Aging 1995; 16(5):765–71.

145. Hu K, van Someren EJ, Shea SA, et al. Reduction of scale-invariance of activity fluctuations with aging and Alzheimer's disease: involvement of the circadian pacemaker. Proc Natl Acad Sci USA 2009; 106(8):2490–4.

146. Cohen-Mansfield J, Garfinkel D, Lipson S. Melatonin for treatment of sundowning in elderly persons with dementia—a preliminary study. Arch Gerontol Geriatr 2000;31(1):65–76.

147. McDuff T, Sumi SM. Subcortical degeneration in Alzheimer's disease. Neurology 1985;35(1):123–6.

148. Swaab DF, Fliers E, Partiman TS. The suprachiasmatic nucleus of the human brain in relation to sex, age and senile dementia. Brain Res 1985; 342(1):37–44.

149. Selkoe DJ. Cell biology of protein misfolding: the examples of Alzheimer's and Parkinson's diseases. Nat Cell Biol 2004;6(11):1054–61.

150. Zhou JN, Hofman MA, Swaab DF. VIP neurons in the human SCN in relation to sex, age and Alzheimer Disease. Neurology of Aging 1995;16(4):571–6.

151. Liu RY, Zhou JN, Hoogendijk WJ, et al. Decreased vasopressin gene expression in the biological clock of Alzheimer disease patients with and without depression. J Neuropathol Exp Neurol 2000;59(4):314–22.

152. Maywood ES, Reddy AB, Wong GK, et al. Synchronization and maintenance of timekeeping in suprachiasmatic circadian clock cells by neuropeptidergic signaling. Curr Biol 2006;16(6): 599–605.

153. Sheward WJ, Maywood ES, French KL, et al. Entrainment to feeding but not to light: circadian phenotype of VPAC2 receptor-null mice. J Neurosci 2007;27(16):4351–8.

154. Wu YH, Feenstra MG, Zhou JN, et al. Molecular changes underlying reduced pineal melatonin levels in Alzheimer disease: alterations in preclinical and clinical stages. J Clin Endocrinol Metab 2003;88(12):5898–906.

155. Wu YH, Fischer DF, Kalsbeek A, et al. Pineal clock gene oscillation is disturbed in Alzheimer's disease, due to functional disconnection from the "master clock". Faseb J 2006;20(11):1874–6.

156. Wang JZ, Wang ZF. Role of melatonin in Alzheimer-like neurodegeneration. Acta Pharmacol Sin 2006; 27(1):41–9.

157. Lahiri DK. Melatonin affects the metabolism of the beta-amyloid precursor protein in different cell types. J Pineal Res 1999;26(3):137–46.

158. Song W, Lahiri DK. Melatonin alters the metabolism of the beta-amyloid precursor protein in the neuroendocrine cell line PC12. J Mol Neurosci 1997;9(2): 75–92.

159. Zhang YC, Wang ZF, Wang Q, et al. Melatonin attenuates beta-amyloid–induced inhibition of neurofilament expression. Acta Pharmacol Sin 2004; 25(4):447–51.

160. Arendt J. Melatonin and the mamallian pineal gland. 1st edition. London: Chapman and Hall; 1995.

161. Cardinali DP, Brusco LI, Liberczuk C, et al. The use of melatonin in Alzheimer's disease. Neuro Endocrinol Lett 2002;23(Suppl 1):20–3.

162. Cardinali DP, Brusco LI, Lloret SP, et al. Melatonin in sleep disorders and jet-lag. Neuro Endocrinol Lett 2002;23(Suppl 1):9–13.

163. Sasaki M, Jordan P, Joh T, et al. Melatonin reduces TNF-a induced expression of MAdCAM-1 via inhibition of NF-kappaB. BMC Gastroenterol 2002;2:9.

164. Pei Z, Cheung RT. Pretreatment with melatonin exerts anti-inflammatory effects against ischemia/reperfusion injury in a rat middle cerebral artery occlusion stroke model. J Pineal Res 2004;37(2):85–91.

165. Feng Z, Chang Y, Cheng Y, et al. Melatonin alleviates behavioral deficits associated with apoptosis and cholinergic system dysfunction in the APP 695 transgenic mouse model of Alzheimer's disease. J Pineal Res 2004;37(2):129–36.

166. Feng Z, Cheng Y, Zhang JT. Long-term effects of melatonin or 17 beta-estradiol on improving spatial memory performance in cognitively impaired, ovariectomized adult rats. J Pineal Res 2004; 37(3):198–206.

167. Riemersma-van der Lek RF, Swaab DF, Twisk J, et al. Effect of bright light and melatonin on cognitive and noncognitive function in elderly residents of group care facilities: a randomized controlled trial. JAMA 2008;299(22):2642–55.

168. Ayas NT, White DP, Manson JE, et al. A prospective study of sleep duration and coronary heart disease in women. Arch Intern Med 2003;163(2):205–9.

169. Harrison Y, Horne JA. The impact of sleep deprivation on decision making: a review. J Exp Psychol Appl 2000;6(3):236–49.

170. Knutson KL, Van Cauter E. Associations between sleep loss and increased risk of obesity and diabetes. Ann N Y Acad Sci 2008;1129:287–304.

171. Monk TH. Shift work: basic principles. In: Kryger MRT, Dement WC, editors. Principles and practice of sleep medicine. 4th edition. Philadelphia: WB Saunders Co; 2005. p. 673–80.

172. Gander PH, Gregory KB, Miller DL, et al. Flight crew fatigue V: long-haul air transport operations. Aviat Space Environ Med 1998;69(Suppl 9):B37–48.

173. Mitler MM, Miller JC, Lipsitz JJ, et al. The sleep of long-haul truck drivers. N Engl J Med 1997; 337(11):755–61.

174. Kawachi I, Colditz GA, Stamfer MJ, et al. Prospective study of shift work and risk of coronary heart disease in women. Circulation 1996;92:3178–82.

175. Karlsson B, Alfredsson L, Knutsson A, et al. Total mortality and cause-specific mortality of Swedish shift- and dayworkers in the pulp and paper industry in 1952-2001. Scand J Work Environ Health 2005;31(1):30–5.

176. Boggild H, Suadicani P, Hein HO, et al. Shift work, social class, and ischaemic heart disease in middle aged and elderly men; a 22 year follow up in the Copenhagen Male Study. Occup Environ Med 1999;56(9):640–5.

177. Oishi M, Suwazono Y, Sakata K, et al. A longitudinal study on the relationship between shift work and the progression of hypertension in male Japanese workers. J Hypertens 2005;23(12):2173–8.

178. Inoue M, Morita H, Inagaki J, et al. Influence of differences in their jobs on cardiovascular risk factors in male blue-collar shift workers in their fifties. Int J Occup Environ Health 2004;10(3):313–8.

179. Knutsson A, Akerstedt T, Jonsson BG, et al. Increased risk of ischaemic heart disease in shift workers. Lancet 1986;328(8498):89–92.

180. Tuchsen F, Hannerz H, Burr H. A 12 year prospective study of circulatory disease among Danish shift workers. Occup Environ Med 2006;63(7):451–5.

181. Sgoifo A, Buwalda B, Roos M, et al. Effects of sleep deprivation on cardiac autonomic and pituitary-adrenocortical stress reactivity in rats. Psychoneuroendocrinology 2006;31(2):197–208.

182. Yamasaki F, Schwartz JE, Gerber LM, et al. Impact of shift work and race/ethnicity on the diurnal rhythm of blood pressure and catecholamines. Hypertension 1998;32(3):417–23.

183. Kitamura T, Onishi K, Dohi K, et al. Circadian rhythm of blood pressure is transformed from a dipper to a non-dipper pattern in shift workers with hypertension. J Hum Hypertens 2002;16(3): 193–7.

184. Ishizaki M YM, Nakagawa H, Honda R, et al. The influence of work characteristics on body mass index and waist to hip ratio in Japanese employees. Ind Health 2004;42:41–9.

185. Niedhammer I, Lert F, Marne MJ. Prevalence of overweight and weight gain in relation to night work in a nurses' cohort. Int J Obes Relat Metab Disord 1996;20(7):625–33.

186. Karlsson B, Knutsson A, Lindahl B. Is there an association between shift work and having a metabolic syndrome? Results from a population based study of 27,485 people. Occup Environ Med 2001;58(11):747–52.

187. Nagaya T, Yoshida H, Takahashi H, et al. Markers of insulin resistance in day and shift workers aged 30–59 years. Int Arch Occup Environ Health 2002;75(8):562–8.

188. Mikuni E, Ohoshi T, Hayashi K, et al. Glucose intolerance in an employed population. Tohoku J Exp Med 1983;141(Suppl):251–6.

189. Kroenke CH, Spiegelman D, Manson J, et al. Work characteristics and incidence of type 2 diabetes in women. Am J Epidemiol 2007;165(2):175–83.

190. Buxton Om SK, Van Cauter E. Modulation of endocrine function and metabolism by sleep and sleep loss. In: Lee-Chiong M, Carskadon M, Sateia M, editors. Sleep medicine. Philadelphia: Hanley& Belfus, Inc; 2002. p. 59–69.

191. Chaput JP, Despres JP, Bouchard C, et al. Short sleep duration is associated with reduced leptin levels and increased adiposity: results from the Quebec family study. Obesity (Silver Spring) 2007;15(1):253–61.

192. Spiegel K, Tasali E, Penev P, et al. Brief communication: sleep curtailment in healthy young men is associated with decreased leptin levels, elevated ghrelin levels, and increased hunger and appetite. Ann Intern Med 2004;141(11):846–50.

193. Mullington JM, Chan JL, Van Dongen HP, et al. Sleep loss reduces diurnal rhythm amplitude of leptin in healthy men. J Neuroendocrinol 2003; 15(9):851–4.

194. Spiegel K, Leproult R, L'Hermite-Baleriaux M, et al. Leptin levels are dependent on sleep duration: relationships with sympathovagal balance, carbohydrate regulation, cortisol, and thyrotropin. J Clin Endocrinol Metab 2004;89(11):5762–71.

195. Muoio DM, Lynis Dohm G. Peripheral metabolic actions of leptin. Best Pract Res Clin Endocrinol Metab 2002;16(4):653–66.

196. Lichnovska R, Gwozdziewiczova S, Hrebicek J. Gender differences in factors influencing insulin resistance in elderly hyperlipemic non-diabetic subjects. Cardiovasc Diabetol 2002;1:4.

197. Saad MF, Khan A, Sharma A, et al. Physiological insulinemia acutely modulates plasma leptin. Diabetes 1998;47(4):544–9.

198. Shea SA, Hilton MF, Orlova C, et al. Independent circadian and sleep/wake regulation of adipokines and glucose in humans. J Clin Endocrinol Metab 2005;90(5):2537–44.

199. Gavrila A, Peng CK, Chan JL, et al. Diurnal and ultradian dynamics of serum adiponectin in healthy men: comparison with leptin, circulating soluble leptin receptor, and cortisol patterns. J Clin Endocrinol Metab 2003;88(6):2838–43.

200. Oliver P, Ribot J, Rodriguez AM, et al. Resistin as a putative modulator of insulin action in the daily feeding/fasting rhythm. Pflugers Arch 2006; 452(3):260–7.

201. Ariyasu H, Takaya K, Tagami T, et al. Stomach is a major source of circulating ghrelin, and feeding state determines plasma ghrelin-like immunoreactivity levels in humans. J Clin Endocrinol Metab 2001;86(10):4753–8.

202. Tritos NA, Mun E, Bertkau A, et al. Serum ghrelin levels in response to glucose load in obese subjects post-gastric bypass surgery. Obes Res 2003;11(8):919–24.

203. Yannielli PC, Molyneux PC, Harrington ME, et al. Ghrelin effects on the circadian system of mice. J Neurosci 2007;27(11):2890–5.

204. Taheri S, Lin L, Austin D, et al. Short sleep duration is associated with reduced leptin, elevated ghrelin, and increased body mass index. PLoS Med 2004; 1(3):e62.

205. Scheer FA, Hilton MF, Mantzoros CS, et al. Adverse metabolic and cardiovascular consequences of circadian misalignment. Proc Natl Acad Sci U S A 2009;106(11):4453–8.

206. Taylor PJ, Pocock SJ. Mortality of shift and day workers 1956-68. Br J Ind Med 1972;29(2):201–7.

207. Schernhammer ES, Laden F, Speizer FE, et al. Rotating night shifts and risk of breast cancer in women participating in the nurses' health study. J Natl Cancer Inst 2001;93(20):1563–8.

208. Tynes T, Hannevik M, Andersen A, et al. Incidence of breast cancer in Norwegian female radio and telegraph operators. Cancer Causes Control 1996;7(2):197–204.

209. Hansen J. Increased breast cancer risk among women who work predominantly at night. Epidemiology 2001;12(1):74–7.

210. Schernhammer ES, Laden F, Speizer FE, et al. Night-shift work and risk of colorectal cancer in the nurses' health study. J Natl Cancer Inst 2003; 95(11):825–8.

211. Krstev S, Baris D, Stewart PA, et al. Risk for prostate cancer by occupation and industry: a 24-state death certificate study. Am J Ind Med 1998;34(5):413–20.

212. Demers PA, Checkoway H, Vaughan TL, et al. Cancer incidence among firefighters in Seattle and Tacoma, Washington (United States). Cancer Causes Control 1994;5(2):129–35.

213. Hill SM, Blask DE. Effects of the pineal hormone melatonin on the proliferation and morphological characteristics of human breast cancer cells (MCF-7) in culture. Cancer Res 1988;48(21):6121–6.

214. Cos S, Fernandez R, Guezmes A, et al. Influence of melatonin on invasive and metastatic properties of MCF-7 human breast cancer cells. Cancer Res 1998;58(19):4383–90.

215. Cos S, Mediavilla MD, Fernandez R, et al. Does melatonin induce apoptosis in MCF-7 human breast cancer cells in vitro? J Pineal Res 2002;32: 90–6.

216. Mediavilla MD, Cos S, Sanchez-Barcelo EJ. Melatonin increases p53 and p21WAF1 expression in MCF-7 human breast cancer cells in vitro. Life Sci 1999;65(4):415–20.

217. Tamarkin L, Cohen M, Roselle D, et al. Melatonin inhibition and pinealectomy enhancement of 7,12-dimethylbenz(a)anthracene–induced mammary tumors in the rat. Cancer Res 1981;41(11): 4432–6.

218. Tam CW, Mo CW, Yao KM, et al. Signaling mechanisms of melatonin in antiproliferation of hormone refractory 22rv1 human prostate cancer cells: implications for prostate cancer chemoprevention. J Pineal Res 2007;42(2):191–202.

219. Zhu Y, Brown HN, Zhang Y, et al. Period3 structural variation: a circadian biomarker associated with breast cancer in young women. Cancer Epidemiol Biomarkers Prev 2005;14(1):268–70.

220. Challet E, Poirel VJ, Malan A, et al. Light exposure during daytime modulates expression of Per1 and Per2 clock genes in the suprachiasmatic nuclei of mice. J Neurosci Res 2003;72(5):629–37.

221. Caldelas I, Poirel VJ, Sicard B, et al. Circadian profile and photic regulation of clock genes in the suprachiasmatic nucleus of a diurnal mammal Arvicanthis ansorgei. Neuroscience 2003;116(2): 583–91.

222. Segawa K, Nakazawa S, Tsukamoto Y, et al. Peptic ulcer is prevalent among shift workers. Dig Dis Sci 1987;32(5):449–53.

223. Rubin NH, Singh P, Alinder G, et al. Circadian rhythms in gastrin receptors in rat fundic stomach. Dig Dis Sci 1988;33(8):931–7.

224. Larsen KR, Dayton MT, Moore JG. Circadian rhythm in gastric mucosal blood flow in fasting rat stomach. J Surg Res 1991;51(4):275–80.

225. Larsen KR, Moore JG, Dayton MT. Circadian rhythms of gastric mucus efflux and residual mucus

gel in the fasting rat stomach. Dig Dis Sci 1991; 36(11):1550–5.

226. Moore JG, Mitchell MD, Larsen KR, et al. Circadian rhythm in prostacyclin activity in gastric tissue of the fasting rat. Am J Surg 1992; 163(1):19–22.

227. Moore JG, Goo RH. Day and night aspirin-induced gastric mucosal damage and protection by ranitidine in man. Chronobiol Int 1987;4(1):111–6.

228. Larsen KR, Moore JG, Dayton MT, et al. Circadian rhythm in aspirin (ASA)-induced injury to the stomach of the fasted rat. Dig Dis Sci 1993;38(8): 1435–40.

229. Goo RH, Moore JG, Greenberg E, et al. Circadian variation in gastric emptying of meals in humans. Gastroenterology 1987;93(3):515–8.

230. Kumar D, Wingate D, Ruckebusch Y. Circadian variation in the propagation velocity of the migrating motor complex. Gastroenterology 1986; 91(4):926–30.

231. Moore JG, Halberg F. Circadian rhythm of gastric acid secretion in men with active duodenal ulcer. Dig Dis Sci 1986;31(11):1185–91.

232. Larsen KR, Moore JG, Dayton MT. Circadian rhythms of acid and bicarbonate efflux in fasting rat stomach. Am J Physiol 1991;260(4 Pt 1):G610–4.

233. Axelsson G, Rylander R, Molin I. Outcome of pregnancy in relation to irregular and inconvenient work schedules. Br J Ind Med 1989;46(6):393–8.

234. Mamelle N, Laumon B, Lazar P. Prematurity and occupational activity during pregnancy. Am J Epidemiol 1984;119(3):309–22.

Effect of Light on Human Circadian Physiology

Jeanne F. Duffy, MBA, PhD*, Charles A. Czeisler, PhD, MD

KEYWORDS

- Biological rhythm • Core body temperature
- Illuminance • Melatonin • Phase-response curve

Circadian rhythms are variations in physiology and behavior that persist with a cycle length close to 24 hours even in the absence of periodic environmental stimuli. It is hypothesized that this system evolved to predict and therefore optimally time the behavior and physiology of the organism to the environmental periodicity associated with the earth's rotation. Because the cycle length, or period, of this endogenous timing system is near, but not exactly, 24 hours in most organisms, circadian rhythms must be synchronized or entrained to the 24-hour day on a regular basis. In most

The studies reviewed here were supported by National Institutes of Health grants MH45130, AG06072, AG09975, HL077453, HL08978, AT002571; by National Aeronautics and Space Administration grants NAG9-524, NAGW-4033, NAG5-3952; by National Aeronautics and Space Administration Cooperative Agreement NCC9-58 with the National Space Biomedical Research Institute; and by Air Force Office of Scientific Research grant F49620-94. Many of these studies were conducted in the General Clinical Research Center at Brigham and Women's Hospital, supported by National Institutes of Health grant RR02635. Dr. Duffy reports no conflicts of interest. Dr. Czeisler has received consulting fees from or has served as a paid member of scientific advisory boards for Actelion, Ltd.; Avera Pharmaceuticals, Inc.; Axon Labs, Inc.; Cephalon, Inc.; Delta Airlines; Eli Lilly and Co.; Fedex Kinko's; Garda Inspectorate, Republic of Ireland; Fusion Medical Education, LLC; Hypnion, Inc.; Morgan Stanley; Sanofi-Aventis, Inc.; the Portland Trail Blazers; Sleep Multimedia, Inc.; Sleep Research Society (for which Dr. Czeisler served as president); Respironics, Inc.; Koninklijke Philips Electronics, N.V.; Sepracor, Inc.; Somnus Therapeutics, Inc.; Takeda Pharmaceuticals; Vanda Pharmaceuticals, Inc., Vital Issues in Medicine and Warburg-Pincus. Dr. Czeisler also owns an equity interest in Axon Labs, Inc.; Lifetrac, Inc.; Somnus Therapeutics, Inc.; and Vanda Pharmaceuticals, Inc. Dr. Czeisler has received lecture fees from the Accreditation Council of Graduate Medical Education; Alfresa; Cephalon, Inc.; Clinical Excellence Commission (Australia); Dalhousie University; Duke University Medical Center; Institute of Sleep Health Promotion (NPO); London Deanery; Morehouse School of Medicine; Sanofi-Aventis, Inc.; Takeda; Tanabe Seiyaku Co., Ltd.; Tokyo Electric Power Company (TEPCO). Dr. Czeisler has also received clinical trial research contracts from Cephalon, Inc.; Merck & Co., Inc.; and Pfizer, Inc.; an investigator-initiated research grant from Cephalon, Inc.; and his research laboratory at the Brigham and Women's Hospital has received unrestricted research and education funds and/or support for research expenses from Cephalon, Inc.; Koninklijke Philips Electronics, N.V.; ResMed; and the Brigham and Women's Hospital. The Harvard Medical School Division of Sleep Medicine (HMS/DSM), which Dr. Czeisler directs, has received unrestricted research and educational gifts and endowment funds from Boehringer Ingelheim Pharmaceuticals, Inc.; Cephalon, Inc.; George H. Kidder, Esq.; Gerald McGinnis; GlaxoSmithKline; Herbert Lee; Hypnion; Jazz Pharmaceuticals; Jordan's Furniture; Merck & Co., Inc.; Peter C. Farrell, PhD; Pfizer; ResMed; Respironics, Inc.; Sanofi-Aventis, Inc.; Sealy, Inc.; Sepracor, Inc.; Simmons; Sleep Health Centers LLC; Spring Aire; Takeda Pharmaceuticals; Tempur-Pedic; Aetna US Healthcare; Alertness Solutions, Inc.; Axon Sleep Research Laboratories, Inc.; Boehringer Ingelheim Pharmaceuticals, Inc.; Bristol-Myers Squibb; Catalyst Group; Cephalon, Inc.; Clarus Ventures; Comfortaire Corporation; Committee for Interns and Residents; Farrell Family Foundation; George H. Kidder, Esq.; GlaxoSmithKline; Hypnion, Inc.; Innovative Brands Group; Nature's Rest; Jordan's Furniture; King Koil Sleep Products; King Koil, Division of Blue Bell Mattress; Land and Sky; Merck Research Laboratories; MPM Capital; Neurocrine Biosciences, Inc.; Orphan Medical/Jazz Pharmaceuticals; Park Place Corporation; Pfizer Global Pharmaceuticals; Pfizer Healthcare Division, Pfizer, Inc.; Pfizer/Neurocrine Biosciences, Inc.; Purdue Pharma L.P.; ResMed, Inc.; Respironics, Inc.; Sanofi-Aventis, Inc.; Sanofi-Synthelabo; Sealy Mattress Company; Sealy, Inc.; Sepracor, Inc.; Simmons Co.; Sleep Health Centers LLC; Spring Air Mattress Co.; Takeda Pharmaceuticals; Tempur-Pedic Medical Division; Total Sleep Holdings; Vanda Pharmaceuticals, Inc.; and the Zeno Group, together with gifts from many individuals and organizations through an annual benefit dinner. The Harvard Medical School Division of Sleep Medicine Sleep and Health Education Program has received educational grant funding from Cephalon, Inc.; Takeda Pharmaceuticals; Sanofi-Aventis, Inc.; and Sepracor, Inc. Dr. Czeisler is the incumbent of an endowed professorship provided to Harvard University by Cephalon, Inc. and holds a number of process patents in the field of sleep/circadian rhythms (eg, photic resetting of the human circadian pacemaker). Since 1985, Dr. Czeisler has also served as an expert witness on various legal cases related to sleep and/or circadian rhythms.

Division of Sleep Medicine, Department of Medicine, Brigham & Women's Hospital, and Division of Sleep Medicine, Harvard Medical School, Boston, MA 02115, USA

* Corresponding author.

E-mail address: jduffy@hms.harvard.edu (J.F. Duffy).

Sleep Med Clin 4 (2009) 165–177
doi:10.1016/j.jsmc.2009.01.004

organisms, this process of entrainment occurs through regular exposure to light and darkness.

Early reports from studies of human circadian rhythms had suggested that humans were unlike other organisms, being relatively insensitive to light and more sensitive to social cues to entrain their circadian systems. However, subsequent studies, and reanalysis of results from those early studies, have found that the human circadian system is like that of other organisms in its organization and in its response to light, and is as sensitive to light as the circadian systems of other diurnal organisms. In this article, we review the results of studies over the past 25 years conducted in our laboratory and in those of others investigating the effects of light on the human circadian timing system.

NEUROANATOMY OF THE MAMMALIAN CIRCADIAN SYSTEM

Studies published in the early 1970s established the suprachiasmatic nucleus of the hypothalamus as the central circadian pacemaker in mammals.[1–5] This pacemaker is composed of individual cells that, when isolated, can oscillate independently with a near-24-hour period.[5,6] The suprachiasmatic nucleus receives direct input from the retina,[7–9] providing a mechanism by which entrainment to light-dark cycles occurs. Investigators have recently described a subset of retinal ganglion cells that serve as photoreceptors for circadian and other non–image-forming responses (NIFs).[10–12] These specialized retinal ganglion cells are distributed throughout the retina, project to the suprachiasmatic nucleus, are photosensitive, and contain melanopsin as their photopigment.[13,14] While the photosensitive retinal ganglion cells can mediate circadian responses to light, evidence suggests that rod and cone photoreceptors can also play a role in circadian responses to light.[15,16] The relative contribution of different photoreceptors to circadian responses is not yet well understood and is an area of intense research. It is likely that the intensity, spectral distribution, and temporal pattern of light can all affect the relative contribution of different photoreceptors to circadian responses. The same neuroanatomical features of the circadian system described in mammals are also present in humans.[17–24]

PHASE-DEPENDENT RESPONSE OF THE HUMAN CIRCADIAN SYSTEM TO LIGHT

Studies of the effects of light on the circadian system of insects, plants, and animals conducted from the late 1950s through the 1970s demonstrated that the timing of a light stimulus has an important influence on the direction and magnitude of response to that stimulus.[25–28] Those studies indicated that the circadian system of both nocturnal and diurnal organisms is most sensitive to light during the biological night. Because humans sleep throughout most of their biological night, testing the influence of light on the human circadian system requires that in the sleep-wake cycle be shifted to deliver the light stimulus at the time of highest expected sensitivity. Because of prior reports suggesting that social cues influenced human circadian rhythms, that manipulation of sleep-wake timing was a concern in the earliest human light studies.[29,30]

For those reasons, we therefore conducted one of our earliest studies of the effect of light on the human circadian system on a subject whose circadian temperature rhythm had an unusual phase relationship to her sleep-wake cycle.[31] We identified a subject whose sleep-wake cycle timing was fairly normal, but whose circadian core body temperature rhythm was several hours earlier than normal, resulting in much of her biological night occurring before the time she went to bed. In the experiment we conducted, the subject was exposed to several hours of light every evening for a week, and the timing of her rhythms of core body temperature and plasma cortisol were assessed before and after that week of evening light exposure. Both rhythms were shifted by approximately 6 hours, and examination of temperature data collected throughout the experiment suggested that the shift had already occurred after only 2 days.

This finding that light could have this rapid and strong effect on the timing of human circadian rhythms led us to conduct a series of studies in normal young adults to whom we applied a series of light stimuli over 2 to 3 days.[32,33] In those studies performed in the late 1980s, we held the intensity, spectral distribution, and duration of the light stimulus constant, but varied the time at which the initial stimulus was applied. To do this, we had to shift the timing of the sleep-wake cycle so as to be able to present light stimuli across the entire 24-hour circadian cycle. In the course of doing these initial experiments, we were attempting to produce a phase-response curve (PRC).[28]

Our results were not surprising in some ways, but surprising in others. We found that humans, like other organisms, are most sensitive to light stimuli during the biological night, and far less sensitive to light in the middle of the biological day.[32,34] We also found that when humans are exposed to a light stimulus in the late-biological-day/

early-biological-night, that stimulus produces a phase-delay shift (a shift to a later hour), and light stimuli presented in the late-biological-night/early-biological-day produce phase-advance shifts (shifts to an earlier hour).

What was somewhat unexpected in those studies was the large magnitude (up to 12 hours) of the phase shifts we were able to achieve, and the PRC that was developed from those three-cycle light stimuli was a type 0 (strong) PRC. A type 0 PRC is characterized by large phase shifts of 12 hours forward or backward, with no "cross-over" point between maximal delays and maximal advances.[35] Type 0 resetting also implied that the phase shift had been produced via changing the amplitude of oscillation of the underlying pacemaker.[36–39] When we subsequently conducted additional experiments to test the phase shifts that could be achieved with a two-cycle stimulus, we found that in some studies we could markedly reduce the amplitude of the core body temperature and cortisol rhythms.[40] This finding suggested that the stimulus affected the amplitude of the underlying pacemaker, lending additional support to the idea that the phase shifts to the strong three-cycle stimulus were type 0.[41]

Since describing that PRC to a strong light stimulus, we and others have conducted PRCs to stimuli consisting of one light pulse.[42–45] In the late 1990s, we constructed a human PRC study to a single 6.7-hour light stimulus.[42] Results from those studies indicated a type 1 PRC, with a shape and magnitude consistent with type 1 PRCs from other organisms. Type 1 PRCs are characterized by a lower amplitude than type 0 with smaller maximal phase shifts, as well as by a crossover point between maximal delays and advances. In the human PRC to the 6.7-hour stimulus, the maximal phase shifts were 2 to 3 hours. There was a phase-delay region in the late-biological-day/early-biological-night, a phase-advance region in the early biological day, small phase shifts during the middle of the biological day, and a transition point toward the end of the biological night (**Fig. 1**).

Evidence from studies in insects shows that both type 0 and type 1 PRCs are possible in the same species, with the PRC type dependent on the strength of the light stimulus, and the organisms in which type 0 resetting has been demonstrated also show type 1 resetting to a weaker stimulus.[35,38,39] In fact, the type 1 and type 0 PRCs of humans are remarkably similar to those of mosquitoes[46] (see article by Czeisler and Wright[47] for illustration of the human and mosquito PRCs).

Additional studies and analyses conducted in our laboratory have also revealed additional features of

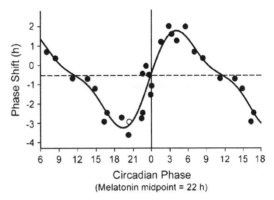

Fig. 1. PRC to a single 6.5-hour episode of bright light in young adults. Phase shifts (in hours) of the plasma melatonin rhythm are plotted with respect to the circadian phase at which the center of the 6.5-hour light stimulus was presented. By convention, phase-delay shifts (shifts to a later hour) are plotted as negative numbers, while phase-advance shifts (shifts to an earlier hour) are plotted as positive numbers. Phase-shift magnitude was determined by assessing phase before and after the light stimulus. Circadian phase of the light stimulus was defined relative to the midpoint of the plasma melatonin rhythm (defined as 22 hours) assessed just before the stimulus. Data from circadian phase 6 through 18 are double-plotted for better visualization. The open circle represents a subject whose phase shift was determined using salivary melatonin. The solid line represents a best-fit dual harmonic function to the data points. The dashed horizontal line represents the assumed 0.54-hour average phase-delay drift of the human circadian pacemaker between the pre- and poststimulus phase assessments. (*From* Khalsa SBS, Jewett ME, Cajochen C, et al. A phase response curve to single bright light pulses in human subjects. J Physiol (Lond) 2003;549(Pt 3):945–52; with permission.)

the human phase-dependent response to light. We have found that humans, like other diurnal species,[48] are sensitive to light throughout the biological day,[34] with little evidence of a so-called "dead zone" (a segment of the PRC during the biological day when no responses are observed). Our analyses have also found that phase shifts to light in humans appear to occur rapidly, with little evidence of transients.[34,49] Together, these studies of the phase-dependent response of humans to light have reinforced the idea that the human circadian system is like that of other organisms.[50]

INTENSITY-DEPENDENT RESPONSE OF THE HUMAN CIRCADIAN SYSTEM TO LIGHT

Reports from studies in nonhuman organisms indicated that the circadian system showed intensity-dependent responses to light stimuli,[25,51–57] in addition to its phase-dependent responses to light. Investigation of the intensity-response relationship to light is typically done by applying light stimuli of varying intensities but of the same duration and spectral composition at a fixed circadian phase. Early reports from human studies had demonstrated that varying the intensity of a light stimulus would produce different amounts of suppression of the pineal hormone melatonin.[58–61] Based on this animal and human evidence, we conducted a series of studies, beginning in the late 1980s,[62] to test the ability of different intensities of light to phase shift the human circadian system.

In the first series of studies, we applied a three-cycle 5-hour light stimulus in the early biological day (the phase-advance portion of the PRC), and studied groups of subjects at several different illuminance levels (0, 12, 180, 600, 1260, and 9500 lux; **Fig. 2**). In those studies,[63–65] we found that the groups exposed to light greater than room-light level showed a significant phase-advance shift, while the groups exposed to darkness or dim light (the 12-lux group) for the same three-cycle 5-hour stimulus timing drifted to a later phase consistent with the longer-than-24-hour period of the human circadian system.[66] The 0-lux and 12-lux control groups also confirmed that the phase shifts produced by the light were mainly due to the light exposure itself, and not to the shift in the timing of the rest-activity schedule.[67]

Subsequently, we conducted another study testing the effect that a single light-exposure would have on the human circadian system when the illuminance was varied.[68] In this study, we used a 6.5-hour light stimulus ranging from 3 to 9100 lux, applied in the late-biological-day/early-biological-night, so as to produce phase-delay shifts. We found that the resetting response and melatonin suppression was related in a nonlinear way to illuminance, with minimal responses below 100 lux and saturating responses above approximately 1000 lux. The best model fit to the data was from a four-parameter logistic model, which predicted a half-maximal response of approximately 100 lux, in the range of normal indoor light.[68] A similar study conducted in healthy older subjects found similar responses to low and high levels of illumination, with a suggestion of slightly less sensitivity in the older subjects compared with that in the younger adults.[69]

In the one-pulse study in young adults, we also examined the relationship between illuminance and measures of alertness, and found that brighter light had greater effects on subjective and objective measures of alertness.[70]

Findings from all of these studies indicate that the human circadian system can be sensitive to rather dim levels of light, including candlelight.[71] In fact, in the one-pulse study by Zeitzer and colleagues,[68] phase shifts of 50% magnitude of the maximal shift (obtained with a 9100-lux stimulus) were obtained with stimuli of only about 1% of that intensity ($\sim$100 lux). However, we should note that the light stimuli in these studies were presented after exposure to many hours of very dim light or darkness, and, as we discuss below, this prior exposure to dim light likely sensitized the system. Thus, while an approximately 100-lux light pulse applied after several hours of very dim light

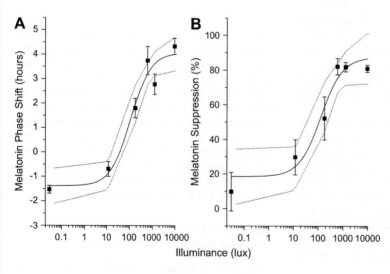

Fig. 2. Phase shifts (A) and melatonin suppression (B) in response to a three-cycle 5-hour light stimulus in young adults. The magnitude of the phase shift (in hours) is plotted with respect to the illuminance of the light stimulus (in lux). Symbols represent mean ($\pm$ standard error of the mean) responses from each group of seven to nine subjects. The solid line represents a three-parameter logistic curve fit to the data, and the upper and lower 95% confidence intervals of this fit are shown in the dashed lines. (From Zeitzer JM, Khalsa SB, Boivin DB, et al. Temporal dynamics of late-night photic stimulation of the human circadian timing system. Am J Physiol 2005;289(3):R839–44; with permission.)

does have a significant phase-shifting and mela-tonin-suppressing effect in humans, the same light pulse applied against a brighter background would likely produce a smaller effect.

RESPONSE OF THE HUMAN CIRCADIAN SYSTEM TO INTERMITTENT BRIGHT-LIGHT EXPOSURE

Studies of light effects in mammals had demon-strated that brief pulses of light could affect the circadian system, and that the system appeared to integrate brief light pulses applied in sequence.[46,55,72] We conducted experiments to explore whether the human circadian system is responsive to short-duration stimuli, and if the human circadian system is capable of integrating short-light stimuli.[73,74] In the first such experi-ment,[73] we used a three-cycle light stimulus applied in the phase-advance region (late-biolog-ical-night/early-biological-day) of the PRC, and tested two different light-stimulus patterns. The first pattern used four periods of light stimuli, each about 46 minutes, alternating with episodes of darkness, each about 44 minutes, so the entire pattern took 5 hours. The second light-stimulus pattern used briefer stimuli, with 13 5.3-minute periods of light stimuli alternating with 19.7-minute episodes of darkness. We compared the results of these two intermittent-light patterns with results from two groups in which we used a continuous 5-hour bright-light stimulus or a continuous 5-hour darkness stimulus.[67] Even though the dura-tion of bright light in the two intermittent-light groups was only 63% or 31% of that for the contin-uous-light group, respectively, we still observed significant phase-advance shifts (**Fig. 3**). The inter-mittent-light group that received 63% of the light duration showed phase shifts that were not signif-icantly different from those for the continuous–bright-light group, with a response approximately 88% of that of the continuous-light group. The intermittent-light group with the shorter light dura-tion (31%) showed phase advances that were approximately 70% of the magnitude of the continuous-light group. These findings demon-strated that humans were responsive to shorter durations of bright-light exposure than had been previously recognized, and that the magnitude of the response was related in a nonlinear way to the duration of light contained within the stimulus.[75,76]

We also conducted an experiment testing the effects of an intermittent-light stimulus using a one-cycle light stimulus.[74] In that study, we used a 6.5-hour stimulus presented in the phase-delay region (early biological night), and compared subjects exposed to continuous bright light,

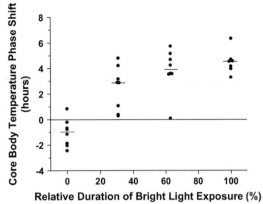

Fig. 3. Phase-resetting responses to a three-cycle 5-hour stimulus in young adults. The magnitude of the phase shift (in hours) is plotted with respect to the relative duration of the bright-light exposure. The 0% group was exposed to complete darkness throughout the 5-hour stimulus and the 100% group was exposed to continuous bright light throughout the stimulus. Two groups received intermittent bright-light exposure during the 5-hour stimulus: 5.3 minutes of bright light alternating with 19.7 minutes of darkness (31% relative-duration group); or 46 minutes of bright light alternating with 44 minutes of darkness (63% relative-duration group). Each point represents the response from one subject, and the horizontal bars represent the median phase shift for the group. (*From* Rimmer DW, Boivin DB, Shanahan TL, et al. Dynamic resetting of the human circadian pacemaker by intermittent bright light. Am J Physiol 2000;279(5):R1574–9; with permission.)

continuous very dim light, and intermittent light. The intermittent-light pattern consisted of six 15-minute bright-light pulses separated by 60 minutes of very dim light, and therefore contained 23% of the duration of the continuous bright-light stim-ulus. We found that both groups exposed to light phase delay shifted by a significant amount, and that the magnitude of the phase delay was not significantly different between the two groups, with approximately 75% of the resetting response achieved with 23% of the bright-light duration. When suppression of melatonin by the intermit-tent-light stimuli was examined, we found that melatonin was suppressed within 5 minutes of the start of each light stimulus, that each subse-quent light pulse suppressed melatonin by a similar percentage, and that melatonin levels began to increase within 10 minutes after each light pulse ended.[77]

The finding from these studies—that the human circadian system is responsive to very short pulses of light—has many practical implications. It suggests that light treatments can be shortened or interrupted without reducing their effectiveness, and it also suggests that brief exposures to bright light may greatly influence entrainment to the 24-hour day.[34,78] In fact, studies of natural light exposure in humans living in a number of different cities have found that most people get relatively little bright-light exposure.[79–83] How such patterns of brief and intermittent exposure to outdoor levels of light influence phase angle of entrainment in modern humans is currently not well understood, but available evidence suggests that prolonged exposure to outdoor light each day can have a significant influence on both sleep timing and the timing of hormonal secretion.[84–86]

Intermittent bright-light stimuli have been tested as a method to adapt the circadian rhythms of shift workers to a night-work–day-sleep schedule. Reports from such studies have indicated that intermittent bright light during night work can aid in adjusting the circadian system to a night work schedule,[87,88] although the bright-light groups in those studies were also required to be in darkness at specified daytime sleep times. Given that the scheduling of daytime darkness/sleep can itself aid in adaptation to a night work schedule,[89,90,91] it is not clear whether it was the intermittent bright light, or the combination of intermittent light and scheduled sleep/darkness that produced better adjustment to the night work schedule.

WAVELENGTH SENSITIVITY OF THE HUMAN CIRCADIAN SYSTEM

Photic resetting of the circadian system is part of a larger class of NIFs to retinal light exposure that have been observed in both humans and in other mammals. After studies in animals had suggested a role for a nonrod, noncone photoreceptor in circadian responses to light, melanopsin was identified as the photopigment present in those specialized photoreceptors.[10–13,23,92–95] Studies of light suppression of melatonin secretion in humans had identified a short-wavelength peak in spectral sensitivity of that response,[96,97] suggesting that human NIF responses were also mediated by a melanopsinlike photopigment. In fact, several years earlier, we had reported that some blind humans could show NIF responses to light, retaining an ability to show melatonin suppression in response to ocular light exposure at night,[98] and that light could phase-shift the circadian rhythms in some blind individuals.[99]

To explore whether human phase-shifting to light would show a short-wavelength sensitivity, a study was conducted in our laboratory in which a 6.5-hour exposure to monochromatic light was applied in the phase-delay region in sighted human subjects.[100] Responses to monochromatic light of 460 nm and 555 nm of equal photon density were compared, and we observed that both phase-shifting and melatonin suppression were significantly greater in the subjects exposed to 460-nm light than in those who received 555-nm light. We also found that during the 6.5-hour light exposure, subjects exposed to the 460-nm light rated themselves as significantly more alert and showed faster reaction times, fewer lapses of attention, less electroencephalographic delta power, and more electroencephalographic high-alpha power than subjects exposed to 555-nm light. This was consistent with a greater alerting effect of the short-wavelength light.[101] More recently, a study conducted in our laboratory reported that NIFs to light in two blind individuals was short-wavelength sensitive.[24]

While these studies provide additional evidence that the human circadian system includes a short-wavelength–sensitive photoreceptor, as in other mammals, they do not rule out the role of visual photoreceptors in mediating circadian responses to light in humans.[15,16,102,103] The relative contribution of different photoreceptors to circadian light responses is not yet well understood, and may depend on the intensity and duration of exposure.

ADAPTATION OF THE HUMAN CIRCADIAN SYSTEM TO PRIOR LIGHT-DARK EXPOSURE

Studies in humans and animals have provided evidence that prior exposure to light and darkness influences the response of the circadian system to light.[104–110] We have conducted several recent studies to examine systematically how the duration and relative intensity of prior light exposure affect the subsequent response to a light pulse.[111,112] In a study we conducted recently, we exposed subjects to a 6.5-hour 200-lux light stimulus during the biological nighttime, and measured the degree of melatonin suppression. Before the light stimulus, subjects were in a background light that was very dim (~0.5 lux) or of room intensity (200 lux, the same intensity as the light stimulus) for 15 hours. Exposure to the dim background resulted in significantly greater melatonin suppression in response to the 200-lux light stimulus than did exposure to 200-lux background light.[111] The design of that study did not allow for an estimate of phase-shifting response, but a subsequent study conducted in our laboratory using a modified design has examined both melatonin suppression and phase-shifting responses to a light stimulus following a dim-light or a room-light background. Preliminary results from that recent study[112] show phase-shifting results consistent with the melatonin-suppression findings from our earlier report.[111]

Studies in circadian photoreceptors suggest a mechanism by which the response observed in human studies may occur. Those studies have demonstrated that the response of those photoreceptors is influenced by prior light history, demonstrating larger responses to light stimuli after dim-light exposure, and reduced responsiveness to light stimuli after bright background-light exposure.[110]

Together, these findings suggest that the overall 24-hour pattern of light and darkness to which humans are exposed plays a role in subsequent sensitivity to light exposure, and thus in entrainment. These findings also suggest that the circadian system of individuals who get little bright-light exposure may become more sensitive to moderate levels of light.[105] Given that most studies show that modern humans get relatively little bright-light exposure and instead spend most of their waking day in light of indoor intensity,[79–83] these findings may have very important practical relevance for most humans.

ENTRAINMENT OF THE HUMAN CIRCADIAN SYSTEM BY LIGHT

As we outlined above, regular exposure to light and darkness is the primary synchronizer of the human circadian system to the solar day. On average, the period of the human circadian system is longer than 24 hours.[66,71,78,113–119] This means that for the circadian system to remain in synchrony with the external environment, it must for most people be reset by a small phase-advance shift each day. For individuals whose circadian period is shorter than 24 hours, entrainment is achieved through a phase-delay shift.[120]

Entrainment theory states that the range of entrainment is related to the strength of the synchronizing signal, meaning that a weak synchronizer will be able to entrain individuals whose periods are very close to 24 hours, but a stronger synchronizer is required to entrain those individuals whose periods are further over or under 24 hours.[35,121] Furthermore, this theory holds that the phase angle of entrainment is related to the strength of the synchronizing signal, and evidence for this had been obtained in animals.[121–123]

By the late 1990s, studies by our group and those of others had demonstrated that humans show a range of circadian periods close to, but on average slightly longer than, 24 hours,[66,113–117] and also that humans show differences in phase angle of entrainment.[124–126] We had also reported that in young humans there is a relationship

between circadian period and phase angle of entrainment,[127] in accordance with entrainment theory. We therefore embarked on several studies to explore entrainment in humans.

In the first such study, we examined whether humans could entrain to a very weak synchronizer (light of ~1.5 lux in the angle of gaze), and tested that ability using three different day lengths.[71] We found that most (five of six) subjects tested could entrain to a 24.0–hour day in this very weak synchronizer, but that subjects studied on a 23.5- or 24.5-hour day length did not remain entrained.

We also conducted two other studies in which we examined how phase angle of entrainment in humans is related to circadian period, and how light intensity affects this relationship.[78,119] In the first of these studies, phase angle was assessed following a variety of routines, including a normal routine at home with uncontrolled lighting, following exposure to a very strong synchronizer throughout the waking day for 5 days, and after 24 hours in very dim (~1.5 lux in the angle of gaze) light. We found, as in our prior study,[127] that phase angle of entrainment is significantly associated with circadian period, such that individuals with shorter periods have a longer interval between evening melatonin onset and usual bedtime than those individuals with longer periods.[119] We also found that when a very strong synchronizer was applied, the range of phase angles was reduced, but the relationship between phase angle and period was still present.

In a subsequent entrainment study, we examined the ability of synchronizers of different strengths to entrain human circadian rhythms to a longer-than-24-hour day.[78] In this study, we first assessed the period of each subject, and then randomized them to one of three groups, each with a different synchronizer strength. The synchronizers were then applied during a month when the each subject was scheduled to a day length 1 hour longer than the subject's circadian period, so that the entrainment challenge was the same for all subjects. We found that most (three of four) subjects living in 25 lux of light were unable to entrain to the imposed day that was 1 hour longer than their circadian period, but all subjects living under 100 lux of light were able to entrain. As would be predicted by entrainment theory, the subjects who entrained to the longer day showed a phase angle that was different from the one they had at the beginning of the study.

Together, these entrainment studies demonstrated that the human circadian system is much like that of other organisms, and that light strongly influences the phase angle of entrainment in humans. This information has implications for understanding and developing treatments for circadian-rhythm sleep disorders.[128,129]

SUMMARY

As we have outlined above, over the past 3 decades studies in our laboratory and elsewhere have revealed a wealth of information about how light affects the human circadian system. Knowledge from these studies has improved our understanding of entrainment of human circadian rhythms to the 24-hour environment, has revealed important insights into circadian-rhythm sleep disorders, and has allowed for the design of light-treatment regimens for night workers, jet travelers, and patients with circadian-rhythm sleep disorders.[89,90,130–135]

Additional laboratory and field studies are still necessary to better understand some features of the human circadian response to light. We are only beginning to understand how prior exposure to light affects the subsequent response to a light stimulus, and our understanding of how light exposure can affect the period of the human circadian system is also limited.[136] In addition, little is known about individual differences in circadian sensitivity to light, nor do we understand how polymorphisms in so-called "clock genes" (or other genes) affect sensitivity to light. Furthermore, while some of our knowledge has been translated into light-treatment regimens for circadian-rhythm disorders, many of the current treatments are impractical, and development and testing of lighting devices and treatment plans that optimize outcomes with shorter and more effective exposures are required. Such studies are time consuming and expensive to conduct in human subjects, but additional well-controlled laboratory-based studies where light-response phenotyping and genotyping are conducted in tandem are still necessary to fully understand the effects of light on the human circadian system and to translate this knowledge into optimized light treatments.

ACKNOWLEDGMENTS

The authors wish to thank the many subjects who participated in the studies reviewed here; the dedicated subject recruitment, technical, and administrative staff of our laboratory whose efforts have made this work possible; the Brigham and Women's Hospital General Clinical Research Center, where many of the studies were conducted; J.M. Ronda and E.N. Brown; and the many current and former members of the Division of Sleep Medicine who contributed to the work reviewed here, including J.S. Allan, D.B. Boivin, C. Cajochen, A.M. Chang, D.J. Dijk, J.J. Gooley, C. Gronfier, M.E. Jewett, S.B.S. Khalsa, E.B. Klerman, S.W. Lockley, D.W. Rimmer, M.W. Schoen, N. Santhi, T.L. Shanahan, K.A. Smith, K.P. Wright, Jr., and J.M. Zeitzer. We also wish to thank Professor R.E. Kronauer for his many important contributions to this work, which cannot be overstated.

REFERENCES

1. Moore RY, Lenn NJ. A retinohypothalamic projection in the rat. J Comp Neurol 1972;146:1–14.
2. Stephan FK, Zucker I. Circadian rhythms in drinking behavior and locomotor activity of rats are eliminated by hypothalamic lesions. Proc Natl Acad Sci U S A 1972;69:1583–6.
3. Ralph MR, Foster RG, Davis FC, et al. Transplanted suprachiasmatic nucleus determines circadian period. Science 1990;247:975–8.
4. Klein DC, Moore RY, Reppert SM, editors. Suprachiasmatic nucleus: the mind's clock. New York: Oxford University Press; 1991.
5. Weaver DR. The suprachiasmatic nucleus: a 25-year retrospective. J Biol Rhythms 1998;13(2):100–12.
6. Welsh DK, Logothetis DE, Meister M, et al. Individual neurons dissociated from rat suprachiasmatic nucleus express independently phased circadian firing rhythms. Neuron 1995;14:697–706.
7. Moore RY. Retinohypothalamic projection in mammals: a comparative study. Brain Res 1973;49:403–9.
8. Sadun AA, Schaechter JD, Smith LEH. A retinohypothalamic pathway in man: light mediation of circadian rhythms. Brain Res 1984;302:371–7.
9. Moore RY, Speh JC, Card JP. The retinohypothalamic tract originates from a distinct subset of retinal ganglion cells. J Comp Neurol 1995;352:351–66.
10. Berson DM, Dunn FA, Takao M. Phototransduction by retinal ganglion cells that set the circadian clock. Science 2002;295:1070–3.
11. Hattar S, Liao H-W, Takao M, et al. Melanopsin-containing retinal ganglion cells: architecture, projections, and intrinsic photosensitivity. Science 2002;295:1065–70.
12. Hattar S, Lucas RJ, Mrosovsky N, et al. Melanopsin and rod-cone photoreceptive systems account for all major accessory visual functions in mice. Nature 2003;424(6944):76–81.
13. Gooley JJ, Lu J, Chou TC, et al. Melanopsin in cells of origin of the retinohypothalamic tract. Nat Neurosci 2001;4(12):1165.

14. Berson DM. Phototransduction in ganglion-cell photoreceptors. Pflügers Arch 2007;454(5): 849–55.

15. Revell VL, Skene DJ. Light-induced melatonin suppression in humans with polychromatic and monochromatic light. Chronobiol Int 2007;24(6): 1125–37.

16. Güler AD, Ecker JL, Lall GS, et al. Melanopsin cells are the principal conduits for rod-cone input to non-image-forming vision. Nature 2008;453(7191): 102–5.

17. Lydic R, Schoene WC, Czeisler CA, et al. Suprachiasmatic region of the human hypothalamus: homolog to the primate circadian pacemaker? Sleep 1980;2(3):355–61.

18. Stopa EG, King JC, Lydic R, et al. Human brain contains vasopressin and vasoactive intestinal polypeptide neuronal subpopulations in the suprachiasmatic region. Brain Res 1984;297: 159–63.

19. Friedman DI, Johnson JK, Chorsky RL, et al. Labeling of human retinohypothalamic tract with the carbocyanine dye, DiI. Brain Res 1991;560: 297–302.

20. Moore RY, Speh JC. A putative retinohypothalamic projection containing substance P in the human. Brain Res 1994;659:249–53.

21. Dai J, Swaab DF, Buijs RM. Distribution of vasopressin and vasoactive intestinal polypeptide (VIP) fibers in human hypothalamus with special emphasis on suprachiasmatic nucleus efferent projections. J Comp Neurol 1997;383: 397–414.

22. Dai J, van der Vliet J, Swaab DF, et al. Human retinohypothalamic tract as revealed by in vitro post-mortem tracing. J Comp Neurol 1998;397:357–70.

23. Provencio I, Rodriguez IR, Jiang G, et al. A novel human opsin in the inner retina. J Neurosci 2000; 20(2):600–5.

24. Zaidi FH, Hull JT, Peirson SN, et al. Short-wavelength light sensitivity of circadian, pupillary, and visual awareness in humans lacking an outer retina. Curr Biol 2007;17(24):2122–8.

25. Hastings JW, Sweeney BM. A persistent diurnal rhythm of luminescence in Gonyaulax polyedra. Biol Bull 1958;115:440–58.

26. DeCoursey PJ. Daily light sensitivity rhythm in a rodent. Science 1960;131:33–5.

27. Pittendrigh CS. Circadian rhythms and the circadian organization of living systems. Cold Spring Harb Symp Quant Biol 1960;25:159–84.

28. Daan S, Pittendrigh CS. A functional analysis of circadian pacemakers in nocturnal rodents. II. The variability of phase response curves. J Comp Physiol [A] 1976;106:253–66.

29. Wever R. Zur Zeitgeber-Stärke eines Licht-Dunkel-Wechsels für die circadiane Periodik des Menschen [Strength of a light-dark cycle as a zeitgeber for circadian rhythms in man]. Pfluegers Arch 1970;321:133–42 [in German].

30. Aschoff J, Fatranská M, Giedke H, et al. Human circadian rhythms in continuous darkness: entrainment by social cues. Science 1971;171:213–5.

31. Czeisler CA, Allan JS, Strogatz SH, et al. Bright light resets the human circadian pacemaker independent of the timing of the sleep-wake cycle. Science 1986;233:667–71.

32. Czeisler CA, Kronauer RE, Allan JS, et al. Bright light induction of strong (type 0) resetting of the human circadian pacemaker. Science 1989;244: 1328–33.

33. Allan JS, Czeisler CA. Persistence of the circadian thyrotropin rhythm under constant conditions and after light-induced shifts of circadian phase. J Clin Endocrinol Metab 1994;79:508–12.

34. Jewett ME, Rimmer DW, Duffy JF, et al. Human circadian pacemaker is sensitive to light throughout subjective day without evidence of transients. Am J Physiol 1997;273:R1800–9.

35. Johnson CH. Phase response curves: What can they tell us about circadian clocks?. In: Hiroshige T, Honma K, editors. Circadian clocks from cell to human. Sapporo: Hokkaido Univ. Press; 1992. p. 209–49.

36. Winfree AT. Integrated view of resetting a circadian clock. J Theor Biol 1970;28:327–74.

37. Winfree AT. Resetting the amplitude of Drosophila's circadian chronometer. J Comp Physiol 1973;85: 105–40.

38. Winfree AT. The geometry of biological time. New York: Springer-Verlag; 1980.

39. Kronauer RE, Jewett ME, Czeisler CA. Commentary: the human circadian response to light—strong and weak resetting. J Biol Rhythms 1993;8:351–60.

40. Jewett ME, Kronauer RE, Czeisler CA. Light-induced suppression of endogenous circadian amplitude in humans. Nature 1991;350:59–62.

41. Lakin-Thomas PL. Commentary: strong or weak phase resetting by light pulses in humans? J Biol Rhythms 1993;8(4):348–50.

42. Khalsa SBS, Jewett ME, Cajochen C, et al. A phase response curve to single bright light pulses in human subjects. J Physiol 2003;549(Pt 3):945–52.

43. Lockley SW, Gooley JJ, Kronauer RE, et al. Phase response curve to single one-hour pulses of 10,000 lux bright white light in humans [abstract]. 10th Meeting of the Society for Research on Biological Rhythms. Sandestin (FL), May 2006.

44. Minors DS, Waterhouse JM, Wirz-Justice A. A human phase-response curve to light. Neurosci Lett 1991;133:36–40.

45. Honma K, Honma S. A human phase response curve for bright light pulses. Jpn J Psychiatry Neurol 1988;42(1):167–8.

46. Peterson EL. A limit cycle interpretation of a mosquito circadian oscillator. J Theor Biol 1980; 84:281–310.

47. Czeisler CA, Wright KP Jr. Influence of light on circadian rhythmicity in humans. In: Turek FW, Zee PC, editors. Neurobiology of Sleep and Circadian Rhythms. New York: Marcel Dekker, Inc; 1999. p. 149–80.

48. Pohl H. Characteristics and variability in entrainment of circadian rhythms to light in diurnal rodents. In: Aschoff J, Daan S, Groos GA, editors. Vertebrate circadian systems: structure and physiology. Berlin: Springer-Verlag; 1982. p. 339–46.

49. Khalsa SBS, Jewett ME, Duffy JF, et al. The timing of the human circadian clock is accurately represented by the core body temperature rhythm following phase shifts to a three-cycle light stimulus near the critical zone. J Biol Rhythms 2000;15(6):524–30.

50. Johnson CH. An atlas of phase response curves for circadian and circatidal rhythms. Nashville (TN): Department of Biology, Vanderbilt University; 1990.

51. Brainard GC, Richardson BA, King TS, et al. The suppression of pineal melatonin content and N-acetyltransferase activity by different light irradiances in the Syrian hamster: a dose-response relationship. Endocrinology 1983;113(1):293–6.

52. Takahashi JS, DeCoursey PJ, Bauman L, et al. Spectral sensitivity of a novel photoreceptive system mediating entrainment of mammalian circadian rhythms. Nature 1984;308:186–8.

53. Joshi D, Chandrashekaran MK. Light flashes of different durations (0.063-3.33 msec) phase shift the circadian flight activity of a bat. J Exp Zool 1985;233:187–92.

54. Nelson DE, Takahashi JS. Comparison of visual sensitivity for suppression of pineal melatonin and circadian phase-shifting in the golden hamster. Brain Res 1991;554:272–7.

55. Nelson DE, Takahashi JS. Sensitivity and integration in a visual pathway for circadian entrainment in the hamster (Mesocricetus auratus). J Physiol 1991;439:115–45.

56. Bauer MS. Irradiance responsivity and unequivocal type-1 phase responsivity of rat circadian activity rhythms. Am J Physiol 1992;263:R1110–4.

57. Sharma VK, Chandrashekaran MK, Singaravel M, et al. Relationship between light intensity and phase resetting in a mammalian circadian system. J Exp Zool 1999;283:181–5.

58. Lewy AJ, Wehr TA, Goodwin FK, et al. Light suppresses melatonin secretion in humans. Science 1980;210:1267–9.

59. Bojkowski CJ, Aldhous ME, English J, et al. Suppression of nocturnal plasma melatonin and 6-sulphatoxymelatonin by bright and dim light in man. Horm Metab Res 1987;19:437–40.

60. Brainard GC, Lewy AJ, Menaker M, et al. Dose-response relationship between light irradiance and the suppression of plasma melatonin in human volunteers. Brain Res 1988;454:212–8.

61. McIntyre IM, Norman TR, Burrows GD, et al. Human melatonin suppression by light is intensity dependent. J Pineal Res 1989;6:149–56.

62. Allan JS, Czeisler CA, Duffy JF, et al. Non-linear dose response of the human circadian pacemaker to light. 154th Annual AAAS Meeting. Boston, February 11–15, 1988.

63. Zeitzer JM, Khalsa SB, Boivin DB, et al. Temporal dynamics of late-night photic stimulation of the human circadian timing system. Am J Physiol 2005;289(3):R839–44.

64. Boivin DB, Duffy JF, Kronauer RE, et al. Sensitivity of the human circadian pacemaker to moderately bright light. J Biol Rhythms 1994;9(3–4):315–31.

65. Boivin DB, Duffy JF, Kronauer RE, et al. Dose-response relationships for resetting of human circadian clock by light. Nature 1996;379:540–2.

66. Czeisler CA, Duffy JF, Shanahan TL, et al. Stability, precision, and near-24-hour period of the human circadian pacemaker. Science 1999; 284:2177–81.

67. Duffy JF, Kronauer RE, Czeisler CA. Phase-shifting human circadian rhythms: influence of sleep timing, social contact and light exposure. J Physiol (Lond) 1996;495(1):289–97.

68. Zeitzer JM, Dijk DJ, Kronauer RE, et al. Sensitivity of the human circadian pacemaker to nocturnal light: melatonin phase resetting and suppression. J Physiol 2000;526(3):695–702.

69. Duffy JF, Zeitzer JM, Czeisler CA. Decreased sensitivity to phase-delaying effects of moderate intensity light in older subjects. Neurobiol Aging 2007; 28:799–807.

70. Cajochen C, Zeitzer JM, Czeisler CA, et al. Dose-response relationship for light intensity and ocular and electroencephalographic correlates of human alertness. Behav Brain Res 2000;115(1):75–83.

71. Wright KP Jr, Hughes RJ, Kronauer RE, et al. Intrinsic near-24-h pacemaker period determines limits of circadian entrainment to a weak synchronizer in humans. Proc Natl Acad Sci U S A 2001; 98(24):14027–32.

72. van den Pol AN, Cao V, Heller HC. Circadian system of mice integrates brief light stimuli. Am J Physiol 1998;275:R654–7.

73. Rimmer DW, Boivin DB, Shanahan TL, et al. Dynamic resetting of the human circadian pacemaker by intermittent bright light. Am J Physiol 2000;279(5):R1574–9.

74. Gronfier C, Wright KP Jr, Kronauer RE, et al. Efficacy of a single sequence of intermittent bright light pulses for delaying circadian phase in humans. Am J Physiol 2004;287:E174–81.

75. Kronauer RE, Forger DB, Jewett ME. Quantifying human circadian pacemaker response to brief, extended, and repeated light stimuli over the photopic range. J Biol Rhythms 1999;14(6): 500–15.

76. Kronauer RE, Forger DB, Jewett ME. Errata: quantifying human circadian pacemaker response to brief, extended, and repeated light stimuli over the photopic range. J Biol Rhythms 2000;15(2):184–6.

77. Gronfier C, Wright KP Jr, Czeisler CA. Time course of melatonin suppression in response to intermittent bright light exposure in humans. J Sleep Res 2002;11(Suppl 1):86–7.

78. Gronfier C, Wright KP Jr, Kronauer RE, et al. Entrainment of the human circadian pacemaker to longer-than-24h days. Proc Natl Acad Sci U S A 2007;104(21):9081–6.

79. Cole RJ, Kripke DF, Wisbey J, et al. Seasonal variation in human illumination exposure at two different latitudes. J Biol Rhythms 1995;10(4): 324–34.

80. Hébert M, Dumont M, Paquet J. Seasonal and diurnal patterns of human illumination under natural conditions. Chronobiol Int 1998;15(1):59–70.

81. Laffan AM, Duffy JF. Light exposure patterns in healthy young and older adults. Sleep 2002;25: A307–8.

82. Kawinska A, Dumont M, Selmaoui B, et al. Are modifications of melatonin circadian rhythm in the middle years of life related to habitual patterns of light exposure? J Biol Rhythms 2005;20(5): 451–60.

83. Scheuermaier K, Laffan AM, Duffy JF. Light exposure patterns in healthy older people living in New England, USA. J Sleep Res 2006;15(Suppl 1):94.

84. Illnerová H, Buresová M, Nedvídková J, et al. Maintenance of a circadian phase adjustment of the human melatonin rhythm following artificial long days. Brain Res 1993;626:322–6.

85. Vondrasová D, Hájek I, Illnerová H. Exposure to long summer days affects the human melatonin and cortisol rhythms. Brain Res 1997;759:166–70.

86. Louzada F, Inacio AM, Souza FHM, et al. Exposure to light versus way of life: effects on sleep patterns of a teenager-case report. Chronobiol Int 2004; 21(3):497–9.

87. Baehr EK, Fogg LF, Eastman CI. Intermittent bright light and exercise to entrain human circadian rhythms to night work. Am J Physiol 1999;277(6 Pt 2):R1598–604.

88. Smith MR, Cullnan EE, Eastman CI. Shaping the light/dark pattern for circadian adaptation to night shift work. Physiol Behav 2008;95(3):449–56.

89. Horowitz TS, Cade BE, Wolfe JM, et al. Efficacy of bright light and sleep/darkness scheduling in alleviating circadian maladaptation to night work. Am J Physiol 2001;281:E384–91.

90. Santhi N, Duffy JF, Horowitz TS, et al. Scheduling of sleep/darkness affects the circadian phase of night shift workers. Neurosci Lett 2005;384(3):316–20.

91. Santhi N, Duffy JF, Horowitz TS, et al. Erratum to "Scheduling of sleep/darkness affects the circadian phase of night shift workers". Neurosci Lett 2005;390:187.

92. Foster RG, Provencio I, Hudson D, et al. Circadian photoreception in the retinally degenerate mouse (rd/rd). J Comp Physiol [A] 1991;169:39–50.

93. Freedman MS, Lucas RJ, Soni B, et al. Regulation of mammalian circadian behavior by non-rod, non-cone, ocular photoreceptors. Science 1999; 284:502–4.

94. Lucas RJ, Freedman MS, Muñoz M, et al. Regulation of the mammalian pineal by non-rod, non-cone, ocular photoreceptors. Science 1999;284: 505–7.

95. Lucas RJ, Foster RG. Neither functional rod photoreceptors nor rod or cone outer segments are required for the photic inhibition of pineal melatonin. Endocrinology 1999;140(4):1520–4.

96. Thapan K, Arendt J, Skene DJ. An action spectrum for melatonin suppression: evidence for a novel non-rod, non-cone photoreceptor system in humans. J Physiol 2001;535(1):261–7.

97. Brainard GC, Hanifin JP, Greeson JM, et al. Action spectrum for melatonin regulation in humans: evidence for a novel circadian photoreceptor. J Neurosci 2001;21(16):6405–12.

98. Czeisler CA, Shanahan TL, Klerman EB, et al. Suppression of melatonin secretion in some blind patients by exposure to bright light. N Engl J Med 1995;332(1):6–11.

99. Klerman EB, Shanahan TL, Brotman DJ, et al. Photic resetting of the human circadian pacemaker in the absence of conscious vision. J Biol Rhythms 2002;17:548–55.

100. Lockley SW, Brainard GC, Czeisler CA. High sensitivity of the human circadian melatonin rhythm to resetting by short wavelength light. J Clin Endocrinol Metab 2003;88(9):4502–5.

101. Lockley SW, Evans EE, Scheer FAJL, et al. Short-wavelength sensitivity for the direct effects of light on alertness, vigilance, and the waking electroencephalogram in humans. Sleep 2006;29(2): 161–8.

102. Zeitzer JM, Kronauer RE, Czeisler CA. Photopic transduction implicated in human circadian entrainment. Neurosci Lett 1997;232:135–8.

103. Czeisler CA, Gooley JJ. Sleep and circadian rhythms in humans. Cold Spring Harb Symp Quant Biol 2007;72:579–97.

104. Meijer JH, Rusak B, Ganshirt G. The relation between light-induced discharge in the suprachiasmatic nucleus and phase shifts of hamster circadian rhythms. Brain Res 1992;598:257–63.

105. Owen J, Arendt J. Melatonin suppression in human subjects by bright and dim light in Antarctica: time and season-dependent effects. Neurosci Lett 1992;137:181–4.

106. Nelson DE, Takahashi JS. Integration and saturation within the circadian photic entrainment pathway of hamsters. Am J Physiol 1999;277(46): R1351–61.

107. Aggelopoulos NC, Meissl H. Responses of neurones of the rat suprachiasmatic nucleus to retinal illumination under photopic and scotopic conditions. J Physiol 2000;523(1):211–22.

108. Refinetti R. Dark adaptation in the circadian system of the mouse. Physiol Behav 2001;74:101–7.

109. Hébert M, Martin SK, Lee C, et al. The effects of prior light history on the suppression of melatonin by light in humans. J Pineal Res 2002;33:198–203.

110. Wong KY, Dunn FA, Berson DM. Photoreceptor adaptation in intrinsically photosensitive retinal ganglion cells. Neuron 2005;48(6):1001–10.

111. Smith KA, Schoen MW, Czeisler CA. Adaptation of human pineal melatonin suppression by recent photic history. J Clin Endocrinol Metab 2004;89: 3610–4.

112. Chang A-M, Scheer FA, Czeisler CA. Adaptation of the human circadian system by prior light history. Sleep 2008;31(Suppl):A45–6.

113. Wyatt JK, Ritz-De Cecco A, Czeisler CA, et al. Circadian temperature and melatonin rhythms, sleep, and neurobehavioral function in humans living on a 20-h day. Am J Physiol 1999;277:R1152–63.

114. Waterhouse J, Minors D, Folkard S, et al. Light of domestic intensity produces phase shifts of the circadian oscillator in humans. Neurosci Lett 1998;245:97–100.

115. Kelly TL, Neri DF, Grill JT, et al. Nonentrained circadian rhythms of melatonin in submariners scheduled to an 18-hour day. J Biol Rhythms 1999; 14(3):190–6.

116. Carskadon MA, Labyak SE, Acebo C, et al. Intrinsic circadian period of adolescent humans measured in conditions of forced desynchrony. Neurosci Lett 1999;260:129–32.

117. Middleton B, Arendt J, Stone BM. Human circadian rhythms in constant dim light (8 lux) with knowledge of clock time. J Sleep Res 1996;5:69–76.

118. Wyatt JK, Cajochen C, Ritz-De Cecco A, et al. Low-dose, repeated caffeine administration for circadian-phase-dependent performance degradation during extended wakefulness. Sleep 2004;27(3): 374–81.

119. Wright KP Jr, Gronfier C, Duffy JF, et al. Intrinsic period and light intensity determine the phase relationship between melatonin and sleep in humans. J Biol Rhythms 2005;20(2):168–77.

120. Duffy JF, Wright KP Jr. Entrainment of the human circadian system by light. J Biol Rhythms 2005; 20(4):326–38.

121. Pittendrigh CS, Daan S. A functional analysis of circadian pacemakers in nocturnal rodents. IV. Entrainment: pacemaker as clock. J Comp Physiol [A] 1976;106:291–331.

122. Hoffmann K. Zur beziehung zwischen phasenlage und spontanfrequenz bei der endogenen tagesperiodik [On the relationship between the phase position and the spontaneous frequency of endogenous daily periodicity]. Z Naturforsch 1963;18: 154–7 [in German].

123. Sharma VK, Chandrashekaran MK, Singaravel M. Relationship between period and phase angle differences in Mus booduga under abrupt versus gradual light-dark transitions. Naturwissenschaften 1998;85:183–6.

124. Duffy JF, Dijk DJ, Klerman EB, et al. Later endogenous circadian temperature nadir relative to an earlier wake time in older people. Am J Physiol 1998;275:R1478–87.

125. Duffy JF, Dijk DJ, Hall EF, et al. Relationship of endogenous circadian melatonin and temperature rhythms to self-reported preference for morning or evening activity in young and older people. J Investig Med 1999;47:141–50.

126. Baehr EK, Revelle W, Eastman CI. Individual differences in the phase and amplitude of the human circadian temperature rhythm: with an emphasis on morningness-eveningness. J Sleep Res 2000; 9:117–27.

127. Duffy JF, Rimmer DW, Czeisler CA. Association of intrinsic circadian period with morningness-eveningness, usual wake time, and circadian phase. Behav Neurosci 2001;115(4):895–9.

128. Jones CR, Campbell SS, Zone SE, et al. Familial advanced sleep-phase syndrome: a short-period circadian rhythm variant in humans. Nat Med 1999;5(9):1062–5.

129. Wyatt JK, Stepanski EJ, Kirkby J. Circadian phase in delayed sleep phase syndrome: predictors and temporal stability across multiple assessments. Sleep 2006;29(8):1075–80.

130. Czeisler CA, Johnson MP, Duffy JF, et al. Exposure to bright light and darkness to treat physiologic maladaptation to night work. N Engl J Med 1990; 322:1253–9.

131. Terman M, Lewy AJ, Dijk DJ, et al. Light treatment for sleep disorders: consensus report. IV. Sleep phase and duration disturbances. J Biol Rhythms 1995;10(2):135–47.

132. Boulos Z, Campbell SS, Lewy AJ, et al. Light treatment for sleep disorders: consensus report. VII. Jet lag. J Biol Rhythms 1995;10(2):167–76.

133. Eastman CI, Boulos Z, Terman M, et al. Light treatment for sleep disorders: consensus report. VI. Shift work. J Biol Rhythms 1995;10(2):157–64.

134. Sack RL, Auckley D, Auger RR, et al. Circadian rhythm sleep disorders: part I, basic principles, shift work and jet lag disorders. An American Academy of Sleep Medicine review. Sleep 2007; 30(11):1460–83.

135. Cain SW, Rimmer DW, Duffy JF, et al. Exercise distributed across day and night does not alter circadian period in humans. J Biol Rhythms 2007; 22(6):534–41.

136. Scheer FA, Wright KP Jr, Kronauer RE, et al. Plasticity of the intrinsic period of the human circadian timing system. PLoS ONE 2007;2(8): e721;10.1371/journal.pone. 0000721.

Melatonin and Melatonin Analogues

Shantha M.W. Rajaratnam, PhD[a,b,c,*], Daniel A. Cohen, MD[b,d,e],
Naomi L. Rogers, PhD[f]

KEYWORDS

- Melatonin • Melatonin agonist • Circadian rhythm • Sleep
- Ramelteon • Tasimelteon • Agomelatine • PD-6735

Over the past 25 years, there has been substantial growth in the field of melatonin and melatonin analogues.[1] Following the first demonstration that exogenous melatonin can entrain the mammalian circadian system[2] and the discovery of the phase-shifting and sleep-promoting properties of the hormone in humans,[3] several groups have demonstrated the potential for melatonin to be used as a treatment for circadian rhythm sleep disorders (CRSDs). Clinical development of melatonin agonists for sleep and psychiatric disorders has also provided significant momentum to this field. There is increasing interest in the use of melatonin-like compounds in the treatment of primary insomnia; however, the mechanisms underlying these effects remain unclear. Herein we review the role of melatonin and melatonin receptors in the circadian regulation of sleep, the phase-shifting and sleep-promoting properties of exogenous melatonin, and some of the melatonin agonists that have been developed or are under development for the treatment of primary insomnia, CRSDs, and major depression.

ENDOGENOUS MELATONIN

The hormone melatonin (5-methoxy-N-acetyltryptamine) is synthesized and secreted by the pineal gland under the control of the circadian timing system. In normally entrained individuals, melatonin secretion into the bloodstream occurs primarily at night, with negligible levels secreted during the day. The circadian pacemaker, located in the suprachiasmatic nuclei (SCN) of the anterior hypothalamus, mediates melatonin secretion via GABAergic inhibition and glutamatergic stimulation of the paraventricular nucleus and sympathetic noradrenergic stimulation of the pineal gland.[4–7]

The physiologic roles of melatonin are not fully understood; however, it is widely recognized that melatonin modulates the circadian system, and it has been implicated in the control of the sleep-wake system as well as a range of other processes.[8] The role of melatonin in mediating photoperiodic responses is well characterized but is not discussed herein.

Melatonin administration is associated with changes in SCN neural activity, energy metabolism, and intrinsic cellular processes. Several years ago it was demonstrated that SCN-lesioned animals do not entrain to daily injections of melatonin,[9] indicating that the SCN is necessary for entrainment. A single in vivo administration of melatonin to rats phase shifted the rhythm of light-induced c-fos expression in the SCN,[10]

[a] School of Psychology, Psychiatry and Psychological Medicine, Monash University, Building 17, Clayton, Victoria 3800, Australia
[b] Division of Sleep Medicine, Department of Medicine, Brigham and Women's Hospital, 221 Longwood Avenue, Boston, MA 02115, USA
[c] Division of Sleep Medicine, Harvard Medical School, 221 Longwood Avenue, Boston, MA 02115, USA
[d] Harvard Medical School, 25 Shattuck Street, Boston, MA 02215, USA
[e] Department of Neurology, Beth Israel Deaconess Medical Center, 330 Brookline Avenue, KS 450, Boston, MA 02215, USA
[f] Brain and Mind Research Institute, University of Sydney, 94 Mallett Street, Building F, Level 5, Camperdown NSW 2050, Australia
* Corresponding author. School of Psychology, Psychiatry and Psychological Medicine, Monash University, Building 17, Clayton, Victoria 3800, Australia.
E-mail address: shantha.rajaratnam@med.monash.edu.au (S.M.W. Rajaratnam).

Sleep Med Clin 4 (2009) 179–193
doi:10.1016/j.jsmc.2009.02.007

indicating that melatonin administration immediately resets SCN rhythmicity. Melatonin injections also affect levels of 2-deoxyglucose uptake in the SCN, with the direction of the response depending on the circadian time of administration.[11] Pituitary adenylate cyclase-activating polypeptide (PACAP)-induced phosphorylation of the transcription factor Ca2+/cAMP responsive element binding protein (CREB), an immediate light-induced cellular response in the SCN, is inhibited by coapplication of melatonin.[12,13]

The circadian effects of melatonin are mediated by the activation of at least two high-affinity melatonin receptors, MT1 (Mel_{1a}) and MT2 (Mel_{1b}),[14] co-localized within the SCN. The so-called "MT3 receptor" is an enzyme, quinone reductase, and is not considered in this review. The precise role of MT1 and MT2 receptors in mediating the phase-shifting and sleep-promoting effects of melatonin are not clear. Neuronal firing rate rhythms recorded from SCN slices of wild-type mice are phase shifted by exposure to melatonin, and this response is only modestly attenuated in homozygous mutant MT1 receptor-deficient mice.[15] Furthermore, the selective MT2 melatonin receptor antagonist, 4P-PDOT, blocks melatonin-induced phase advances of rat SCN neuronal activity rhythms[16] and phase advances of circadian activity rhythms of mice.[17] These results support the role of MT2 receptors in mediating the phase-shifting response to exogenous melatonin; however, melatonin-induced behavioral phase shifts are reported in wild-type mice but not in MT1-deficient mice,[18] and the inhibition of PACAP-induced CREB phosphorylation in SCN cells by melatonin appears to be mediated through MT1 receptors.[19] Dubocovich proposes that possible interactions between the MT1 and MT2 receptors, together with the differential response of melatonin receptors to physiologic and supraphysiologic melatonin levels, may explain these apparently inconsistent findings.[20]

In addition to its phase-shifting effects, melatonin acutely inhibits SCN neuronal activity in vitro in a concentration-dependent manner.[21] This inhibitory effect is abolished in homozygous mutant MT1 receptor–deficient mice[15] but not in MT2 receptor–deficient mice.[22] These data suggest that the MT1 receptor has a role in mediating the acute inhibitory effect of melatonin on SCN neuronal firing, which may be linked to the direct, sleep-promoting effects of the hormone.

EXOGENOUS MELATONIN

Melatonin has been administered to humans in a variety of preparations, including oral tablets and capsules, intravenous solutions, intranasal sprays, transbuccal patches, and transdermal creams. The most common route of administration is oral, with both immediate acting and sustained release formulations available. The doses of melatonin administered vary widely, ranging from high pharmacologic (several hundred milligrams[23]) to low pharmacologic (0.5–10 mg[24,25]) and physiologic (0.05 mg[26,27]). Recent meta-analyses have concluded that melatonin is safe, at least with occasional or short-term use.[28–30] The most commonly reported adverse events were headaches, dizziness, nausea, and drowsiness; however, the occurrence of these events was similar for melatonin- and placebo-treated participants.[28,30]

Following ingestion, melatonin is absorbed from the small intestine and transported by the portal circulation to the liver, where partial metabolism to 6-hydroxymelatonin occurs followed by renal excretion. The nonmetabolized portion of melatonin travels through the systemic circulation to various peripheral tissues, as well as crossing the blood-brain barrier to bind in the brain. Peak levels of administered melatonin are observed in the periphery within about 30 to 60 minutes after ingestion,[31] or 60 to 150 minutes after larger doses,[32] with a serum half-life of between 30 and 50 minutes.

Phase-Shifting Effects of Exogenous Melatonin

Exogenous melatonin phase shifts circadian rhythms of rats, mice, and humans according to a phase response curve (PRC); that is, the magnitude and direction of the observed shift depend on the circadian time of administration.[33] Phase-dependent sensitivity to exogenous melatonin has also been demonstrated in vitro in neuronal firing rhythms of rat SCN,[34] and the density of SCN melatonin-binding sites varies according to the circadian time of day.[33]

In humans, several melatonin PRCs have been published,[35–38] although the methodologies used have differed between studies. Lewy and colleagues[37] described a four-pulse PRC (0.5 mg, orally) from six entrained humans and reported phase-advancing effects of melatonin when taken in the late subjective day and phase-delaying effects when taken in the late subjective night and early subjective day. More recently, Burgess and colleagues[36] reported a three-pulse PRC to melatonin (3 mg, orally) in free-running healthy subjects. When compared with placebo, melatonin induced maximal phase advances about 5 hours before the time of the dim light melatonin onset (afternoon/evening) and maximal phase delays about 11 hours after the dim light melatonin onset (morning). These findings suggest that, in individuals who show the normal temporal relationship between the sleep-wake cycle and the endogenous melatonin rhythm, melatonin administration just before habitual bedtime would be expected to induce relatively modest phase shifts (∼0.5 hours). A single administration of melatonin (5 mg) in the morning (07:00 hours) did not phase delay the endogenous melatonin rhythm,[39] suggesting that multiple doses are required to elicit this effect.[36]

In addition to the melatonin PRCs, several studies have reported that single or repeated doses of exogenous melatonin can phase shift the endogenous melatonin rhythm,[3,40–45] with some evidence of a dose-response relationship.[26,44] To examine the hypothesis that exogenous melatonin simultaneously shifts multiple endogenous circadian rhythms in humans, the authors examined the phase-shifting effects of melatonin (0.5 mg, surge-sustained release, 8 days, at 16:00 hours) on rhythms of plasma melatonin and cortisol,[45] heart rate and heart rate variability,[46] and polysomnographic sleep.[47] The magnitude of phase advances induced by exogenous melatonin was similar for all of the variables assessed including sleep, suggesting that melatonin shifts a central circadian pacemaker (**Fig. 1**).

The well-established phase-shifting properties of melatonin suggest that appropriately timed melatonin treatment might be beneficial for patients with CRSDs. In blind patients with non–24 hour sleep wake disorder, daily melatonin treatment entrains endogenous circadian rhythms.[48–52] Beneficial effects have also been reported in patients with delayed sleep phase syndrome (DSPS), shiftworkers, and transmeridian travelers (jet lag),[53–57] although not in all cases.[58,59] Recent meta-analyses conclude that melatonin is effective in the treatment of jet lag,[29] and there is some evidence of its efficacy in treating DSPS;[30] however, another meta-analysis concluded that melatonin is not efficacious in treating secondary sleep disorders or CRSDs such as jet lag and shift-work disorder.[28] The latter conclusion is the subject of some debate.[60]

Sleep-Promoting Effects of Exogenous Melatonin

A close relationship has been reported between the endogenous melatonin rhythm and the rhythm of sleep propensity in both sighted and blind individuals.[61–65] Sleep efficiency is reported to be decreased in patients who show absence of nocturnal melatonin secretion due to cervical spinal cord injury (n = 3) when compared with healthy controls (n = 10) and patients with thoracic spinal cord injury who show normal melatonin rhythms (n = 2).[66] Administration of melatonin, particularly daytime administration, is widely reported to increase sleep propensity and sleepiness.[67] This sleep-promoting effect has been observed following various doses of melatonin and with administration occurring via several different routes, including oral, intravenous, intranasal, and transbuccal.

Early studies investigated the effects of high doses of melatonin administered intravenously. Cramer and colleagues[68] reported sleep-inducing effects of 50 mg of intravenous melatonin, and Anton-Tay and colleagues[69] reported that melatonin administration of 0.25 to 1.25 mg/kg reduced sleep latency. Doses of immediately acting oral melatonin (0.1–100 mg) administered during the daytime or several hours before habitual bedtime have also been reported to significantly reduce sleep latency when individuals were presented with a sleep opportunity following ingestion,[27,70–74] or when using the multiple sleep latency test paradigm.[72,75,76]

Changes in polysomnographic sleep parameters have been observed following melatonin administration. For example, increased sleep efficiency or total sleep time[27,47,71,73,74,77–79] and decreased wake after sleep onset[71] have been reported following melatonin administration. Some studies report sleep disturbance following melatonin when compared with placebo, but these effects may be attributable to the phase-advancing effect of the hormone causing increased wakefulness in the latter part of the sleep episode,[80,81] or to the hypothesis that melatonin administered at a specific circadian time in the evening may uncouple circadian oscillators.[82] Other changes to sleep architecture that are reported include increased non-rapid eye movement (NREM) sleep stage 2,[71,73,78,83,84] increased total NREM sleep,[79] increased REM sleep,[80] decreased latency to REM sleep,[70] increased latency to REM sleep,[79] and decreased slow-wave sleep.[62,71,85] Daytime administration of melatonin also influences sleep stage–specific electroencephalogram characteristics.[47,83,86] However, not all studies report significant improvements in sleep, particularly those in which melatonin was administered before nocturnal sleep.

When melatonin (0.3 or 5.0 mg) was administered during the biologic day, the time when endogenous levels of the hormone are low, but not during the biologic night, a significant increase in sleep efficiency was observed in healthy young men studied in a forced desynchrony protocol.[77]

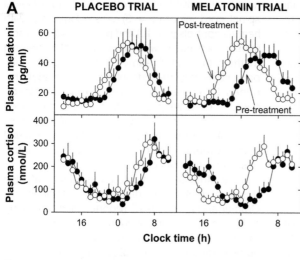

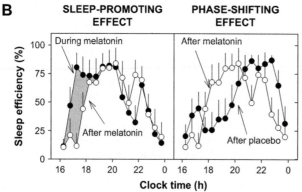

A

PLACEBO TRIAL   MELATONIN TRIAL

Post-treatment

Pre-treatment

Plasma melatonin (pg/ml)

Plasma cortisol (nmol/L)

Clock time (h)

B

SLEEP-PROMOTING EFFECT   PHASE-SHIFTING EFFECT

During melatonin   After melatonin

After melatonin   After placebo

Sleep efficiency (%)

Clock time (h)

Fig. 1. (*A*) Melatonin administration phase advances endogenous melatonin and cortisol rhythms. Healthy male subjects (n = 8) were exposed to a phase-advanced, extended sleep opportunity (16 hour) protocol with melatonin (1.5 mg) or placebo administered in a within-subjects crossover design. Mean (± standard error of the mean, SEM) profiles of plasma melatonin and plasma cortisol for the placebo trial (*left*) and melatonin trial (*right*) pretreatment (*closed circles*) and post-treatment (*open circles*) are shown. Clock time is shown on the horizontal axis. The phase advances induced in both melatonin and cortisol rhythms following melatonin treatment were significantly larger than those induced following placebo ($P<.05$). (*From* Rajaratnam SM, Dijk DJ, Middleton B, et al. Melatonin phase shifts human circadian rhythms with no evidence of changes in the duration of endogenous melatonin secretion or the 24-hour production of reproductive hormones. J Clin Endocrinol Metab 2003;88(9):4303–9; with permission. Copyright © 2003, The Endocrine Society.) (*B*) Sleep-promoting and phase-shifting effects of melatonin administration. Mean (± SEM) sleep efficiency levels (percent per hour) derived from polysomnographic data recorded in the same subjects as described for **Fig. 1**A are shown. The direct, sleep-promoting effect of melatonin (*left panel*) is illustrated by a comparison between sleep efficiency profiles on the last day of melatonin treatment (treatment day 8, *closed circles*) and sleep efficiency on the washout day (posttreatment day 1, *open circles*). Increased sleep efficiency is observed for the first 2 to 3 hours during melatonin treatment (*gray shaded area*). The phase-shifting effect of melatonin on sleep (*right panel*) is illustrated by a comparison of sleep efficiency profiles on posttreatment day 1, which was the day after melatonin (*closed circles*) or placebo (*open circles*) treatment. A shift in the distribution of sleep can be observed after melatonin treatment, with the major bout of sleep occurring earlier in the sleep opportunity. On the corresponding day after placebo, the major bout of sleep occurred later in the sleep opportunity, although an initial rise in sleep efficiency is noted at around the commencement of the sleep opportunity. (*From* Rajaratnam SM, Middleton B, Stone BM, et al. Melatonin advances the circadian timing of EEG sleep and directly facilitates sleep without altering its duration in extended sleep opportunities in humans. J Physiol 2004;561(Pt 1):339–51; with permission.)

Similarly, melatonin administered before nocturnal sleep (23:30 hours) was found to have little effect, but when administered before evening sleep (18:00 hour) melatonin increased total sleep time and sleep efficiency.[87] These findings suggest that exogenous melatonin is efficacious in improving sleep efficiency when administered during times of the day when endogenous melatonin levels are low and when sleep propensity is low.

Rajaratnam and colleagues[47] examined the sleep-promoting effects of exogenous melatonin in healthy young males maintained in a 16:8 dark-light and sleep-wake cycle for nine days,

with randomized treatment (melatonin, 1.5 mg, or placebo) taken just before bedtime. In this protocol, bedtime was advanced by 7 hours and the sleep opportunity was extended to 16 hours to assess possible photoperiodic responses in humans and to unmask the sleep-wake cycle. When compared with placebo, melatonin increased total sleep time by 2 hours during the first half of the sleep opportunity (16:00 to 0:00 hours), but the total sleep time across the entire 16-hour sleep opportunity was the same in both conditions. These results suggest that afternoon or evening administration of melatonin shifted the timing of sleep and promoted sleep during the circadian wake maintenance zone or forbidden zone for sleep.[88,89] These findings add further support to the hypothesis that melatonin is most effective in improving sleep efficiency when it is administered and when the sleep episode occurs during the biologic day (see **Fig. 1**).

Several studies have investigated the potential use of melatonin as a sleep-promoting agent in the treatment of "insomnia", with mixed results. Although in some studies a positive effect of melatonin on sleep latency and sleep efficiency was reported,[90–94] in others no effect of melatonin[25,95,96] or a negative effect[81] was found. When looking at the various studies investigating exogenous melatonin administration in insomnia, there are large interstudy differences, including in the definition of insomnia used, the type of insomnia (eg, sleep onset versus sleep maintenance), the duration of insomnia, patient ages, and the preparations and doses of melatonin administered. In addition, the definition and method of assessment of sleep benefit differs between studies.

One type of "insomnia" for which melatonin has repeatedly been demonstrated to have a beneficial effect is in the treatment of delayed sleep phase type.[97] This success is likely due to the phase-shifting action of melatonin and possibly the sleep-promoting action. The underlying mechanisms of action for melatonin's effects on sleep are not yet fully understood, although a number of possible mechanisms have been proposed.

One possibility is that melatonin acts via reducing the circadian drive for wakefulness generated by the SCN. As mentioned previously, binding of melatonin to SCN MT1 receptors has been demonstrated to reduce SCN activity. It has been proposed that this information is then relayed to brain areas involved in the regulation of sleep (eg, ventrolateral preoptic area[98,99]) or wakefulness (eg, the locus caeruleus[100] or orexin/hypocretin neurons in the lateral hypothalamus[101–103]).

Another possible explanation is that the sleep-promoting and hypothermic effects of melatonin are causally related.[104] To date, a temporal relationship between an increase in circulating melatonin levels, an increase in sleep propensity, and a decrease in core temperature has been demonstrated; however, a causal relationship has not been fully established.

Hypothermic and Neurobehavioral Effects of Exogenous Melatonin

The nocturnal increase in endogenous melatonin levels is temporally associated with the nocturnal decline in core body temperature.[105] It has been hypothesized that the timing of these two events is related not only temporally but also causally. Melatonin onset precedes the decrease in heat production and increase in heat loss measured by the distal-to-proximal skin temperature gradient; this thermoregulatory cascade seems to be the most reliable predictor for rapid initiation of sleep.[106] Further support for this theory comes from observations of the hypothermic effect induced by diurnal melatonin administration,[67] and the observed increase in core temperature when melatonin levels are suppressed via bright light exposure[107–110] or administration of the β1-adrenergic antagonist atenolol.[111,112]

It would appear that the magnitude of the hypothermic effects of melatonin administration are equivalent for doses of melatonin greater than 10 mg,[113,114] with no evidence of a dose-response effect at these high doses. Some differences in hypothermic response have been reported for oral doses of melatonin between 0.1 and 10 mg.[27,71,115] Rather than being a dose-response effect, it would appear that a minimum dose of melatonin is required to induce a hypothermic response, and that, at low doses, interindividual differences in pharmacokinetics may account for differences in the hypothermic response. Similar findings have also been reported with intravenous administration of melatonin.[116]

Following the daytime administration of melatonin, reductions in alertness and various measures of neurocognitive function have been reported.[117–119] These deficits were evident following a range of doses administered (0.1–240 mg) and on a number of neurocognitive tasks; however, not all facets of neurocognitive functioning appear to be affected.[67] For example, decreased performance levels have been reported on tasks assessing reaction time,[23,27,113,117,120] unpredictable tracking,[117] vigilance,[27,113,118,121] and spatial memory.[118] In contrast, no significant effects of melatonin administration were reported on memory,[23] digit symbol substitution,[23,113] dual attention,[113] auditory tracking,[117] letter cancellation,[121] or driving performance.[119] Some studies have suggested that there may be a dose-dependent effect of melatonin administration on neurocognitive performance.[26,27] The increased subjective sleepiness induced by melatonin administration during the daytime was reflected in spectral electroencephalographic changes (higher theta/alpha).[122] These effects were found to be posture dependent; orthostasis counteracted the soporific effect.

The potential "hangover" effects of melatonin have also been investigated in a number of studies in which melatonin administration occurred before a sleep episode (either a nap or nocturnal sleep period) and neurocognitive functioning was assessed post sleep. In one study, 0.3 or 1.0 mg of melatonin administered at 21:00 hours followed by a normal nocturnal sleep period had no effect on neurocognitive functioning assessed the following morning.[74,123] In another study, 3 mg of melatonin given before sleep had no effect on subjective sleepiness or neurocognitive functioning following a 2-hour nap; however, subjective sleepiness levels were elevated following a 30-minute nap.[124]

MELATONIN ANALOGUES

The rationale for the development of melatonin analogues is not immediately obvious given that the naturally occurring hormone is available; however, melatonin formulations vary substantially, and in the United States, the potency, purity, and safety of melatonin are not regulated by the Food and Drug Administration. Large scale clinical trials confirming the efficacy of melatonin for CRSDs are lacking. It is possible that the analogues will be more potent and have more clinically useful pharmacokinetic profiles than melatonin itself. Because each of the currently available analogues have different chemical structures and binding affinities, comparative data from a range of compounds may elucidate the role of the MT1 and MT2 melatonin receptors in mediating the effects of melatonin on sleep and circadian rhythms. The discussion herein reviews four of the melatonin agonists that have been developed or are under development—ramelteon, agomelatine, tasimelteon, and PD-6735.

Ramelteon

Ramelteon, (S)-N-[2-(1,6,7,8-tetrahyrdo-2H-indeno-[5,4-b]furan-8-yl)ethyl]propionamide (TAK-375), is a high-affinity selective MT1/MT2 receptor agonist that shows approximately four times greater potency at the MT1 receptor and 17 times greater potency at the MT2 receptor when compared with melatonin, with low affinity for binding to the MT3 receptor or other neurotransmitter receptor systems.[125] Ramelteon's pharmacologic effects at the MT1/MT2 receptors may be mediated by a cAMP-dependent signal transduction cascade. It is rapidly absorbed, with peak plasma concentrations occurring within approximately 20 to 60 minutes, although absorption is delayed following a high-fat meal.[126–128] At least 84% of the parent compound is absorbed, but it undergoes extensive first-pass liver metabolism primarily by the CYP1A2 isozyme of the hepatic cytochrome P450 system.[126,127] Strong CYP1A2 inhibitors such as the selective serotonin reuptake

inhibitor fluvoxamine as well as severe hepatic impairment may cause marked elevation in serum ramelteon concentrations; therefore, ramelteon should not be used in these circumstances.[126] The active monohydroxylated metabolite, M-II, is approximately 20-fold less potent than the parent compound but circulates with at least a 20-fold higher serum concentration; therefore, may contribute to the clinical effect.[127,128] The elimination half-life of the parent compound is 1 to 2 hours and that of the active metabolite 2 to 4 hours; therefore, by 24 hours, the concentrations of both compounds are undetectable. However, in elderly patients, serum clearance is reduced by up to 40% when compared with younger subjects. There do not appear to be gender differences in pharmacokinetics, and ramelteon does not affect the metabolism of other drugs. The recommended nightly dose for the treatment of adults with insomnia is 8 mg.

In contrast to traditional hypnotic agents, safety data from animal models suggest that ramelteon has a low risk of cognitive impairment and physiologic dependence. Relatively high doses of ramelteon up to 30 mg/kg did not impair learning and memory for the water maze and delayed matching to position tasks in rats;[129,130] ramelteon up to 30 mg/kg did not impair motor coordination on the rota-rod task in mice and, unlike melatonin, did not exacerbate the motor impairment induced by diazepam.[131] Monkeys treated with large daily doses of ramelteon for 1 year showed no indication of any abnormal clinical behavior or alterations in operant behavior related to intermittent discontinuation of treatment.[132] There was no evidence of rewarding properties in the conditioned place-preference test in rats, suggesting low abuse potential.[129,133]

Animal models have demonstrated acute sleep-promoting effects of ramelteon. Cats treated with 0.1 mg/kg of ramelteon achieved a 20% reduction in the percentage of time spent in wakefulness with an almost 20% increase in the amount of slow-wave sleep and a small increase in REM sleep.[130] There was a nonsignificant statistical trend for decreased sleep onset latency of about 30 minutes. In this study, the sleep-inducing effect of ramelteon was about 10 times greater in potency than that of melatonin, and the effect of ramelteon lasted about 6 hours compared with 2 hours for melatonin. In macaque monkeys, ramelteon decreased sleep latency and slow-wave sleep latency and increased total sleep time; spectral analysis power densities were indistinguishable from natural sleep, whereas zolpidem and benzodiazepines decrease low-frequency and increase high-frequency power density spectra.[134] In rats, ramelteon caused an approximately 50% reduction in the NREM sleep latency.[135]

Ramelteon can phase advance circadian rhythms. When rats were subjected to an 8-hour phase advance of the light-dark cycle, re-entrainment of wheel running behavior took approximately 3 days less with ramelteon administered before the new lights out time when compared with the vehicle control.[129] Re-entrainment was achieved by phase advances with ramelteon as opposed to phase delays seen in the control condition. The advance region of the ramelteon PRC in mice is broader than for melatonin.[136] Precise circadian phase information is seldom readily available in the clinic when treating patients with DSPS, and a wider phase advance region could increase the chances of achieving desired phase advances with ramelteon versus melatonin.

Limited data exist regarding the ability of ramelteon to promote phase shifts in humans. A total of 110 volunteers with a history of jet lag sleep disturbances were randomized to placebo or ramelteon, 1 mg, 4 mg, or 8 mg, after flying eastward across five time zones. Across four treatment days, the latency to persistent sleep was reduced by only 7 to 10 minutes when compared with placebo. There was no dose-response relationship, and only the 1-mg dose achieved statistical significance.[137] In a laboratory study imposing a 5-hour advance of the sleep-wake cycle, ramelteon administered 30 minutes before bedtime caused a progressive advance of a circadian phase marker (salivary dim light melatonin offset) by up to 90 minutes compared with only 7 minutes with placebo. There was no clear dose-response effect between ramelteon given in doses of 1, 2, 4, and 8 mg, and the 28-minute phase advance in the 8-mg group did not reach statistical significance. Surprisingly, despite the phase advance of the circadian pacemaker seen in the ramelteon groups, there was no significant change in subjective or objective sleep parameters in comparison with placebo.[138]

Two multicenter, randomized, placebo-controlled, single-dose trials were conducted to determine the efficacy of ramelteon in a transient insomnia model in which healthy volunteers were required to sleep in a novel (laboratory) environment. In the first study, 375 participants received placebo or ramelteon, 16 or 64 mg, administered 30 minutes before habitual bedtime. There were no clinically significant differences between the two doses of ramelteon on polysomnographic sleep parameters or waking performance on the digit symbol substitution test (DSST), suggesting a flat dose-response curve. Ramelteon improved the latency to persistent sleep by approximately 10 minutes, and total sleep time increased by roughly 12 minutes, largely due to shortened sleep latencies. The amount of wake after sleep onset, the number of awakenings, and the distribution of sleep stages did not differ between groups.[139] Using a similar methodology, 289 adults were randomized to placebo or ramelteon, 8 or 16 mg. When compared with placebo, the 8-mg ramelteon dose decreased sleep latency by 7.5 minutes; the 16-mg dose decreased sleep latency by 5 minutes, which was not statistically significant. There was a similar increase in total sleep time of approximately 17 minutes in both ramelteon dose conditions.[140]

Several multicenter, randomized, placebo-controlled trials were conducted in adults with primary chronic insomnia. Two studies used a crossover design in which subjects received placebo or several doses of ramelteon for 2 days each separated by a 5- to 12-day washout period. In the first study, adult subjects received, in randomized order, placebo and ramelteon in doses of 4, 8, 16, and 32 mg. All of the ramelteon doses resulted in comparable reductions of sleep latency ranging from 38 minutes in the placebo condition to roughly 24 minutes in the ramelteon conditions. Total sleep time increased from 400 minutes in the placebo condition to approximately 413 minutes across all ramelteon conditions, without a clear dose-response effect. Ramelteon was associated with a slight reduction in the percentage of slow-wave sleep, attributed to an increase in the total light NREM sleep time.[141] Elderly insomnia patients aged 65 to 83 years were studied in a similar crossover design comparing placebo with ramelteon in doses of 4 mg and 8 mg. The polysomnographic latency to persistent sleep decreased by 10 minutes, and total sleep time increased by about 10 minutes when compared with placebo, without a dose-response relationship.[142]

Two trials studied the efficacy of ramelteon over 5 weeks in patients with primary chronic insomnia. Adults aged 18 to 64 years were randomized to placebo or ramelteon in doses of 8 or 16 mg. Ramelteon reduced sleep latency by 11 to 19 minutes (average, 15 minutes) and increased total sleep time by 5 to 22 minutes (average, 12 minutes) when compared with placebo, with the most robust difference seen in the first week. The decline in differences across the study seen between the ramelteon and placebo groups was attributable to the progressive improvement in sleep parameters in the placebo group.[143] Elderly subjects greater than 65 years old were studied in a 5-week active treatment protocol with either placebo or ramelteon in doses of 4 or 8 mg, with subjective sleep measures used as the primary outcome variables. Subjective sleep latency was reduced by 8 to 13 minutes, and patient-reported total sleep time increased by approximately 9 minutes across the study without a dose-response effect.[144] No withdrawal effects or rebound worsening of sleep symptoms was detected in either study using a placebo run-out phase after the 5-week treatment protocol.

In all of the clinical studies described previously, adverse event profiles for the various doses of ramelteon were comparable with those for placebo. Cognitive performance measured after an 8-hour sleep opportunity on tasks such as the DSST was generally similar to that with placebo. The low risk of cognitive side effects or abuse potential was highlighted by a study that used supratherapeutic doses of ramelteon. Fourteen subjects aged 18 to 60 years with a past or current history of psychoactive substance abuse or dependence were studied in a crossover design comparing 16, 80, or 160 mg of ramelteon, 0.25, 0.5, 0.75 mg of triazolam, and placebo. Cognitive measures included tests of balance, motor coordination, the DSST, and declarative memory; subjective measures included questions related to abuse potential. Triazolam induced dose-related impairments of the cognitive measures when compared with placebo, with deficits lasting approximately 4 hours; there were no significant differences between any ramelteon dose and placebo. Triazolam was associated with subjective ratings indicative of abuse potential, whereas ramelteon was not.[145] Safety studies have also been conducted in the setting of sleep-related breathing disorders. In 26 patients with mild-to-moderate obstructive sleep apnea, ramelteon did not worsen the apnea-hypopnea index when compared with placebo in a crossover design.[146] Ramelteon in doses of 8 to 16 mg did not have adverse effects on oxygen saturation during sleep in the setting of mild-to-moderate and moderate-to-severe chronic obstructive pulmonary disease (COPD).[147,148] Interestingly, in the COPD studies, ramelteon was associated with a 27- to 41-minute increase in total sleep time when compared with placebo, an effect generally greater than that seen in the insomnia trials.

In summary, ramelteon has a flat dose-response curve at doses greater than the recommended 8 mg, provides modest reductions in sleep latency and increases in total sleep time, has generally comparable adverse effect profiles when compared with placebo, is associated with minimal next-day cognitive impairment, does not have known abuse potential, and appears to lack the rebound worsening of insomnia associated with traditional hypnotic agents.

Agomelatine

Agomelatine (S20098), a napthalenic analogue of melatonin (N-[2-(7-methoxy-1-naphthyl)ethyl]acetamide), is a selective MT1 and MT2 agonist with a ratio of binding affinities (KiMT1/KiMT2) of 2.0.[20] It is also an antagonist at 5-HT2B and 5-HT2C serotonin receptors.[149] Studies in animal models have demonstrated that agomelatine is able to accelerate the re-entrainment of activity rhythms after a shift in the light-dark cycle and dose dependently inhibit SCN neuronal firing.[150] Furthermore, like melatonin, agomelatine is able to entrain free-running rhythms of rats, and this effect is abolished by SCN lesions.[150]

In humans, administration of agomelatine (5 mg, 100 mg) and melatonin (5 mg) 5 hours before bedtime to eight healthy young men phase advanced the circadian system, as assessed by core body temperature, melatonin, and heart rate decline.[43] Sleep termination and REM propensity were also phase advanced, but no effects were observed on NREM sleep parameters.[80] Daily administration of agomelatine (50 mg) to healthy elderly men approximately 4.5 hours before their bedtime for 15 days phase advanced rhythms of core body temperature and cortisol but did not significantly affect sleep parameters.[151] These findings indicate that, like melatonin, agomelatine has phase-shifting properties.

Agomelatine is unique among the current melatonin analogues in that it not only is an agonist at the MT1 and MT2 receptors but also an antagonist at the 5-HT2C receptor.[149] In addition, administration of agomelatine has been reported to increase dopamine and noradrenaline levels in the prefrontal cortex.[149] This effect is likely due to the antagonism of the 5-HT2C receptors. Because of these properties, several studies have investigated the antidepressant effects of this compound in addition to its phase-shifting and sleep-promoting effects.

It is widely accepted that disruption to the circadian system is common in many affective disorders, including major depressive disorder.[152] The type of disruption is not consistent, with differing changes in phase (eg, some individuals display phase advances whereas other experience phase delays) and reductions in the amplitude of circadian rhythms reported.[153] Although melatonin administration to patients with depression has been reported to improve sleep and sleep-wake timing, its antidepressant efficacy, per se, appears to be mild.[154] In contrast, agomelatine has been reported to produce antidepressant effects[155] as well as anxiolytic effects in animal models.[156] To date, a small number of randomized control trials in humans have reported significant antidepressant effects of agomelatine.[157-160] Although the mechanisms underlying the antidepressant and anxiolytic properties of agomelatine have not yet been elucidated, it is hypothesized that the combined binding of agomelatine at the melatonin (MT1 and MT2) and the 5-HT2C receptors may produce this action.

Tasimelteon

Tasimelteon (VEC-162, previously known as BMS-214,778) ((1R-trans)-N-[[2-(2,3-dihydro-4-benzofuranyl)cyclopropyl] methyl] propanamide) is a melatonin receptor agonist with high affinity for both the human MT1 (pKi = 9.45 ± 0.04 [0.35 nM]) and MT2 receptor (pKi = 9.8 ± 0.07 [0.17 nM]).[161] Studies in animal models report that tasimelteon has similar phase-shifting properties to melatonin.[162] Two recent randomized controlled trials (phase II and III) demonstrated that tasimelteon dose dependently improved the initiation and maintenance of sleep after a 5-hour phase advance of the sleep-wake and light-dark cycle, and that these effects occurred simultaneously with a phase advance of the plasma melatonin rhythm.[161] Because tasimelteon is able to alleviate the sleep disturbance induced by an abrupt shift of the sleep episode, the authors suggest that the compound has therapeutic potential for CRSDs. A phase III trial of the compound for primary insomnia has also recently been completed.

PD-6735

PD-6735 (R(-N-[2-(6-chloro-5-methoxy-1H-indol-3-yl)propyl]acetamide)), previously known as LY-156,735, is a beta-substituted melatonin analogue that is selective for MT1 and MT2 melatonin receptors (KiMT1/KiMT2 of 2.0^{20}). Potentially important differences are reported in the pharmacokinetics of PD-6735 and melatonin; with oral dosing, the area under the curve for PD-6735 is sixfold higher and the bioavailability ninefold higher than for melatonin.[163] A laboratory study in healthy male volunteers reported that PD-6735 (5 mg) accelerated the re-entrainment of several circadian rhythms (core body temperature, cortisol, potassium, sodium, and chloride acrophases) to a 9-hour phase advance of the light-dark and sleep-wake cycles.[163] Importantly, on two wake-time performance tests, PD-6735 significantly attenuated the impairment caused by the simulated time zone shift.

The compound appears to be safe and well tolerated at doses up to 100 mg and does not appear to be associated with hypothermia (assessed by tympanic temperature), bradycardia, or hypotension.[164] A randomized controlled trial of beta-methyl-6-chloromelatonin (PD-6735) (20 mg, 50 mg, 100 mg) was conducted in primary insomnia patients.[165] Beta-methyl-6-chloromelatonin reduced the latency to persistent sleep by 31%, 32%, and 41% in the 20-mg, 50-mg, and 100-mg dose groups, respectively. Subjective sleep latency was also reduced by beta-methyl-6-chloromelatonin. As is true for the other melatonin agonists studied, this compound shows efficacy in the treatment of primary insomnia.

SUMMARY AND FUTURE DIRECTIONS

Melatonin and melatonin agonists are well suited as therapeutic agents for CRSDs. The phase-shifting effects of melatonin are well characterized; phase advances are achieved by melatonin treatment in the late subjective day (afternoon or evening), and phase delays are achieved with melatonin treatment in the early subjective day (morning). The sleep-promoting effects of melatonin appear to be maximal when melatonin is administered just before a sleep episode occurring during the biologic day. Although melatonin agonists may have advantages to the naturally occurring compound, PRCs to inform treatment timing are lacking. Despite the obvious potential for these compounds in CRSDs, no large trials of melatonin agonists have been published in patients with chronic CRSDs.

The clinical utility of melatonin and melatonin agonists may extend well beyond the realm of sleep disorders. Melatonin appears to exert effects on many physiologic processes in the organism through its receptors in the hippocampus and other brain areas, the eye, cardiovascular and immune systems, and in cancer cells.[8]

Although it is becoming generally accepted that sleep promotes neuroplasticity and memory consolidation,[166-169] several lines of evidence suggest that the circadian phase may directly modulate neuroplasticity and that this effect may be mediated by the melatonin receptor system. For example, in both diurnal and nocturnal species of Aplysia, long-term memory for associative learning (ie, whether potential food was edible or inedible) was better when consolidation occurred over phases corresponding to each species' usual active period, independent of the experimental rest-activity cycle;[170] in vivo recordings in anesthetized rats have demonstrated a circadian rhythm in the capacity to induce long-term potentiation (LTP) in the rat hippocampus;[171] in vitro slice preparations in mice have demonstrated an intrinsic circadian oscillator governing hippocampal LTP;[172] and gene expression profiles in *Drosophila* have demonstrated a circadian rhythm in the transcription of several molecules believed to be involved in synaptic plasticity.[173] Ramelteon has recently been shown to increase the translation of brain-derived neurotrophic factor and to activate neuronal extracellular-signal-regulated kinase (ERK), important molecules for neuroplasticity, learning, and memory.[174,175] Knock-out mice were used to confirm that the activation of ERK by ramelteon was mediated by the MT1/MT2 receptor system. These studies open the door to clinical trials testing the effect of melatonin and melatonin analogues on learning and memory consolidation in humans.

ACKNOWLEDGMENTS

The authors thank Ms. Ahuva Segal, Caroline Bambrick, and Reena Kaur for editorial assistance.

REFERENCES

1. Arendt J, Rajaratnam SM. Melatonin and its agonists: an update. Br J Psychiatry 2008;193(4):267–9.
2. Redman J, Armstrong S, Ng KT. Free-running activity rhythms in the rat: entrainment by melatonin. Science 1983;219:1089–91.
3. Arendt J, Bojkowski C, Folkard S, et al. Some effects of melatonin and the control of its secretion in humans. Ciba Found Symp 1985;117:266–83.
4. Perreau-Lenz S, Kalsbeek A, Garidou ML, et al. Suprachiasmatic control of melatonin synthesis in rats: inhibitory and stimulatory mechanisms. Eur J Neurosci 2003;17:221–8.
5. Perreau-Lenz S, Kalsbeek A, Pevet P, et al. Glutamatergic clock output stimulates melatonin synthesis at night. Eur J Neurosci 2004;19:318–24.
6. Reppert SM, Perlow MJ, Ungerleider LG, et al. Effects of damage to the suprachiasmatic area of the anterior hypothalamus on the daily melatonin and cortisol rhythms in the rhesus monkey. J Neurosci 1981;1:1414–25.
7. Klein DC, Moore RY. Pineal N-acetyltransferase and hydroxyindole-O-methyltransferase: control by the retinohypothalamic tract and the suprachiasmatic nucleus. Brain Res 1979;174:245–62.
8. Pandi-Perumal SR, Trakht I, Srinivasan V, et al. Physiological effects of melatonin: role of melatonin receptors and signal transduction pathways. Prog Neurobiol 2008;85(3):335–53.
9. Cassone VM, Chesworth MJ, Armstrong SM. Entrainment of rat circadian rhythms by daily injection of melatonin depends upon the hypothalamic suprachiasmatic nuclei. Physiol Behav 1986;36:1111–21.
10. Sumova A, Illnerova H. Melatonin instantaneously resets intrinsic circadian rhythmicity in the rat suprachiasmatic nucleus. Neurosci Lett 1996;218(3):181–4.
11. Cassone VM, Roberts MH, Moore RY. Effects of melatonin on 2-deoxy-[1-14C] glucose uptake within rat suprachiasmatic nucleus. Am J Phys 1988;255:R332–7.
12. von Gall C, Duffield GE, Hastings MH, et al. CREB in the mouse SCN: a molecular interface coding the phase-adjusting stimuli light, glutamate, PACAP, and melatonin for clockwork access. J Neurosci 1998;18(24):10389–97.
13. Kopp M, Meissl H, Korf HW. The pituitary adenylate cyclase-activating polypeptide-induced phosphorylation of the transcription factor CREB (cAMP response element binding protein) in the rat suprachiasmatic nucleus is inhibited by melatonin. Neurosci Lett 1997;227(3):145–8.
14. Reppert SM, Weaver DR, Godson C. Melatonin receptors step into the light: cloning and classification of subtypes. Trends Pharmacol Sci 1996;17(3):100–2.
15. Liu C, Weaver DR, Jin X, et al. Molecular dissection of two distinct actions of melatonin on the suprachiasmatic circadian clock. Neuron 1997;19(1):91–102.
16. Hunt AE, Al-Ghoul WM, Gillette MU, et al. Activation of MT(2) melatonin receptors in rat suprachiasmatic nucleus phase advances the circadian clock. Am J Physiol Cell Physiol 2001;280(1):C110–8.
17. Dubocovich ML, Yun K, Alghoul WM, et al. Selective MT2 melatonin receptor antagonists block melatonin-mediated phase advances of circadian rhythms. FASEB J 1998;12(12):1211–20.
18. Dubocovich ML, Hudson RL, Sumaya IC, et al. Effect of MT1 melatonin receptor deletion on melatonin-mediated phase shift of circadian rhythms in the C57BL/6 mouse. J Pineal Res 2005;39(2):113–20.
19. von Gall C, Weaver DR, Kock M, et al. Melatonin limits transcriptional impact of phosphoCREB in the mouse SCN via the Mel1a receptor. Neuroreport 2000;11(9):1803–7.
20. Dubocovich ML. Melatonin receptors: role on sleep and circadian rhythm regulation. Sleep Med 2007;8(Suppl 3):34–42.
21. Shibata S, Cassone VM, Moore RY. Effects of melatonin on neuronal activity in the rat suprachiasmatic nucleus in vitro. Neurosci Lett 1989;97(1–2):140–4.
22. Jin X, von Gall C, Pieschl RL, et al. Targeted disruption of the mouse Mel(1b) melatonin receptor. Mol Cell Biol 2003;23(3):1054–60.
23. Lieberman HR, Waldhauser F, Garfield G, et al. Effects of melatonin on human mood and performance. Brain Res 1984;323(2):201–7.

24. Rogers NL, Dinges DF, Kennaway DJ, et al. Potential action of melatonin in insomnia. Sleep 2003; 26(8):1058–9.

25. Hughes RJ, Sack RL, Lewy AJ. The role of melatonin and circadian phase in age-related sleep-maintenance insomnia: assessment in a clinical trial of melatonin replacement. Sleep 1998;21(1): 52–68.

26. Deacon S, Arendt J. Melatonin-induced temperature suppression and its acute phase-shifting effects correlate in a dose-dependent manner in humans. Brain Res 1995;688(1–2):77–85.

27. Dollins AB, Zhdanova IV, Wurtman RJ, et al. Effect of inducing nocturnal serum melatonin concentrations in daytime on sleep, mood, body temperature, and performance. Proc Natl Acad Sci U S A 1994;91:1824–8.

28. Buscemi N, Vandermeer B, Hooton N, et al. Efficacy and safety of exogenous melatonin for secondary sleep disorders and sleep disorders accompanying sleep restriction: meta-analysis. BMJ 2006;332(7538):385–93.

29. Herxheimer A, Petrie KJ. Melatonin for the prevention and treatment of jet lag (Cochrane Review). Cochrane Database Syst Rev 2002;(2):CD001520.

30. Buscemi N, Vandermeer B, Hooton N, et al. The efficacy and safety of exogenous melatonin for primary sleep disorders: a meta-analysis. J Gen Intern Med 2005;20(12):1151–8.

31. Aldhous M, Franey C, Wright J, et al. Plasma concentrations of melatonin in man following oral absorption of different preparations. Br J Clin Pharmacol 1985;19(4):517–21.

32. Waldhauser F, Waldhauser M, Lieberman HR, et al. Bioavailability of oral melatonin in humans. Neuroendocrinology 1984;39(4):307–13.

33. Redman JR. Circadian entrainment and phase shifting in mammals with melatonin. J Biol Rhythms 1997;12(6):581–7.

34. McArthur AJ, Hunt AE, Gillette MU. Melatonin and signal transduction in the rat suprachiasmatic circadian clock: activation of protein kinase C at dawn and dusk. Endocrinology 1997;138:627–34.

35. Arendt J, Middleton B, Stone B, et al. Complex effects of melatonin: evidence for photoperiodic responses in humans? Sleep 1999;22(5):625–35.

36. Burgess HJ, Revell VL, Eastman CI. A three pulse phase response curve to three milligrams of melatonin in humans. J Physiol 2008;586(2):639–47.

37. Lewy AJ, Bauer VK, Ahmed S, et al. The human phase response curve (PRC) to melatonin is about 12 hours out of phase with the PRC to light. Chronobiol Int 1998;15(1):71–83.

38. Zaidan R, Geoffriau M, Brun J, et al. Melatonin is able to influence its secretion in humans: description of a phase response curve. Neuroendocrinology 1994;60:105–12.

39. Wirz-Justice A, Werth E, Renz C, et al. No evidence for a phase delay in human circadian rhythms after a single morning melatonin administration. J Pineal Res 2002;32(1):1–5.

40. Sack RL, Lewy AJ, Hoban TM. Free-running melatonin rhythms in blind people: phase shifts with melatonin and triazolam administration. In: Rensing L, van der Heiden U, Mackey MC, editors. Temporal disorder in human oscillatory systems. Heidelberg: Springer-Verlag; 1987. p. 219–24.

41. Deacon S, English J, Arendt J. Acute phase-shifting effects of melatonin associated with suppression of core body temperature in humans. Neurosci Lett 1994;178(1):32–4.

42. Attenburrow MEJ, Dowling BA, Sargent PA, et al. Melatonin phase advances circadian rhythm. Psychopharmacology (Berl) 1995;121(4):503–5.

43. Krauchi K, Cajochen C, Mori D, et al. Early evening melatonin and S-20098 advance circadian phase and nocturnal regulation of core body temperature. Am J Phys 1997;272(4 Pt 2):R1178–88.

44. Sharkey KM, Eastman CI. Melatonin phase shifts human circadian rhythms in a placebo-controlled simulated night-work study. Am J Physiol Regul Integr Comp Physiol 2002;282(2):R454–63.

45. Rajaratnam SM, Dijk DJ, Middleton B, et al. Melatonin phase shifts human circadian rhythms with no evidence of changes in the duration of endogenous melatonin secretion or the 24-hour production of reproductive hormones. J Clin Endocrinol Metab 2003;88(9):4303–9.

46. Vandewalle G, Middleton B, Rajaratnam SM, et al. Robust circadian rhythm in heart rate and its variability: influence of exogenous melatonin and photoperiod. J Sleep Res 2007;16(2):148–55.

47. Rajaratnam SM, Middleton B, Stone BM, et al. Melatonin advances the circadian timing of EEG sleep and directly facilitates sleep without altering its duration in extended sleep opportunities in humans. J Physiol 2004;561(Pt 1):339–51.

48. Lockley SW, Skene DJ, James K, et al. Melatonin administration can entrain the free-running circadian system of blind subjects. J Endocrinol 2000; 164:R1–6.

49. Sack RL, Brandes RW, Kendall AR, et al. Entrainment of free-running circadian rhythms by melatonin in blind people. N Engl J Med 2000;343(15):1070–7.

50. Lewy AJ, Emens JS, Sack RL, et al. Low, but not high, doses of melatonin entrained a free-running blind person with a long circadian period. Chronobiol Int 2002;19(3):649–58.

51. Hack LM, Lockley SW, Arendt J, et al. The effects of low-dose 0.5-mg melatonin on the free-running circadian rhythms of blind subjects. J Biol Rhythms 2003;18(5):420–9.

52. Lewy AJ, Emens JS, Lefler BJ, et al. Melatonin entrains free-running blind people according to

a physiological dose-response curve. Chronobiol Int 2005;22(6):1093–106.

53. Sharkey KM, Fogg LF, Eastman CI. Effects of melatonin administration on daytime sleep after simulated night shift work. J Sleep Res 2001; 10(3):181–92.

54. Dahlitz MJ, Alvarez B, Vignau J, et al. Delayed sleep phase syndrome: response to melatonin. Lancet 1991;337:1121–4.

55. Folkard S, Arendt J, Clark M. Can melatonin improve shift workers' tolerance of the night shift? Some preliminary findings. Chronobiol Int 1993; 10(5):315–20.

56. Arendt J, Skene DJ, Middleton B, et al. Efficacy of melatonin treatment in jet lag, shift work, and blindness. J Biol Rhythms 1997;12(6):604–17.

57. Nagtegaal JE, Kerkhof GA, Smits MG, et al. Delayed sleep phase syndrome: a placebo-controlled crossover study on the effects of melatonin administered five hours before the individual dim light melatonin onset. J Sleep Res 1998;7(2):135–43.

58. Dawson D, Encel N, Lushington K. Improving adaptation to simulated night shift: timed exposure to bright light versus daytime melatonin administration. Sleep 1995;18(1):11–21.

59. Spitzer RL, Terman M, Williams JB, et al. Jet lag: clinical features, validation of a new syndrome-specific scale, and lack of response to melatonin in a randomized, double-blind trial. Am J Psychiatry 1999;156(9):1392–6.

60. Arendt J. Does melatonin improve sleep? Efficacy of melatonin. BMJ 2006;332(7540):550.

61. Nakagawa H, Sack RL, Lewy AJ. Sleep propensity free-runs with the temperature, melatonin and cortisol rhythms in a totally blind person. Sleep 1992;15(4):330–6.

62. Dijk DJ, Cajochen C. Melatonin and the circadian regulation of sleep initiation, consolidation, structure, and the sleep EEG. J Biol Rhythms 1997; 12(6):627–35.

63. Lockley SW, Skene DJ, Tabandeh H, et al. Relationship between napping and melatonin in the blind. J Biol Rhythms 1997;12(1):16–25.

64. Wyatt JK, Ritz-De Cecco A, Czeisler CA, et al. Circadian temperature and melatonin rhythms, sleep, and neurobehavioral function in humans living on a 20-h day. (Regulatory, Integrative and Comparative Physiology). Am J Physiol 1999; 277(46):R1152–63.

65. Wehr TA, Aeschbach D, Duncan WC Jr. Evidence for a biological dawn and dusk in the human circadian timing system. J Physiol 2001;535(Pt 3): 937–51.

66. Scheer FA, Zeitzer JM, Ayas NT, et al. Reduced sleep efficiency in cervical spinal cord injury: association with abolished night time melatonin secretion. Spinal Cord 2006;44(2):78–81.

67. Wright KP Jr, Rogers NL. Endogenous versus exogenous effects of melatonin. In: Pandi-Perumal SR, Cardinali DP, editors. Melatonin: from molecules to therapy. New York: Nova Science Publishers; 2007. p. 547–69.

68. Cramer H, Rudolph J, Consbruch U, et al. On the effects of melatonin on sleep and behavior in man. Adv Biochem Psychopharmacol 1974;11:187–91.

69. Anton-Tay F, Diaz JL, Fernandez-Guardiola A. On the effect of melatonin upon human brain: its possible therapeutic implications. Life Sci 1971; 1015:841–50.

70. Cajochen C, Krauchi K, Danilenko KV, et al. Evening administration of melatonin and bright light: interactions on the EEG during sleep and wakefulness. J Sleep Res 1998;7(3):145–57.

71. Hughes RJ, Badia P. Sleep-promoting and hypothermic effects of daytime melatonin administration in humans. Sleep 1997;20(2):124–31.

72. Mishima K, Satoh K, Shimizu T, et al. Hypnotic and hypothermic action of daytime-administered melatonin. Psychopharmacol 1997;133:168–71.

73. Nave R, Peled R, Lavie P. Melatonin improves evening napping. Eur J Pharmacol 1995;275(2): 213–6.

74. Zhdanova IV, Wurtman RJ, Morabito C, et al. Effects of low oral doses of melatonin, given 2-4 hours before habitual bedtime, on sleep in normal young humans. Sleep 1996;19(5):423–31.

75. Reid K, Van den Heuvel C, Dawson D. Day-time melatonin administration: effects on core temperature and sleep onset latency. J Sleep Res 1996; 5(3):150–4.

76. Gilbert SS, Van den Heuvel C, Dawson D. Daytime melatonin and temazepam in young adult humans: equivalent effects on sleep latency and body temperatures. J Physiol 1999;514(Pt 3):905–14.

77. Wyatt JK, Dijk DJ, Ritz-de Cecco A, et al. Sleep-facilitating effect of exogenous melatonin in healthy young men and women is circadian-phase dependent. Sleep 2006;29(5):609–18.

78. Waldhauser F, Saletu B, Trinchard-Lugan I. Sleep laboratory investigations on hypnotic properties of melatonin. Psychopharmacology (Berl) 1990; 100(2):222–6.

79. Attenburrow ME, Cowen PJ, Sharpley AL. Low dose melatonin improves sleep in healthy middle-aged subjects. Psychopharmacology (Berl) 1996; 126(2):179–81.

80. Cajochen C, Krauchi K, Mori D, et al. Melatonin and S-20098 increase REM sleep and wake-up propensity without modifying NREM sleep homeostasis. Am J Phys 1997;272(4 Pt 2):R1189–96.

81. Dawson D, Rogers NL, van den Heuvel CJ, et al. Effect of sustained nocturnal transbuccal melatonin administration on sleep and temperature in elderly insomniacs. J Biol Rhythms 1998;13:532–8.

82. Middleton BA, Stone BM, Arendt J. Melatonin and fragmented sleep patterns. Lancet 1996; 348(9026):551–2.

83. Nave R, Herer P, Haimov I, et al. Hypnotic and hypothermic effects of melatonin on daytime sleep in humans: lack of antagonism by flumazenil. Neurosci Lett 1996;214(2–3):123–6.

84. Tzischinsky O, Lavie P. Melatonin possesses time-dependent hypnotic effects. Sleep 1994;17(7): 638–45.

85. Zhdanova IV, Wurtman RJ. Efficacy of melatonin as a sleep-promoting agent. J Biol Rhythms 1997; 12(6):644–50.

86. Dijk DJ, Roth C, Landolt HP, et al. Melatonin effect on daytime sleep in men: suppression of EEG low frequency activity and enhancement of spindle frequency activity. Neurosci Lett 1995;201(1):13–6.

87. Stone BM, Turner C, Mills SL, et al. Hypnotic activity of melatonin. Sleep 2000;23(5):663–9.

88. Lavie P. Ultrashort sleep-waking schedule. III. 'Gates' and 'forbidden zones' for sleep. Electroencephalogr Clin Neurophysiol 1986;63(5):414–25.

89. Strogatz SH, Kronauer RE, Czeisler CA. Circadian regulation dominates homeostatic control of sleep length and prior wake length in humans. Sleep 1986;9(2):353–64.

90. Garfinkel D, Laudon M, Nof D, et al. Improvement of sleep quality in elderly people by controlled-release melatonin. Lancet 1995;346(8974):541–4.

91. Haimov I, Lavie P, Laudon M, et al. Melatonin replacement therapy of elderly insomniacs. Sleep 1995;18(7):598–603.

92. MacFarlane JG, Cleghorn JM, Brown GM, et al. The effects of exogenous melatonin on the total sleep time and daytime alertness of chronic insomniacs: a preliminary study. Biol Psychiatry 1991;30:371–6.

93. Wurtman RJ, Zhdanova I. Improvement of sleep quality by melatonin. Lancet 1995;346(8988):1491.

94. Zhdanova IV, Wurtman RJ, Regan MM, et al. Melatonin treatment for age-related insomnia. J Clin Endocrinol Metab 2001;86(10):4727–30.

95. Ellis CM, Lemmens G, Parkes JD. Melatonin and insomnia. J Sleep Res 1996;5(1):61–5.

96. James SP, Sack DA, Rosenthal NE, et al. Melatonin administration in insomnia. Neuropsychopharmacology 1990;3:19–23.

97. Dagan Y. Circadian rhythm sleep disorders (CRSD) in psychiatry: a review. Isr J Psychiatry Relat Sci 2002;39(1):19–27.

98. Chou TC, Bjorkum AA, Gaus SE, et al. Afferents to the ventrolateral preoptic nucleus. J Neurosci 2002; 22:977–90.

99. Deurveilher S, Semba K. Indirect projections from the suprachiasmatic nucleus to major arousal-promoting cell groups in rat: implications for the circadian control of behavioural state. Neurosci 2005;130:165–83.

100. Aston-Jones G, Chen S, Zhu Y, et al. A neural circuit for circadian regulation of arousal. Nat Neurosci 2001;4:732–8.

101. Deboer T, Overeem S, Visser NA, et al. Convergence of circadian and sleep regulatory mechanisms on hypocretin-1. Neuroscience 2004;129: 727–32.

102. Zeitzer JM, Buckmaster CL, Parker KJ, et al. Circadian and homeostatic regulation of hypocretin in a primate model: implications for the consolidation of wakefulness. J Neurosci 2003;23:3555–60.

103. Zhang S, Zeitzer JM, Yoshida Y, et al. Lesions of the suprachiasmatic nucleus eliminate the daily rhythm of hypocretin-1 release. Sleep 2004;27:619–27.

104. Cajochen C, Krauchi K, Wirz-Justice A. Role of melatonin in the regulation of human circadian rhythms and sleep. J Neuroendocrinol 2003; 15(4):432–7.

105. Cagnacci A, Elliott JA, Yen SS. Melatonin: a major regulator of the circadian rhythm of core temperature in humans. J Clin Endocrinol Metab 1992;75: 447–52.

106. Krauchi K, Cajochen C, Werth E, et al. Warm feet promote the rapid onset of sleep. Nature 1999; 401(6748):36–7.

107. Burgess HJ, Sletten T, Savic N, et al. Effects of bright light and melatonin on sleep propensity, temperature, and cardiac activity at night. J Appl Phys 2001;91:1214–22.

108. Cagnacci A, Soldani R, Yen SSC. The effect of light on core body temperature is mediated by melatonin in women. J Clin Endocrinol Metab 1993; 76(4):1036–8.

109. Wright KP, Badia P, Myers BL, et al. Caffeine and light effects on nighttime melatonin and temperature levels in sleep-deprived humans. Brain Res 1997;747:78–84.

110. Wright KP Jr, Myers BL, Plenzler SC, et al. Acute effects of bright light and caffeine on nighttime melatonin and temperature levels in women taking and not taking oral contraceptives. Brain Res 2000; 873:310–7.

111. Cagnacci A, Soldani R, Romagnolo C, et al. Melatonin-induced decrease of body temperature in women: a threshold event. Neuroendocrinology 1994;60(5):549–52.

112. van den Heuvel CJ, Reid KJ, Dawson D. Effect of atenolol on nocturnal sleep and temperature in young men: reversal by pharmacological doses of melatonin. Physiol Behav 1997;61:795–802.

113. Dollins AB, Lynch HJ, Wurtman RJ, et al. Effect of pharmacological daytime doses of melatonin on human mood and performance. Psychopharmacology 1993;112(4):490–6.

114. Dawson D, Gibbon S, Singh P. The hypothermic effect of melatonin on core body temperature: is more better? J Pineal Res 1996;20(4):192–7.

115. Satoh K, Mishima K. Hypothermic action of exoge-nously administered melatonin is dose dependent in humans. Clin Neuropharmacol 2001;24:334–40.

116. van den Heuvel CJ, Kennaway DJ, Dawson D. Thermoregulatory and soporific effects of very low dose melatonin injection. Am J Physiol 1999;276:E249–54.

117. Rogers NL, Phan O, Kennaway DJ, et al. Effect of daytime oral melatonin administration on neurobehavioral performance in humans. J Pineal Res 1998;25:47–53.

118. Rogers NL, Kennaway DJ, Dawson D. Neurobehavioural performance effects of daytime melatonin and temazepam administration. J Sleep Res 2003;12:207–12.

119. Suhner A, Schlagenhauf P, Tschopp A, et al. Impact of melatonin on driving performance. J Travel Med 1998;5(1):7–13.

120. Wynn VT, Arendt J. Effect of melatonin on the human electrocardiogram and simple reaction time responses. J Pineal Res 1988;5:427–35.

121. Graw P, Werth E, Krauchi K, et al. Early morning melatonin administration impairs psychomotor vigilance. Behav Brain Res 2001;121:167–72.

122. Cajochen C, Kraeuchi K, Wirz-Justice A. The acute soporific action of daytime melatonin administration: effects on the EEG during wakefulness and subjective alertness. J Biol Rhythms 1997;12(6):636–43.

123. Zhdanova IV, Wurtman RJ, Lynch HJ, et al. Sleep-inducing effects of low doses of melatonin ingested in the evening. Clin Pharmacol Ther 1995;57(5): 552–8.

124. Nave R, Iani C, Herer P, et al. Residual effects of daytime administration of melatonin on performance relevant to flight. Behav Brain Res 2002; 131:87–95.

125. Kato K, Hirai K, Nishiyama K, et al. Neurochemical properties of ramelteon (TAK-375), a selective MT1/MT2 receptor agonist. Neuropharmacology 2005;48(2):301–10.

126. Rozerem, (ramelteon tablets). Package insert. Takeda Pharmaceuticals; 2005.

127. Stevenson S, Cornelissen K, Clarke E, et al. Study of the absorption, metabolism, and excretion of (14C)-ramelteon (TAK-375) [abstract]. Clin Pharmacol Ther 2004;75:22.

128. Karim A, Tolbert D, Cao C. Disposition kinetics and tolerance of escalating single doses of ramelteon, a high-affinity MT1 and MT2 melatonin receptor agonist indicated for treatment of insomnia. J Clin Pharmacol 2006;46(2):140–8.

129. Hirai K, Kita M, Ohta H, et al. Ramelteon (TAK-375) accelerates reentrainment of circadian rhythm after a phase advance of the light-dark cycle in rats. J Biol Rhythms 2005;20(1):27–37.

130. Miyamoto M, Nishikawa H, Doken Y, et al. The sleep-promoting action of ramelteon (TAK-375) in freely moving cats. Sleep 2004;27(7):1319–25.

131. Miyamoto M. Effect of ramelteon (TAK-375), a selective MT1/MT2 receptor agonist, on motor performance in mice. Neurosci Lett 2006;402(3):201–4.

132. France CP, Weltman RH, Koek W, et al. Acute and chronic effects of ramelteon in rhesus monkeys (Macaca mulatta): dependence liability studies. Behav Neurosci 2006;120(3):535–41.

133. Miyamoto M, Nishikawa H, Ohta H, et al. Behavioral pharmacology of ramelteon (TAK-375) in small animals. [abstract] Ann Neurol 2003;54(Suppl 7): S46.

134. Yukuhiro N, Kimura H, Nishikawa H, et al. Effects of ramelteon (TAK-375) on nocturnal sleep in freely moving monkeys. Brain Res 2004;1027(1–2):59–66.

135. Fisher SP, Davidson K, Kulla A, et al. Acute sleep-promoting action of the melatonin agonist, ramelteon, in the rat. J Pineal Res 2008;45(2):125–35.

136. Rawashdeh O, Stepien I, Smith M, et al. Phase response curve for ramelteon in C3H/HeN mice. Society for Biological Rhythms Program and Abstracts 2008;190.

137. Zee P, Richardson G, Wang-Weigand S. Effects of ramelteon on insomnia symptoms induced by rapid, eastward travel. Society for Biological Rhythms Program and Abstracts 2008;70.

138. Richardson GS, Zee PC, Wang-Weigand S, et al. Circadian phase-shifting effects of repeated ramelteon administration in healthy adults. J Clin Sleep Med 2008;4(5):456–61.

139. Roth T, Stubbs C, Walsh JK. Ramelteon (TAK-375), a selective MT1/MT2-receptor agonist, reduces latency to persistent sleep in a model of transient insomnia related to a novel sleep environment. Sleep 2005;28(3):303–7.

140. Zammit G, Schwartz H, Roth T, et al. The effects of ramelteon in a first-night model of transient insomnia. Sleep Med 2009;10(1):55–9.

141. Erman M, Seiden D, Zammit G, et al. An efficacy, safety, and dose-response study of ramelteon in patients with chronic primary insomnia. Sleep Med 2006;7(1):17–24.

142. Roth T, Seiden D, Wang-Weigand S, et al. A 2-night, 3-period, crossover study of ramelteon's efficacy and safety in older adults with chronic insomnia. Curr Med Res Opin 2007;23(5):1005–14.

143. Zammit G, Erman M, Wang-Weigand S, et al. Evaluation of the efficacy and safety of ramelteon in subjects with chronic insomnia. J Clin Sleep Med 2007;3(5):495–504.

144. Roth T, Seiden D, Sainati S, et al. Effects of ramelteon on patient-reported sleep latency in older adults with chronic insomnia. Sleep Med 2006; 7(4):312–8.

145. Johnson MW, Suess PE, Griffiths RR. Ramelteon: a novel hypnotic lacking abuse liability and sedative adverse effects. Arch Gen Psychiatry 2006; 63(10):1149–57.

146. Kryger M, Wang-Weigand S, Roth T. Safety of ramelteon in individuals with mild to moderate obstructive sleep apnea. Sleep Breath 2007; 11(3):159–64.

147. Kryger M, Roth T, Wang-Weigand S, et al. The effects of ramelteon on respiration during sleep in subjects with moderate to severe chronic obstructive pulmonary disease. Sleep Breath 2009;13(1):79–84.

148. Kryger M, Wang-Weigand S, Zhang J, et al. Effect of ramelteon, a selective MT(1)/MT(2)-receptor agonist, on respiration during sleep in mild to moderate COPD. Sleep Breath 2008;12(3):243–50.

149. Millan MJ, Gobert A, Lejeune F, et al. The novel melatonin agonist agomelatine (S20098) is an antagonist at 5-hydroxytryptamine-2C receptors, blockade of which enhances the activity of frontocortical dopaminergic and adrenergic pathways. J Pharmacol Exp Ther 2003;306(3):954–64.

150. Turek FW, Gillette MU. Melatonin, sleep, and circadian rhythms: rationale for development of specific melatonin agonists. Sleep Med 2004;5(6):523–32.

151. Leproult R, Van Onderbergen A, L'Hermite-Baleriaux M, et al. Phase shifts of 24-h rhythms of hormonal release and body temperature following early evening administration of the melatonin agonist agomelatine in healthy older men. Clin Endocrinol (Oxf) 2005;63(3):298–304.

152. Boivin DB. Influence of sleep-wake and circadian rhythm disturbances in psychiatric disorders. J Psychiatry Neurosci 2000;25(5):446–58.

153. Tsujimoto T, Yamada N, Shimoda K, et al. Circadian rhythms in depression. Part II. Circadian rhythms in inpatients with various mental disorders. J Affect Disord 1990;18(3):199–210.

154. Dalton EJ, Rotondi D, Levitan RD, et al. Use of slow-release melatonin in treatment-resistant depression. J Psychiatry Neurosci 2000;25(1):48–52.

155. Zupancic M, Guilleminault C. Agomelatine: a preliminary review of a new antidepressant. CNS Drugs 2006;20(12):981–92.

156. Pandi-Perumal SR, Srinivasan V, Maestroni GJ, et al. Melatonin: nature's most versatile biological signal? FEBS J 2006;273(13):2813–38.

157. Loo H, Hale A, D'Haenen H. Determination of the dose of agomelatine, a melatoninergic agonist and selective 5-HT(2C) antagonist, in the treatment of major depressive disorder: a placebo-controlled dose range study. Int Clin Psychopharmacol 2002; 17(5):239–47.

158. Kennedy SH, Emsley R. Placebo-controlled trial of agomelatine in the treatment of major depressive disorder. Eur Neuropsychopharmacol 2006;16(2): 93–100.

159. Olie JP, Emsley R. Confirmed clinical efficacy of agomelatine (25–50 mg) in major depression: two randomized, double-blind, placebo-controlled studies. Eur Neuropsychopharmacol 2005;15(Suppl 3):S416.

160. Olie JP, Kasper S. Efficacy of agomelatine, a MT1/MT2 receptor agonist with 5-HT2C antagonistic properties, in major depressive disorder. Int J Neuropsychopharmacol 2007;10(5):661–73.

161. Rajaratnam SM, Rajaratnam MH, Fisher DM, et al. Melatonin agonist tasimelteon (VEC-162) for transient insomnia after sleep-time shift: two randomised controlled trials. Lancet 2009;373(9662):482–91.

162. Vachharajani NN, Yeleswaram K, Boulton DW. Preclinical pharmacokinetics and metabolism of BMS-214778, a novel melatonin receptor agonist. J Pharm Sci 2003;92(4):760–72.

163. Nickelsen T, Samel A, Vejvoda M, et al. Chronobiotic effects of the melatonin agonist LY 156735 following a simulated 9 h time shift: results of a placebo-controlled trial. Chronobiol Int 2002;19(5):915–36.

164. Mulchahey JJ, Goldwater DR, Zemlan FP. A single blind, placebo controlled, across group dose escalation study of the safety, tolerability, pharmacokinetics and pharmacodynamics of the melatonin analog beta-methyl-6-chloromelatonin. Life Sci 2004;75(15):1843–56.

165. Zemlan FP, Mulchahey JJ, Scharf MB, et al. The efficacy and safety of the melatonin agonist beta-methyl-6-chloromelatonin in primary insomnia: a randomized, placebo-controlled, crossover clinical trial. J Clin Psychiatry 2005;66(3):384–90.

166. Maquet P. The role of sleep in learning and memory. Science 2001;294(5544):1048–52.

167. Walker MP, Stickgold R. Sleep, memory, and plasticity. Annu Rev Psychol 2006;57:139–66.

168. Graves L, Pack A, Abel T. Sleep and memory: a molecular perspective. Trends Neurosci 2001; 24(4):237–43.

169. Stickgold R, Walker MP. Sleep and memory: the ongoing debate. Sleep 2005;28(10):1225–7.

170. Lyons LC, Rawashdeh O, Katzoff A, et al. Circadian modulation of complex learning in diurnal and nocturnal *Aplysia*. Proc Natl Acad Sci U S A 2005;102(35):12589–94.

171. Dana RC, Martinez JL Jr. Effect of adrenalectomy on the circadian rhythm of LTP. Brain Res 1984; 308(2):392–5.

172. Chaudhury D, Wang LM, Colwell CS. Circadian regulation of hippocampal long-term potentiation. J Biol Rhythms 2005;20(3):225–36.

173. Claridge-Chang A, Wijnen H, Naef F, et al. Circadian regulation of gene expression systems in the *Drosophila* head. Neuron 2001;32(4):657–71.

174. Imbesi M, Uz T, Dzitoyeva S, et al. Stimulatory effects of a melatonin receptor agonist, ramelteon, on BDNF in mouse cerebellar granule cells. Neurosci Lett 2008;439(1):34–6.

175. Imbesi M, Uz T, Manev H. Melatonin receptor agonist ramelteon activates the extracellular signal-regulated kinase 1/2 in mouse cerebellar granule cells. Neuroscience 2008;155(4):1160–4.

Non–24-Hour Sleep–Wake Syndrome in Sighted and Blind Patients

Makoto Uchiyama, MD, PhD[a],*, Steven W. Lockley, PhD[b],*

KEYWORDS

- Circadian rhythm sleep disorders
- Non–24-hour sleep–wake disorder
- Free-running type • Non-entrained type
- Hypernychthemeral syndrome • Blindness
- Melatonin

NON–24-HOUR SLEEP–WAKE SYNDROME (CIRCADIAN RHYTHM SLEEP DISORDER, FREE-RUNNING TYPE, NON-ENTRAINED TYPE, HYPERNYCHTHEMERAL SYNDROME)

Non–24-hour sleep–wake syndrome (N24HSWS) is defined as a "complaint of insomnia or excessive sleepiness related to abnormal desynchronization between the 24-hour light/dark cycle and the endogenous circadian rhythm of sleep and wake propensity."[1,2] The daily light/dark cycle is the most powerful environmental time cue for synchronizing the hypothalamic circadian pacemaker to the 24-hour day. Individuals who are physically or biologically isolated from a normal 24-hour light/dark cycle exhibit a sleep/wake cycle that is different from, and usually longer than, 24 hours.[3,4] This non–24-hour cycle leads to progressively later or progressively earlier bedtimes and wake times. N24HSWS is a rare condition in sighted individuals and is characterized by a chronic steady pattern of typically approximately 1-hour delays in spontaneous sleep onset and wake times while living under normal environmental conditions.[1] Because most individuals usually are required to live on a 24-hour social day and maintain a regular sleep–wake schedule, the sufferer displays periodically recurring problems with sleep initiation, sleep maintenance, and rising, as the circadian cycle of wakefulness and sleep propensity moves in and out of synchrony with the fixed social sleep episode.[5] Although the disorder is generally rare in sighted people, there are a considerable number of reports of N24HSWS in sighted subjects,[5,6] and a recent review indicated that the disorder may be more common than previously thought in individuals in their teens and 20s.[6]

N24HSWS is most common in individuals who are totally blind;[1,5,7] as many as half of totally blind patients have this disorder. In these patients, the lack of ocular light information reaching the circadian pacemaker prevents the pacemaker from entraining to the normal 24-hour light/dark cycle.[7] Consequently, the circadian pacemaker reverts to its endogenous non–24-hour period, causing a chronic, cyclic sleep–wake disorder characterized by episodes of good sleep followed by periods of poor sleep and excessive daytime sleepiness, followed by good sleep, ad infinitum. There are some differences, however, between sighted and blind subjects in the etiology and expression of this disorder. This article reviews the clinical aspects and pathophysiology of

S.W.L. was supported in part by the National Institute for Neurological Disorders and Stroke (R01 NS040982).
[a] Department of Psychiatry, Nihon University School of Medicine, Itabashi, 173-8610 Tokyo, Japan
[b] Division of Sleep Medicine, Brigham and Women's Hospital, Harvard Medical School, 221 Longwood Avenue, Boston, MA 02115, USA
* Corresponding authors.
E-mail addresses: maco.uchiyama@nifty.com (M. Uchiyama); slockley@hms.harvard.edu (S. W. Lockley).

sighted and blind patients suffering from N24HSWS.

CLINICAL CHARACTERISTICS OF NON–24-HOUR SLEEP–WAKE SYNDROME IN SIGHTED PATIENTS

The prevalence of N24HSWS in the general population has not been established, but it is assumed to be rare.[1] Systematic clinical examinations of sighted patients who have N24HSWS also are relatively rare, although many single-case reports have been described (**Table 1**).[8–34]

Clinical Features

The basic characteristics of sighted patients who have N24HSWS (eg, sex, age, and age at onset) remain to be elucidated.[1] Hayakawa and colleagues[6] examined 57 consecutively diagnosed sighted patients who had N24HSWS and found that 72% of them were men. This finding is consistent with previous studies listed in **Table 1**, in which 85% of the patients were male. The commencement of a free-running sleep/wake cycle usually occurred when patients were in their teens or 20s (see **Table 1**). Nearly all the patients (98%) had a history of disturbed social functioning resulting from the inability to attend school or work regularly, and about a quarter (28%) had psychiatric disorders.

Sleep Features

By definition, a non–24-hour sleep–wake pattern is characteristic of this disorder and usually is defined by data from daily sleep logs and/or wrist actigraphy collected over several consecutive weeks. Sleep duration tends to be normal to long with a mean (± SD) sleep duration of 9.3 hours (± 1.3 hours) and a median duration of 9.0 hours.[6] Polysomnography typically has not been performed or reported in detail in such patients, because sleep structure and quality on a given single-night recording depend on the phase relationship between internal biologic time and sleep.[35]

Fig. 1 shows representative self-reported sleep–wake records for three patients who had N24HSWS: a 26-year-old woman (see **Fig. 1**A, case 1), a 22-year-old man (see **Fig. 1**B, case 2),[6] and a 30-year-old man (see **Fig. 1**C, case 3).[8] All subjects began exhibiting symptoms in their teens and had difficulty adjusting to school and college schedules. Clinical examinations failed to reveal any abnormalities in routine electroencephalogram, MRI, hematology, or biochemistry tests. Semistructured psychiatric interviews revealed that case 1 had an adjustment disorder

and case 2 suffered from major depression (according to *Diagnostic and Statistical Manual edition 4* criteria). Case 3 had no Axis I or III disorders. Although the sleep/wake cycle clearly has a non–24-hour pattern in all three cases, the behavior is not identical. Case 1 shows a relatively steadily delaying free-running sleep pattern, albeit with some occasional minor changes in sleep duration. This pattern can be expressed only in those patients without strong social commitments (eg, work or school) that would prevent sleep during the daytime hours. Cases 2 and 3 show more typical patterns, although they also result in substantial social isolation. In both cases, the sleep/wake cycle does not simply have a constant non–24-hour pattern; there are at least two distinct components that repeat cyclically. The sleep/wake cycle shows a regular "free run" when sleep is initiated during the night or early morning, close to a normal social sleep time and when natural sunlight is not available, although most sleep episodes still start during the night (see **Fig. 1**C, *middle panel*). Once the sleep onset has delayed into the morning hours, the sleep/wake cycle becomes more disrupted and seems to delay more rapidly or to have a series of delayed-phase "jumps." These jumps tend to occur when sleep onset approaches 8:00 to 10:00 AM; sleep onset rarely occurs between 10:00 AM and 4 PM (see **Fig. 1**B and C).

Such phase jumps occur in about half of patients who have N24HSWS (54%) and result in a longer observed sleep–wake period on average (26.1 ± 0.8 hours) than observed in those who do not exhibit such changes (24.9 ± 0.5 hours). The non-uniform distribution of the sleep–wake behavior and the fact that sleep tends to become more abnormal when it coincides with the light phase of the day suggests that the free-running sleep/wake cycle of these patients is influenced by the timing of the light/dark cycle. As discussed later, several experimental protocols provide support for this conclusion. Rapid changes in the phase of the sleep/wake cycle also are observed in some totally blind subjects who have N24HSWS, however, suggesting a potential role for nonphotic or social cues in altering sleep–wake behavior in these patients.

N24HSWS and delayed sleep phase disorder (DSPD) may share a common pathology, and persistent sleep phase delay may increase the risk of the occurrence of N24HSWS.[21,36] For example, Oren and Wehr[21] reported that two patients who had DSPD had developed N24HSWS after chronotherapy in which their sleep phase was scheduled to be delayed by 3 to 4 hours in an attempt to obtain the desired sleep phase, suggesting that, in patients who have DSPD, an enforced sleep-phase delay may trigger N24HSWS. A review of previous studies (see **Table 1**) shows that persistent sleep-phase delay preceded the symptoms of N24HSWS in 5 of 39 sighted patients (13%). In the study by Hayakawa and colleagues,[6] 26% of the patients had suffered from a persistent sleep-phase delay, which was diagnosed as DSPD, before the onset of N24HSWS. Delayed sleep phase, even in the absence of DSPD, is highly prevalent in adolescents and young adults,[37] which is consistent with the typical age of onset of N24HSWS. As discussed in more detail later, the interaction between environmental light exposure and internal circadian time may contribute to a common pathway underlying both disorders.

Circadian Rhythm Features

Repeated assessments of strongly endogenous circadian rhythms (eg, melatonin, cortisol, core body temperature [BT]) to assess the internal circadian phase or period are rarely performed clinically but may offer a great deal of insight into the origin of the disorder and the optimal timing of potential treatment options. When measured, these rhythms tend to exhibit an observed non–24-hour period approximately parallel, although not identical, to the sleep–wake period. The phase angle between the circadian system and the sleep/wake cycle (ie, the timing of sleep relative to internal circadian phase) may be altered in these patients. For example, the authors' previous studies revealed that sleep timing was delayed relative to the melatonin or core BT rhythm in patients who had N24HSWS, as compared with healthy controls.[38,39] Phase-angle disorders probably contribute to the inappropriate light exposure that may underlie the development of N24HSWS in some patients and may affect other behaviors, such as mood and performance.

Psychiatric Features

There have been several reports of sighted patients who had N24HSWS preceded by schizophrenia, bipolar disorder, depression, obsessive-compulsive disorder, or schizoid personality (see **Table 1**). Of the total cohort in the series of sighted patients studied by Hayakawa and colleagues,[6] 28% had developed psychiatric problems before the onset of N24HSWS. Kokkoris and colleagues[9] reported on a patient in whom onset of N24HSWS was preceded by development of a schizoid-like personality and postulated that this patient's non-entrained sleep–wake pattern was the result of either a primary defect in the mechanism

underlying entrainment or weakened social zeitgebers resulting from the behavioral problems of the personality disorder. Tagaya and colleagues[22] and Wulff and colleagues[40] also have described schizophrenic patients who had N24HSWS. Although it is possible that a major defect that prevents circadian entrainment may underlie the sleep disorder, it is more likely in the majority of cases that exposure to inappropriate light/dark cycles induces the non-entrained sleep cycle. Psychiatric disorders and associated medications may induce social withdrawal, behavioral problems, or altered sleep behavior that in turn reduce patients' daytime activities and deprive them of appropriate exposure to sunlight, and/or expose them to unusual artificial light–dark patterns. As discussed later, self-selected exposure to light can induce a non–24-hour sleep–wake pattern even in healthy subjects.

By contrast, there are indications that N24HSWS may predispose patients to develop psychiatric disorders. In the Hayakawa series,[6] of the patients who had no psychiatric problems before the onset of N24HSWS, 14 (34%) developed major depression thereafter. In five of these patients, the symptoms of depression were exacerbated when they slept during the daytime and were ameliorated slightly when they slept during the night. This observation suggests that desynchronization between the environmental light/dark cycle and the endogenous circadian phase may increase the risk of developing depression in vulnerable patients.[6] Although reports have indicated that depression is a common psychopathology associated with DSPS,[41–43] no reports have described the relationship between N24HSWS and depression systematically. Phase-angle disorders, such as those observed in patients who have N24HSWS,[38,39] have been associated with a number of depressive disorders[44–46] and can determine the time course of mood in healthy, nondepressed subjects.[46–48] The delay of sleep timing relative to the circadian pacemaker may be an etiologic factor of both N24HSWS[38,39] and the depression that can be associated with N24HSWS,[44] and the correction of the delay of sleep timing may be important for long-term treatment of both symptoms.[44]

CLINICAL CHARACTERISTICS OF NON–24-HOUR SLEEP–WAKE SYNDROME IN BLIND PATIENTS

Given the central role of light in entraining the circadian pacemaker to the 24-hour day, it is not surprising that those individuals who cannot detect light experience problems in maintaining entrainment, and sleep and other rhythm disorders

Table 1
Published reports of sighted patients who have non–24-hour sleep–wake syndrome

Author	Year	No.	Sex	Age at First Visit (Years)	Age, at Onset (Years)	Occupational Status at First Visit	Period of Sleep–Wake Cycle (Hours)	Premorbid Psychiatric Problems	Premorbid Sleep Disorder
Eliott	1970	1	M	NA	NA	NA	26		
Kokkoris	1978	1	M	34	26	Unemployed	24.8	Schizoid personality	
Weber	1980	1	M	28	24	College student	25.6		
Kamgar-Parsi	1983	1	M	32	22	Unemployed	25.1		DSPS
Wollman	1986	1	M	26	22	Student	27.4		
Sugita	1987	1	M	25	23	Student	25		
Eastman	1988	1	M	26	High school	NA	25		
Hoban	1989	1	F	40	NA	Artist	25.1		
Moriya	1990	1	M	16	15	Student	24.5–25.0		
Sasaki	1990	1	F	22	21	NA	NA	Bipolar affective disorder	
Ohta	1991	1	M	17	15	Student	24.6		
Oren	1992	2	M	22,28	NA	NA	NA		DSPS
Tagaya	1993	1	M	20	18	Unemployed	25.3	Schizophrenia	
Emens	1994	1	M	31	22	NA	25.2		
Tomoda	1994	1	M	18	17	Student	25		
McArthur	1996	1	M	41	41	Computer programmer	25.1	Depression, social phobia	DSPS

Study	Year	No.	Sex			Occupation		Comorbidity	
Uchiyama	1996	1	M	30	18	Designer	27.2		
Yamadera	1996	13	10M	23.2[a]	19.8[a]	54% students, 23% unemployed, 15% employed, 8% part-time work	NA		DSPS
Nakamura	1997	1	M	26	NA	Student	NA		
Shibui	1998	1	M	43	41	Local government official	25.8		
Hashimoto	1998	1	M	26	26	Student	NA		
Hayakawa	1998	1	M	20	16	Student	25		
Akaboshi	2000	1	M	5	4	Kindergarten	24.9	Mental retardation	
Watanabe	2000	1	M	17	17	NA	NA		
Morinobnu	2002	1	M	22	20	NA	NA	OCD	
Boivin	2003	1	F	39	32	NA	NA		
Hayakawa	2005	57	41M	M 26.3, F 25.8[a]	20.2[a]	35% students, 39% unemployed, 21% employed, 5% part-time work	24.9[a]	28% psychiatric problems, 2% physical problems	26% DSPS

Abbreviations: DSPS, delayed sleep-phase syndrome; NA, not available; OCD, obsessive-compulsive disorders.
[a] Mean.
From Hayakawa T, Uchiyama M, Kamei Y, et al. Clinical analyses of sighted patients with non-24-h sleep–wake syndrome: a study of 57 consecutively diagnosed cases. Sleep. 2005;28(8):949; with permission.

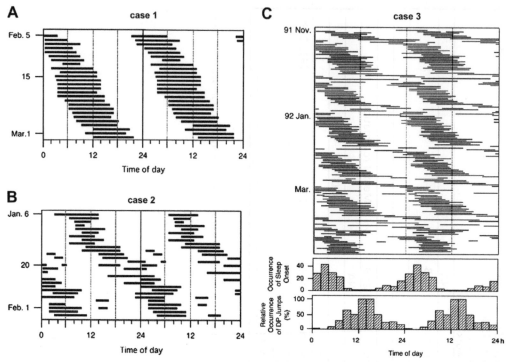

Fig. 1. Non–24-hour sleep–wake syndrome in three sighted patients: (*A*) a 26-year-old woman (case 1), (*B*) a 22-year-old man (case 2), and (*C*) a 30-year-old man (case 3). Sleep episodes (*horizontal black bars*) are double-plotted for clarity according to time of day (abscissa) and study day (ordinate). Case 1 clearly exhibits a non–24-hour sleep rhythm (24.8 hours) that remains relatively consistent. Case 2 also exhibits a non–24-hour sleep rhythm of 24.7 hours on average, although the rhythm becomes more disrupted for about a week in the middle of the data sequence. (*From* Hayakawa T, Uchiyama M, Kamei Y, et al. Clinical analyses of sighted patients with non-24-h sleep–wake syndrome: a study of 57 consecutively diagnosed cases. Sleep 2005;28:948; with permission.) This change in rhythmicity is illustrated more clearly in case 3, who has episodes of regularly free-running sleep (24.6 hours) interspersed regularly (∼ every 4 weeks) with episodes in which the sleep pattern delays more quickly and becomes more disrupted. These phase jumps in the sleep/wake cycle are characteristic of early studies of subjects living in temporal isolation but with access to artificial light (eg, in caves and laboratory experiments) and probably are caused when light exposure occurs at a particular phase of the circadian cycle (see **Fig. 5** and text). Even under this non-entrained condition, the sleep onset occurs most often during the night (case 3, *middle panel*), reflecting the fact that the patient generally attempts to live on a 24-hour social day. The rapid delay in sleep–wake timing (delay phase [DP] jumps) also occurs at a particular circadian phase (case 3, *bottom panel*; see text). (*From* Uchiyama M, Okawa M, Ozaki S, et al. Delayed phase jumps of sleep onset in a patient with non-24-hour sleep-wake syndrome. Sleep 1996:19:638; with permission.)

have been recognized in the blind for more than 60 years.[7] Recent studies show that more than half of those who have no perception of light exhibit nonentrained circadian rhythms of melatonin, cortisol, or temperature.[7,49–51] Many of these patients, but not all, also exhibit non–24-hour sleep–wake rhythms.[52] Although the exact prevalence of N24HSWS diagnosed without additional information on other rhythmic variables is unknown, N24HSWS is likely to afflict between one third and two thirds of the totally blind population. Of the remaining totally blind patients who do not exhibit sleep–wake or other circadian rhythm disorders, most are entrained to the 24-hour social day (not to the 24-hour light/dark cycle) via nonphotic time cues including strict scheduling of

activities, exercise, mealtimes, and social interaction.[50,53,54] In a small proportion of cases (∼ 5%), patients may retain circadian photoreception in the absence of visual function.[55–57] Non–24-hour sleep–wake disorder is rare in visually impaired patients who retain at least minimal light perception; only a handful of such cases have been reported.[7]

Clinical Features

The clinical characteristics of blind patients who have N24HSWS have not been elucidated formally. Most of the reported cases are male,[50,51,58] although this finding may represent subject selection and not a true gender distinction. Onset can occur at any age, from birth onwards,[50,59,60] and usually coincides with or follows shortly after loss of light perception or loss or removal of the eyes.[50] There may be age-related differences in recognizing a cyclical sleep–wake complaint and reporting N24HSWS, however, so that middle-aged adults may tend to recognize the sleep complaint more readily than younger adults.

The type of blindness does not seem to be related to the risk of N24HSWS. Complete loss of visual and circadian photoreceptive function caused by any ocular disorder will abolish light–dark input to the circadian pacemaker and prevent entrainment to the light/dark cycle. A small proportion of totally visually blind subjects can remain entrained to the 24-hour light/dark cycle if they retain functional non-rod, non-cone "nonvisual" photoreception.[55–57] Recent work has shown that light detection for circadian entrainment is mediated primarily by a novel non-rod, non-cone photoreceptor system located in a small number (< 3%) of retinal ganglion cells. These cells are intrinsically photosensitive and are functionally and anatomically distinct from the traditional rod and cone visual photoreceptors in the outer retina (for reviews, see[61,62]). Disruption of rod and cone function that leaves the ganglion cell layer intact can permit continued light detection for entrainment of the circadian system in the absence of any measurable visual responses and does not result in cyclic sleep–wake disorders.[55,57] Eye disorders that damage the ganglion cell layer (eg, glaucoma) or the optic nerve or removal of the eye entirely (eg, retinoblastoma, trauma) probably will prevent circadian entrainment and increase the likelihood of N24HSWS.[7,50,51]

Sleep Features

The main sleep features are similar in sighted and blind patients who have N24HSWS, namely a cyclic non–24-hours sleep–wake pattern when measured over several weeks or months, usually with episodes of relatively good sleep followed by episodes of poor nighttime sleep and excessive daytime napping and sleepiness, followed by a return to good sleep, ad infinitum.[52] The cyclic nature of the sleep disorder results from the patient's attempt to live on a 24-hour social day while the patient's internal circadian system runs on its non–24-hour intrinsic period. The two rhythms run in and out of synchrony with each other so that sleep is relatively good when the internal circadian rhythm of sleepiness coincides with the social night. When the internal circadian rhythm of sleepiness occurs in the social day, poor nighttime sleep and high levels of daytime

sleepiness phase ensue. If the patient lived on a non–24-hour day equal to the internal circadian period, a sleep disorder would not be apparent (**Fig. 2**C, B).

The longitudinal polysomnographic measurements required to observe the cyclic nature of the disruptions to sleep structure typically also have not been performed in totally blind patients. One case study[63] has quantified detailed changes in sleep structure and showed changes consistent with laboratory studies of sleep in healthy sighted subjects at different circadian phases.[35,64] Single-night recordings in some non-entrained totally blind subjects also show changes in sleep structure consistent with their sleeping at an adverse circadian phase,[58,65] although single-night polysomnographic measures are difficult to interpret without additional longitudinal assessments.

When assessed over many weeks or months, the cyclic nature of the sleep disturbance is easier to detect.[52,66] **Fig. 2**A and B shows representative examples of self-reported sleep–wake records in two totally blind patients who have N24HSWS, a 66-year-old man (see case 1, see **Fig. 2**A), and a 35-year-old man (see case 2, see **Fig. 2**B). Cases 1 and 2 had a non-entrained rhythm of 24.68 hours in urinary 6-sulphatoxymelatonin, the major urinary metabolite of melatonin (*open circles* in **Fig. 2**A and B; Subjects 20 and 31, respectively[50]). Their average duration nighttime sleep (6.2 and 5.8 hours, respectively) and total sleep time per 24 hours (7.2 and 6.3 hours, respectively) are typical of blind patients who have N24HSWS and are reduced compared with blind subjects who have normally phased circadian rhythms.[52]

Case 3 (see **Fig. 2**C) represents the first detailed case report of non–24-hour sleep–wake disorder in a blind subject[66] and shows a 28-year-old man who had a 24.9-hour rhythm in sleep, plasma cortisol, and other parameters.[66] The 24.9-hour sleep rhythm is observed clearly when the subject is living freely (see **Fig. 2**C, B) but changes (as seen in cases 1 and 2) when the subject attempts to live on a social 24-hour day (see **Fig. 2**C), with the characteristic changes in nighttime and daytime sleep described earlier.[52] Clear relative coordination of the sleep–wake pattern occurs as the 24-hour social schedule cycles in and out of phase with the internal non–24-hour circadian system.

Fig. 3 shows these rhythmic changes in more detail in a number of subjective sleep parameters and peak activity time.[52,67] Nighttime sleep usually is attempted at a normal social time, and sleep onset and offset times occur across a relatively narrow range (up to 3 hours). Nighttime sleep and daytime nap duration vary reciprocally according the circadian phase at which nighttime

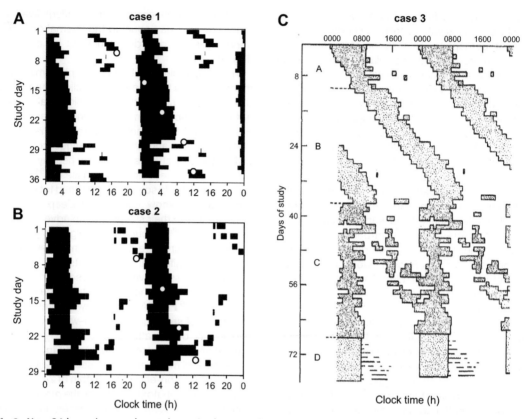

Fig. 2. Non–24-hour sleep–wake syndrome in three totally blind patients, plotted as in **Fig. 1**. The peak time of the urinary 6-sulphatoxymelatonin rhythm, collected each week, is also plotted (*open circles*). (*A*) Case 1 is a 66-year-old man who is totally blind because of ocular trauma. He has one eye and no conscious light perception. He exhibits a non–24-hour sleep/wake cycle and a melatonin rhythm with a period (τ) of 24.68 hours. (*B*) Case 2 is a 35-year-old bilaterally enucleated male (retinoblastoma) who also has a 24.68-hour melatonin rhythm and non–24-hour sleep–wake disorder. Both patients exhibit the characteristic recurrent episodes of disturbed nighttime sleep and many daytime naps when nighttime sleep is attempted at an adverse circadian phase (ie, when melatonin peaks during the day; eg, days 1–8 and 28–35 for case 1). This pattern alternates with episodes of good sleep at night when the circadian phase coincides with nighttime melatonin production (eg, days 10–25 in case 1). (*From* Lockley SW. Sleep, melatonin and other circadian rhythms in the blind [PhD thesis]. Guildford (UK): University of Surrey; 1997. p. 16–31; with permission.) (*C*) Case 3 shows the sleep–wake pattern of a 28-year-old man who lost his light perception at birth because of retinopathy of prematurity (retrolental fibroplasia). Sections A and C represent his sleep while living freely at home, and section B shows sleep during an ad lib inpatient study when the subject was free to sleep as he pleased. During section D, an unsuccessful attempt was made to entrain his cycle via strict 24-hour scheduling of sleep, meals, and activity. While living freely in the laboratory (*B*), his sleep–wake, plasma cortisol, alertness, performance, and urinary electrolyte rhythms all exhibited a circadian period of 24.9 hours. This rhythm persisted when living at home (*C*) but was modulated by attempting to live on a social 24-hour day, as in cases 1 and 2. (*From* Miles LE, Raynal DM, Wilson MA. Blind man living in normal society has circadian rhythms of 24.9 hours. Science 1977;198(4315):422; with permission.)

sleep is attempted. When nighttime sleep coincides with the peak production of melatonin at night (*open bar*), nighttime duration is maximal, and daytime naps are minimal. This situation is reversed when nighttime sleep is attempted when melatonin production occurs during the social day. The melatonin rhythm can be considered a marker of the biologic night or the time at which the circadian drive for sleepiness is maximal. When sleep occurs outside this time,

sleep duration, timing, and quality are impaired, and patients experience daytime dysfunction in their sleepiness, mood, and performance.[68]

Circadian Rhythm Features

As illustrated previously, non–24-hour circadian rhythm disorders in the blind have tended to be confirmed from circadian markers other than sleep, such as melatonin, cortisol, or temperature

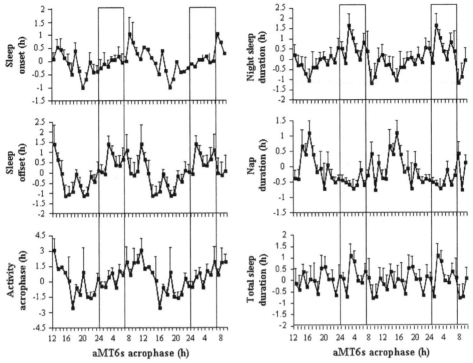

Fig. 3. Cyclic sleep–wake disturbances in totally blind subjects who have non–24-hour sleep–wake syndrome. **Fig. 3** shows the mean (± SEM) sleep parameters for six non-entrained totally blind subjects and the peak in daily activity for four subjects in relation to their urinary 6-sulphatoxymelatonin (aMT6s) peak, or acrophase, time. Data are plotted twice for clarity and are expressed relative to each subject's own mean. The open bars represent the range (mean ± 2 SD) of aMT6s peak times for normally entrained subjects (n = 80, English and Arendt, unpublished results) to illustrate when the circadian melatonin rhythm, a marker of the circadian rhythm in sleep propensity, is occurring at a normal phase, during the night. Most totally blind subjects who have N24HSWS attempt to sleep at night on a normal 24-hour social schedule while their internal circadian system "free-runs" on a non–24-hour day (see text and **Fig. 2**). Consequently, their nighttime sleep episodes vary in timing and duration, depending on the circadian phase at which sleep occurs (here represented by the melatonin rhythm). When the melatonin peak occurs at a relatively early social time (approximately before midnight), sleep onset, offset, and activity peak occur relatively early (*left panels*). As the melatonin rhythm delays progressively, sleep and activity timing also get later and later until the melatonin peak passes into late morning (8:00–12:00). As the melatonin rhythm continues to delay around the clock, the sleep "catches up" at the other end of the day and becomes relatively advanced again (see **Fig. 2**). Similarly, when sleep timing coincides with a normal nighttime melatonin phase (*open bar*), nighttime sleep is maximal in duration, and daytime naps are minimal (*right panels*). When the melatonin rhythm peaks in the day, nighttime sleep duration is reduced, and the incidence and duration of daytime naps are enhanced. (*From* Lockley SW, Skene DJ, Butler LJ, et al. Sleep and activity rhythms are related to circadian phase in the blind. Sleep 1999;22(5):621; with permission.)

rhythms.[7,49–51,69] Collectively, these studies show that circadian rhythms in totally blind subjects can be categorized into four main groups: normal circadian phase, advanced phase, delayed phase, and non-entrained rhythms. Of these, non-entrained subjects are the largest group, representing 50% to 60% of totally blind patients; individual circadian periods range from 23.8 to 25.1 hours. The remainder is divided approximately equally between normal and abnormally phased (advanced or delayed) rhythms. It is possible that some of these subjects are misclassified and actually represent non-entrained

rhythms with a period very close to, and therefore difficult to distinguish from, 24 hours.[55] As discussed earlier, some totally visually blind patients do remain entrained to 24 hours via either nonphotic time cues or intact circadian photoreception.

Given the social restraints on the sleep–wake pattern, the free-running sleep rhythm often is not observed as readily as other non-sleep rhythms.[52] The free-running period of the sleep/wake cycle usually is shorter than that of the hormonal rhythms, if apparent at all. For example, of 16 totally blind subjects who had non-entrained melatonin rhythms (range 24.1–24.8 hours), only 7 had non–24-hour activity rhythms, and only 5 had non–24-hour sleep rhythms (< 24.3 hours) (see **Fig. 1** in Ref[52]). Similarly, a quarter of these patients did not complain of sleep disturbance (as assessed using the Pittsburgh Sleep Quality Index[50]). This apparent inconsistency may occur for several reasons. Most people do not sleep precisely according to their circadian phase, given strong social cues to do otherwise (eg, school, work, family commitments, and other influences) and often use stimulants to overcome this nonoptimal sleep, as illustrated by the widespread use of caffeine. Blind patients who have a short circadian period change their internal circadian phase by only a few minutes per day and may not recognize minor changes to sleep as part of a cyclic sleep disorder. For example, a patient who has a circadian period of 24.1 hours has a 6-minute internal change per day, which may be relatively easy to overcome in the short term. Because it takes a very long number of days to complete a full circadian cycle and free run around-the-clock (121 days, or 4 months, if the circadian period is 24.1 hours), neither patient nor physician would recognize the sleep disorder as cyclic, and the problem might be misdiagnosed as insomnia because of the poor sleep when the patient's circadian period is maximally out of phase with the social day. A patient who has a period of 24.67 hours, however, would have a shift of 40 minutes per day in internal time and a much more noticeable change in the ability to sleep (ie, thirty-five days would be required to complete one circadian cycle.) These patients often recognize that their sleep changes from day to day in a predictable manner and are easier to diagnose as having non–24-hour sleep–wake disorder. Even without a sleep complaint, patients who have non–24-hour circadian rhythms may exhibit cyclic sleep–wake patterns and may benefit from treatment to improve both their sleep and their daytime functioning. These data illustrate the importance of assessing markers in addition to sleep to diagnose non–24-hour sleep–wake disorder correctly. It is not known if there are sighted subjects who also have a similar phenotype, namely a free-running internal pacemaker but a nearly normal sleep/wake cycle. Such subjects would be unlikely to seek treatment and presumably would be relatively rare.

Psychiatric Features

The detailed reports of circadian rhythm sleep disorders in blind patients have excluded those who had psychiatric disorders before study. Therefore little is known about the psychiatric features of blind patients who have N24HSWS. Noncyclic sleep disorders are common in visually impaired patients[70–72] and have been suggested to be caused at least in part by concomitant psychiatric disorders.[72]

BIOLOGIC BASIS AND PATHOGENESIS OF NON–24-HOUR SLEEP–WAKE SYNDROME

N24HSWS occurs because the internal circadian pacemaker and sleep/wake cycle do not remain entrained with the 24-hour light/dark cycle. In totally blind patients, the reason for lack of entrainment to the light/dark cycle is clear. In sighted patients who have N24HSWS, the exact mechanisms responsible for this desynchrony are unknown but probably are multiple in origin. In particular, an abnormal interaction between the endogenous circadian rhythm and the sleep homeostatic process that regulates sleep and wakefulness plays an essential role in the pathophysiology of N24HSWS.[5,73] The biologic factors possibly related to the pathogenesis of N24HSWS are reviewed briefly in the next sections.

Phase-Angle Difference Between the Circadian Pacemaker and Sleep/Wake Cycle

Under normal conditions, most people tend to go to sleep at a particular circadian phase that corresponds to the rising part of the melatonin rhythm and the falling limb of the core BT cycle. If the core BT minimum, or trough, is used as a nominal circadian phase marker, most people tend to initiate sleep onset approximately 4 to 6 hours before and wake 2 to 3 hours after the BT minimum (**Fig. 4**). Under conditions of temporal isolation, but with self-timed access to light, subjects tend to initiate sleep at a later circadian phase, closer to their BT minimum.[4,64] The BT minimum happens to coincide with a particularly sensitive part of the circadian cycle, namely the phase at which light switches from causing a phase delay of the circadian pacemaker (shifting to a later time) to causing a phase advance (shifting to an earlier time). The magnitude and direction of the phase-resetting effects of light are described more fully by several phase-response curves (PRCs).[74–77] By initiating sleep at a later circadian phase, individuals 'expose' more of their PRC to the delaying effects of light and reduce exposure at a time when advances would occur when they close their eyes to sleep or switch off the light, resulting in a net daily phase delay.[5,38,78] Under these conditions, subjects exhibit a long circadian "period", often 25 hours or more, as a result of the daily net delays caused by the self-selected exposure

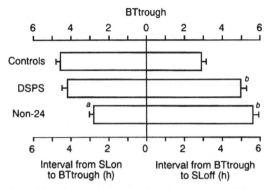

Fig. 4. The phase relationship between sleep and circadian phase in circadian rhythm sleep disorders. **Fig. 4** shows the intervals from sleep onset to BT trough and from BT trough to sleep offset in control subjects, patients who have delayed sleep phase syndrome (DSPS), and patients who have non–24-hour sleep–wake syndrome (N24HSWS). The time interval from sleep onset (SLon) to BT trough is significantly shorter and the time from BT trough to sleep offset (SLoff) is significantly longer in the patients who have N24HSWS than in the controls or in patients who have DSPS, so that patients who have N24HSWS go to sleep and wake later in their circadian cycle. This abnormal phase relationship between the sleep and circadian rhythms exposes patients who have N24HSWS to more light at a time that will cause a phase delay in their circadian pacemaker and reduces light exposure at a time that would cause a corrective phase advance. (*From* Uchiyama M, Okawa M, Shibui K, et al. Altered phase relation between sleep timing and core body temperature rhythm in delayed sleep phase syndrome and non-24-h sleep–wake syndrome in humans. Neurosci Lett 2000;294:103; with permission.)

a common basis between what happens to humans under temporal isolation and the pathophysiology of these circadian rhythm disorders. By sleeping at a relatively late circadian phase and for a relatively long duration,[38] patients both expose themselves to light and avoid light at times that causes a net phase delay each day, inducing a non–24-hour sleep/wake cycle. The underlying cause of this late sleep time may be an inherent internal desynchronization between the sleep–wake homeostat and the circadian system,[73,78] and preliminary studies suggest that patients who have N24HSWS may have difficulty in elevating homeostatic sleep pressure.[39,80] A more likely cause of the disorder is a change in behavior whereby patients choose to sleep later in their circadian cycle and induce a systematic phase delay. This explanation also may account for the observation that DSPD often precedes N24HSWS and that a DSPD-like sleep pattern and a N24HSWS-like sleep pattern can be observed in the same patient.[6] Consistent with this hypothesis, Emens and colleagues[23] reported that a sighted patient suffering from N24HSWS with a sleep/wake cycle of 25.17 hours under a normal 24-hour day–night condition displayed a core BT rhythm of 24.5 hours under a forced desynchrony protocol, suggesting that self-selected access to light artificially lengthened his observed circadian period. The association between N24HSWS and psychiatric disorders further supports the idea that unusual behavior may initiate and then drive the development of N24HSWS.

to light. The resulting sleep–wake pattern is very similar to that exhibited by sighted patients who have N24HSWS, including a long non–24-hour circadian period and recurrent phase delay jumps and long sleep episodes when the sleep timing is initiated at a particular circadian phase (**Fig. 5,** *middle panel*).[78] When subjects are studied in an environment free of time cues but with light–dark exposure scheduled to a 20- or 28-hour day, the circadian period observed is much closer to 24 hours (on average 24.2 hours) (see **Fig. 5**) and probably represents more accurately the intrinsic period of the circadian pacemaker.[78]

Detailed studies of the timing of sleep relative to the BT minimum or melatonin rhythm in patients who have DSPS and N24HSWS[5,6,38,39,79] show that these patients also tend to initiate sleep at a later circadian phase than normal controls and that patients who have N24HSWS initiate sleep later than patients who have DSPS[38] (see **Fig. 4**). The timing of the sleep behavior may indicate

Reduced Circadian Phase Resetting Response to Light

Although the circadian-resetting effect of light is abolished in totally blind patients who have N24HSWS, sighted subjects in theory may suffer from an impaired response to light resetting that prevents appropriate entrainment with the light/dark cycle. A blunted response to a light-induced melatonin suppression test as a proxy marker for sensitivity to circadian light responses has been reported in two single-case studies,[25,27] but an attenuated phase-shifting response has not been confirmed. Differences in individual PRCs, such as a reduced sensitivity in the phase-advancing portion of the PRC, also hypothetically could underlie the disorder, as could impairments in circadian photoreception (eg, melanopsin dysfunction) in the presence of normal vision, although there are no reports of such patients in the literature.

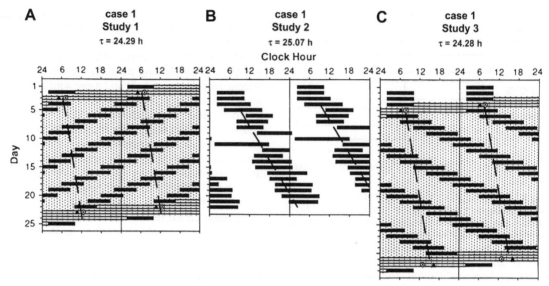

Fig. 5. Effect of self-selected light exposure on circadian period. The timing of the circadian system was studied in a single subject under three different laboratory conditions. In (*A*) study 1 and (*C*) study 3, the subject was scheduled to live on a 20-hour sleep–wake/light–dark cycle (study 1) or a 28-hour sleep–wake/light–dark cycle (study 3), with sleep permitted only for one third of each "day" (*horizontal black bars*). During scheduled wake times, light was kept relatively dim (< 15 lux). These forced desynchrony protocols are outside the limits of entrainment for the circadian pacemaker, and the clock reverts to its endogenous period, as illustrated by the fact that the circadian system has the same period (τ = 24.28, *dashed line*) for the BT rhythm under both the 20- and 28-hour protocols. (*B*) In study 2, when the same subject was allowed to live freely and to choose when to sleep and when to switch on normal room lights (150 lux), the BT rhythm had a longer period (τ = 25.07 h; *dashed line*), and the pattern of the sleep episodes (*horizontal black bars*) resembled that of patients who have non–24-hour sleep–wake syndrome (see **Fig. 1**). The sleep/wake cycle free ran with a long period (27.07 hours) and had characteristic phase jumps as the sleep-onset time approached the morning hours. The gradual change in the timing of sleep relative to the BT minimum (*dashed line*) is clear, with sleep onset occurring closer and closer to the BT minimum. Light exposure before the BT minimum causes a phase delay of the circadian pacemaker (see text) and progressively delays the circadian pacemaker, inducing the non–24-hour sleep–wake disorder. (*From* Czeisler CA, Duffy JF, Shanahan TL, et al. Stability, precision, and near-24-hour period of the human circadian pacemaker. Science 1999;284(5423):2178; with permission.)

Longer Endogenous Circadian Period

In animal studies, mutations of core clock genes that cause expression of an abnormally long or short endogenous circadian period have been shown to be responsible for the alteration of the phase angle between the rest/activity cycle and the 24-hour environmental light/dark cycle.[81,82] No such evidence has been reported for similar intrinsic period abnormalities in humans, nor have there been any observations of sleep–wake problems during the early development in these patients that would be an expected consequence of a congenital abnormality.[6] A number of reports have associated mutations and polymorphisms in circadian clock genes with advanced and delayed sleep phase disorder (reviewed in[83]), including a relatively short circadian period in a woman who had severe advanced sleep phase disorder,[84] but as yet no reports have associated such changes in circadian clock genes with N24HSWS.

TREATMENT STRATEGIES OF NON–24-HOUR SLEEP–WAKE SYNDROME

Therapeutic interventions for N24HSWS should be targeted at entraining the patient's circadian pacemaker at an appropriate phase relative to the environmental light/dark cycle. Although clinical trials to reset the phase of the circadian pacemaker using light exposure or administration of melatonin and its analogues have been reported in healthy subjects and some patient groups, there have been no large-scale controlled trials for treating N24HSWS. At this time treatment options therefore are based largely on case studies.

Light Therapy

In humans and other mammals, appropriately timed exposure to light can reset the phase of circadian rhythms.[74–77] As reviewed earlier, the PRC phase most sensitive to light usually

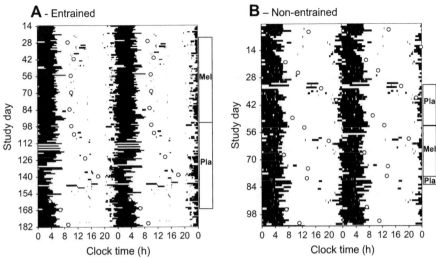

Fig. 6. Melatonin treatment of non–24-hour sleep–wake syndrome in the blind. **Fig. 6** shows the double-plotted sleep timing (*horizontal black bars*) and urinary cortisol peak times (*open circles*) for two totally blind men treated with 5 mg fast-release melatonin administered orally at 21:00 hours for at least one circadian cycle. Sequential study days are plotted on the ordinate, and clock time is quadruple-plotted on the abscissa. The study had a placebo-controlled, single-blind design,[91] and the start and end of placebo (Pla) and melatonin (Mel) treatment are indicated by the adjacent boxes. (*A*) A subject (S17) who was entrained by melatonin treatment exhibited a non-entrained cortisol rhythm (24.3 hours) during placebo treatment but was entrained at a normal circadian phase by the melatonin treatment (mean ± SD cortisol peak time = 9.9 ± 0.7 hours). The entrained sleep/wake cycle observed during melatonin treatment becomes disrupted immediately upon cessation of treatment and reverts to the characteristic non–24-hour cyclic pattern. (*B*) This subject (S45) failed to entrain to 5-mg melatonin treatment despite receiving treatment for nearly two full circadian cycles. The persistent cyclic non–24-hour sleep–wake disorder is clearly apparent throughout both the placebo and melatonin treatment. (*From* Lockley SW, Arendt J, Skene DJ. Visual impairment and circadian rhythm disorders. Dialogs Clin Neurosci. 2007;9(3):310; with permission.)

coincides with the last half of the sleep episode, and therefore the timing of the sleep itself is a major determinant of light input to the pacemaker. If self-selected light exposure is the underlying cause of the disorder, behavioral therapy aimed at correcting unusual sleep–wake behavior may be useful. Direct light therapy for N24HSWS has been used in a number of cases with the aim of inducing a phase advance of the circadian pacemaker to counteract the typical phase delay observed.[13,17,30,32] The initial timing of light therapy relative to the patient's internal circadian pacemaker may be key in ensuring that the light therapy does not exacerbate the adverse circadian phase by causing a phase shift opposite to that required. Light exposure timed to advance the clock should start after the BT minimum, and light should be avoided before BT minimum to reduce phase-delaying effects. Clinical measurement of circadian phase for diagnosis or treatment timing is rarely performed but can be achieved relatively simply using home-based assessments of salivary or urinary melatonin timing or its metabolites.[50,85,86] In the absence of circadian phase information, having

the patient maintain a fixed rise time and perform morning light therapy at the same time for several weeks, so that the light therapy eventually is applied during the phase-advance portion of the PRC, may be successful.

Melatonin Treatment

Appropriately timed melatonin also can phase shift the human circadian pacemaker, with the pattern of the melatonin PRC broadly opposite to that of light. Under normally entrained conditions, melatonin induces a phase advance when administered in the early evening and a phase delay when administered in the early morning.[87] In addition to its ability to shift the circadian pacemaker, melatonin also has sleepiness-inducing properties,[88] and the timing of administration should take this effect into account. Sighted patients who have N24HSWS have been treated successfully in open-label studies of melatonin therapy,[25,30,89] although no controlled clinical trials have been published. As with light therapy, prior knowledge of circadian phase is important to time treatment appropriately. To phase advance the internal pacemaker optimally, melatonin treatment should be administered at or before the onset of the rise in melatonin production (the "dim light melatonin onset"[85,86]). Without prior knowledge of circadian phase, maintaining melatonin treatment at a fixed time in the early evening for several weeks may provide some benefit.

Melatonin treatment for N24HSWS has been studied more extensively in blind patients and remains the most promising therapeutic strategy in this population.[7] Although the soporific properties of melatonin have been shown to stabilize the sleep/wake cycle in blind patients without entraining the circadian pacemaker,[90] entrainment of the circadian pacemaker, and therefore the sleep rhythm, is necessary to treat N24HSWS fully. After the initial demonstrations that a 5-mg[91] or 10-mg[65] dose of melatonin could entrain circadian rhythms in the blind, several studies have shown that lower doses (≤ 0.5 mg) seem to be equally as effective in entraining the clock,[92,93] if not more so, perhaps by providing a more discreet temporal signal than higher doses. Because of melatonin's soporific properties, treatment should be administered at the same time each day close to the desired bedtime to ensure the alignment of the circadian and social day. Regarding the circadian time of administration, although low doses (≤ 0.5 mg) initiated at any circadian phase eventually will cause entrainment of the circadian pacemaker,[92–95] there may be a lag in experiencing beneficial effects until the time of administration coincides with the phase-advance part of the PRC. If treatment can be timed initially to induce a phase advance, entrainment should occur within a few days, and the patient will perceive immediate benefit (**Fig. 6**). The individual's circadian period also may affect the likelihood of entrainment with melatonin,[96] because patients who have periods furthest from 24 hours may be outside the range of entrainment for this relatively weak time cue. Long-term safety data are not available for melatonin, although research studies suggest that it is a relatively safe drug in most patient groups.[97,98]

In summary, more detailed assessments of sleep and circadian rhythms in N24HSWS, under both field and laboratory conditions, will improve the diagnosis and treatment of this disorder. Larger-scale clinical trials are required to establish the risk factors underlying N24HSWS and to establish formal treatment guidelines.

REFERENCES

1. American Academy of Sleep Medicine. International classification of sleep disorders: diagnostic and coding manual. 2nd edition. Westchester (IL): American Academy of Sleep Medicine; 2005.

2. Sack RL, Auckley D, Auger RR, et al. Circadian rhythm sleep disorders: part II, advanced sleep phase disorder, delayed sleep phase disorder, free-running disorder, and irregular sleep-wake rhythm. An American Academy of Sleep Medicine review. Sleep 2007;30(11):1484–501.

3. Moore-Ede MC, Czeisler CA, Richardson GS. Circadian time-keeping in health and disease. I. Basic properties of circadian pacemakers. N Engl J Med 1983;309:469–76.

4. Wever RA. The circadian system of man. In: Topics in environmental physiology and medicine. New York: Springer-Verlag; 1979.

5. Okawa M, Uchiyama M. Circadian rhythm sleep disorders: characteristics and entrainment pathology in delayed sleep phase and non-24-h sleep-wake syndrome. Sleep Med Rev 2007;11(6):485–96.

6. Hayakawa T, Uchiyama M, Kamei Y, et al. Clinical analyses of sighted patients with non-24-h sleep–wake syndrome: a study of 57 consecutively diagnosed cases. Sleep 2005;28:945–52.

7. Lockley SW, Arendt J, Skene DJ. Visual impairment and circadian rhythm disorders. Dialogues Clin Neurosci 2007;9(3):301–14.

8. Uchiyama M, Okawa M, Ozaki S, et al. Delayed phase jumps of sleep onset in a patient with non-24-hour sleep-wake syndrome. Sleep 1996;19: 637–40.

9. Kokkoris CP, Weitzman ED, Pollak CP, et al. Long-term ambulatory temperature monitoring in a subject with a hypernychthemeral sleep-wake cycle disturbance. Sleep 1978;1:177–90.

10. Weber AL, Cary MS, Connor N, et al. Human non-24-hour sleep-wake cycles in an everyday environment. Sleep 1980;2:347–54.

11. Kamgar-Parsi B, Wehr TA, Gillin JC. Successful treatment of human non-24-hour sleep-wake syndrome. Sleep 1983;6:257–64.

12. Wollman M, Lavie P. Hypernychthemeral sleep-wake cycle: some hidden regularities. Sleep 1986;9: 324–34.

13. Hoban TM, Sack RL, Lewy AJ, et al. Entrainment of a free-running human with bright light? Chronobiol Int 1989;6:347–53.

14. Okawa M, Uchiyama M, Shirakawa S, et al. Favourable effects of combined treatment with vitamin B12 and bright light for sleep-wake rhythm disorders. In: Kumar VM, Mallick Nayar U, editors. Sleep-wakefulness. New Delhi: Wiley Eastern Ltd; 1993. p. 71–7.

15. Eliott AL, Mills JN, Waterhouse JM. A man with too long a day. J Physiol 1970;212:30–1.

16. Sugita Y, Ishikawa H, Mikami A, et al. Successful treatment for a patient with hypernychthemeral syndrome. Sleep Res 1987;16:642.

17. Eastman CI, Anagnopoulos CA, Cartwright RD. Can bright light entrain a free-runner? Sleep Res 1988; 17:372.

18. Moriya Y, Yamazaki J, Higuchi T, et al. A case of non-24-hour sleep-wake syndrome. Jpn J Psychiatry Neurol 1990;44:189–90.

19. Sasaki T, Hashimoto O, Honda Y. A case of non-24-hour sleep-wake syndrome preceded by depressive state. Jpn J Psychiatry Neurol 1990;44:191–2.

20. Ohta T, Ando K, Iwata T, et al. Treatment of persistent sleep-wake schedule disorders in adolescents with methylcobalamin (vitamin B12). Sleep 1991;14:414–8.

21. Oren DA, Wehr TA. Hypernyctohemeral syndrome after chronotherapy for delayed sleep phase syndrome. N Engl J Med 1992;327:1762.

22. Tagaya H, Matsuno Y, Atsumi Y. A schizophrenic with non-24-hour sleep-wake syndrome. Jpn J Psychiatry Neurol 1993;47:441–2.

23. Emens JS, Brotman DJ, Czeisler CA. Evaluation of the intrinsic period of the circadian pacemaker in a patient with a non-24-hour sleep-wake schedule disorder. Sleep Res 1994;23:256.

24. Tomoda A, Miike T, Uezono K, et al. A school refusal case with biological rhythm disturbance and melatonin therapy. Brain Dev 1994;16:71–6.

25. McArthur AJ, Lewy AJ, Sack RL. Non 24 hour sleep-wake syndrome in a sighted man: circadian rhythm studies and efficacy of melatonin treatment. Sleep 1996;19:544–53.

26. Yamadera H, Takahashi K, Okawa M. A multicenter study of sleep-wake rhythm disorders: clinical features of sleep-wake rhythm disorders. Psychiatry Clin Neurosci 1996;50:195–201.

27. Nakamura K, Hashimoto S, Honma S, et al. A sighted man with non-24-hour sleep-wake syndrome shows damped plasma melatonin rhythm. Psychiatry Clin Neurosci 1997;51:115–9.

28. Shibui K, Uchiyama M, Iwama H, et al. Periodic fatigue symptoms due to desynchronization in a patient with non-24-hours sleep-wake syndrome. Psychiatry Clin Neurosci 1998;52:477–81.

29. Hashimoto S, Nakamura K, Honma S, et al. Free-running of plasma melatonin rhythm prior to full manifestation of a non-24 hour sleep-wake syndrome. Psychiatry Clin Neurosci 1998;52:264–5.

30. Hayakawa T, Kamei Y, Urata J, et al. Trials of bright light exposure and melatonin administration in a patient with non-24 hour sleep-wake syndrome. Psychiatry Clin Neurosci 1998;52:261–2.

31. Akaboshi S, Inoue Y, Kubota N, et al. Case of a mentally retarded child with non-24 hour sleep-wake syndrome caused by deficiency of melatonin secretion. Psychiatry Clin Neurosci 2000;54:379–80.

32. Watanabe T, Kajimura N, Kato M, et al. Case of a non-24 hours sleep-wake syndrome patient improved by phototherapy. Psychiatry Clin Neurosci 2000;54:369–70.

33. Morinobu S, Yamashita H, Yamawaki S, et al. Obsessive-compulsive disorder with non-24-hour sleep-wake syndrome. J Clin Psychiatry 2002;63:838–40.

34. Boivin DB, James FO, Santo JB, et al. Non-24-hour sleep-wake syndrome following a car accident. Neurology 2003;60:1841–3.

35. Dijk DJ, Czeisler CA. Contribution of the circadian pacemaker and the sleep homeostat to sleep propensity, sleep structure, electroencephalographic slow waves, and sleep spindle activity in humans. J Neurosci 1995;15(5 Pt 1):3526–38.

36. Boivin DB, Caliyurt O, James FO, et al. Association between delayed sleep phase and hypernyctohemeral syndromes: a case study. Sleep 2004;27(3): 417–21.

37. Crowley SJ, Acebo C, Carskadon MA. Sleep, circadian rhythms, and delayed phase in adolescence. Sleep Med 2007;8(6):602–12.

38. Uchiyama M, Okawa M, Shibui K, et al. Altered phase relation between sleep timing and core body temperature rhythm in delayed sleep phase syndrome and non-24-h sleep–wake syndrome in humans. Neurosci Lett 2000;294:101–4.

39. Uchiyama M, Shibui K, Hayakawa T, et al. Larger phase angle between sleep propensity and melatonin rhythms in sighted humans with non-24-hour sleep-wake syndrome. Sleep 2002;25:83–8.

40. Wulff K, Joyce E, Middleton B, et al. The suitability of actigraphy, diary data, and urinary melatonin profiles for quantitative assessment of sleep disturbances in schizophrenia: a case report. Chronobiol Int 2006;23(1–2):485–95.

41. Thorpy MJ, Korman E, Spielman AJ, et al. Delayed sleep phase syndrome in adolescents. J Adolesc Health Care 1988;9:22–7.

42. Regestein QR, Monk TH. Delayed sleep phase syndrome: a review of its clinical aspects. Am J Psychiatry 1995;152:602–8.

43. Wyatt JK. Delayed sleep phase syndrome: pathophysiology and treatment options. Sleep 2004; 27(6):1195–203.

44. Wehr TA, Wirz-Justice A, Goodwin FK, et al. Phase advance of the circadian sleep-wake cycle as an antidepressant. Science 1979;206:710–3.

45. Lewy AJ, Lefler BJ, Emens JS, et al. The circadian basis of winter depression. Proc Natl Acad Sci USA 2006;103(19):7414–9.

46. Boivin DB. Influence of sleep-wake and circadian rhythm disturbances in psychiatric disorders. J Psychiatry Neurosci 2000;25(5):446–58.

47. Boivin DB, Czeisler CA, Dijk DJ, et al. Complex interaction of the sleep-wake cycle and circadian phase modulates mood in healthy subjects. Arch Gen Psychiatry 1997;54(2):145–52.

48. Surridge DM, MacLean A, Coulter ME, et al. Mood change following an acute delay of sleep. Psychiatry Res 1987;22:149–58.

49. Sack RL, Lewy AJ, Blood ML, et al. Circadian rhythm abnormalities in totally blind people: incidence and clinical significance. J Clin Endocrinol Metab 1992; 75:127–34.

50. Lockley SW, Skene DJ, Arendt J, et al. Relationship between melatonin rhythms and visual loss in the blind. J Clin Endocrinol Metab 1997;82:3763–70.

51. Skene DJ, Lockley SW, Thapan K, et al. Effects of light on human circadian rhythms. Reprod Nutr Dev 1999;39:295–304.

52. Lockley SW, Skene DJ, Butler LJ, et al. Sleep and activity rhythms are related to circadian phase in the blind. Sleep 1999;22(5):616–23.

53. Klerman EB, Rimmer DW, Dijk DJ, et al. Nonphotic entrainment of the human circadian pacemaker. Am J Phys 1998;274(4 Pt 2):R991–6.

54. Mistlberger RE, Skene DJ. Nonphotic entrainment in humans? J Biol Rhythms 2005;20(4):339–52.

55. Czeisler CA, Shanahan TL, Klerman EB, et al. Suppression of melatonin secretion in some blind patients by exposure to bright light. N Engl J Med 1995;332(1):6–11.

56. Klerman EB, Shanahan TL, Brotman DJ, et al. Photic resetting of the human circadian pacemaker in the absence of conscious vision. J Biol Rhythms 2002; 17(6):548–55.

57. Zaidi FH, Hull JT, Peirson SN, et al. Short-wavelength light sensitivity of circadian, pupillary, and visual awareness in humans lacking an outer retina. Curr Biol 2007;17(24):2122–8.

58. Leger D, Guilleminault C, Santos C, et al. Sleep/wake cycles in the dark: sleep recorded by polysomnography in 26 totally blind subjects compared to controls. Clin Neurophysiol 2002;113(10): 1607–14.

59. Okawa M, Nanami T, Wada S, et al. Four congenitally blind children with circadian sleep–wake rhythm disorder. Sleep 1987;10:101–10.

60. Wee R, Van Gelder RN. Sleep disturbances in young subjects with visual dysfunction. Ophthalmology 2004;111(2):297–302.

61. Brainard GC, Hanifin JP. Photons, clocks, and consciousness. J Biol Rhythms 2005;20(4):314–25.

62. Peirson S, Foster RG. Melanopsin: another way of signaling light. Neuron 2006;49(3):331–9.

63. Klein T, Martens H, Dijk DJ, et al. Circadian sleep regulation in the absence of light perception: chronic non-24-hour circadian rhythm sleep disorder in a blind man with a regular 24-hour sleep-wake schedule. Sleep 1993;16(4):333–43.

64. Czeisler CA, Weitzman ED, Moore-Ede MC, et al. Human sleep: its duration and organization depend on its circadian phase. Science 1980;210:1264–7.

65. Sack RL, Brandes RW, Kendall AR, et al. Entrainment of free-running circadian rhythms by melatonin in blind people. N Engl J Med 2000;343(15): 1070–7.

66. Miles LE, Raynal DM, Wilson MA. Blind man living in normal society has circadian rhythms of 24.9 hours. Science 1977;198(4315):421–3.

67. Lockley SW, Skene DJ, Arendt J. Comparison between subjective and actigraphic measurement of sleep and sleep rhythms. J Sleep Res 1999; 8(3):175–83.

68. Lockley SW, Dijk DJ, Kosti O, et al. Alertness, mood and performance rhythm disturbances associated with circadian sleep disorders in the blind. J Sleep Res 2008;17(2):207–16.

69. Lewy AJ, Newsome DA. Different types of melatonin circadian secretory rhythms in some blind subjects. J Clin Endocrinol Metab 1983;56:1103–7.

70. Tabandeh H, Lockley SW, Buttery R, et al. Disturbance of sleep in blindness. Am J Ophthalmol 1998;126:707–12.

71. Leger D, Guilleminault C, Defrance R, et al. Prevalence of sleep/wake disorders in persons with blindness. Clin Sci 1999;97:193–9.

72. Moseley MJ, Fouladi M, Jones HS, et al. Sleep disturbance and blindness. Lancet 1996; 348(9040):1514–5.

73. Dijk DJ, Lockley SW. Integration of human sleep-wake regulation and circadian rhythmicity. J Appl Phys 2002;92(2):852–62.

74. Honma K, Honma S. A human phase response curve for bright light pulse. Jpn J Psychiatry Neurol 1988;42:167–8.

75. Minors DS, Waterhouse JM, Wirz-Justice A. A human phase–response curve to light. Neurosci Lett 1991;133:36–40.

76. Czeisler CA, Kronauer RE, Allan JS, et al. Bright light induction of strong (type 0) resetting of the human circadian pacemaker. Science 1989;244(4910): 1328–33.

77. Khalsa SB, Jewell ME, Cajochen C, et al. A phase response curve to single bright light pulses in human subjects. J Physiol 2003;549:945–52.

78. Czeisler CA, Duffy JF, Shanahan TL, et al. Stability, precision, and near-24-hour period of the human circadian pacemaker. Science 1999;284(5423):2177–81.

79. Uchiyama M, Okawa M, Ozaki S, et al. Circadian characteristics of delayed sleep phase syndrome and non-24-hour sleep-wake syndrome. In: Honma K, Honma S, editors. Circadian clocks and entrainment. Sapporo: Hokkaido University Press; 1998. p. 115–30.

80. Uchiyama M, Okawa M, Shibui K, et al. Poor compensatory function for sleep loss as a pathologic factor in patients with delayed sleep phase syndrome. Sleep 2000;23:553–8.

81. Ralph MR, Meneker M. Amutation of the circadian system in golden hamster. Science 1988;241:1225–7.

82. Vitaterna MH, King DP, Chang A, et al. Mutagenesis and mapping of a mouse gene, clock, essential for circadian behavior. Science 1994;264:719–21.

83. Ebisawa T. Circadian rhythms in the CNS and peripheral clock disorders: human sleep disorders and clock genes. J Pharm Sci 2007;103(2):150–4.

84. Jones CR, Campbell SS, Zone SE, et al. Familial advanced sleep-phase syndrome: a short-period circadian rhythm variant in humans. Nat Med 1999; 5(9):1062–5.

85. Wright KP Jr, Drake CL, Lockley SW. Diagnostic tools for circadian rhythm sleep disorders. In: Kushida CA, editor. Handbook of sleep disorders. New York: Taylor & Francis Group, LLC; 2008. p. 147–73.

86. Benloucif S, Burgess HJ, Klerman EB, et al. Measuring melatonin in humans. J Clin Sleep Med 2008;4(1):66–9.

87. Lewy AJ, Ahmed S, Jackson JM, et al. Melatonin shifts human circadian rhythms according to a phase-response curve. Chronobiol Int 1992;9: 380–92.

88. Cajochen C, Kräuchi K, Wirz-Justice A. The acute soporific action of daytime melatonin administration: effects on the EEG during wakefulness and subjective alertness. J Biol Rhythms 1997;12(6): 636–43.

89. Kamei Y, Hayakawa T, Urata J, et al. Melatonin treatment for circadian rhythm sleep disorders. Psychiatry Clin Neurosci 2000;54:381–2.

90. Arendt J, Skene DJ, Middleton B, et al. Efficacy of melatonin treatment in jet lag, shift work, and blindness. J Biol Rhythms 1997;12(6):604–17.

91. Lockley SW, Skene DJ, James K, et al. Melatonin administration can entrain the free-running circadian system of blind subjects. J Endocrinol 2000;164:R1–6.

92. Hack LM, Lockley SW, Arendt J, et al. The effects of low-dose 0.5-mg melatonin on the free-running circadian rhythms of blind subjects. J Biol Rhythms 2003;18(5):420–9.

93. Lewy AJ, Bauer VK, Hasler BP, et al. Capturing the circadian rhythms of free-running blind people with 0.5 mg melatonin. Brain Res 2001;918:96–100.

94. Lewy AJ, Emens JS, Lefler BJ, et al. Melatonin entrains free-running blind people according to a physiological dose-response curve. Chronobiol Int 2005;22(6):1093–106.

95. Lewy AJ, Emens JS, Bernert RA, et al. Eventual entrainment of the human circadian pacemaker by melatonin is independent of the circadian phase of treatment initiation: clinical implications. J Biol Rhythms 2004;19(1):68–75.

96. Lewy AJ, Hasler BP, Emens JS, et al. Pretreatment circadian period in free-running blind people may predict the phase angle of entrainment to melatonin. Neurosci Lett 2001;313:158–60.

97. Arendt J. Safety of melatonin in long-term use (?). J Biol Rhythms 1997;12(6):673–81.

98. Buscemi N, Vandermeer B, Hooton N, et al. Efficacy and safety of exogenous melatonin for secondary sleep disorders and sleep disorders accompanying sleep restriction: meta-analysis. BMJ 2006; 332(7538):385–93.

Circadian Rhythm Sleep Disorder: Irregular Sleep Wake Rhythm

Phyllis C. Zee, MD, PhD[a],*, Michael V. Vitiello, PhD[b]

KEYWORDS

- Circadian • Rhythm • Neurodegeneration
- Alzheimer's disease • Irregular

Most physiologic, hormonal, and behavioral processes, most notably the sleep–wake cycle, exhibit nearly 24-hour (circadian) rhythms. These endogenous circadian rhythms are generated by the suprachiasmatic nucleus (SCN), a paired nucleus in the hypothalamus of the brain.[1–3] In humans, light is the strongest entraining agent for the circadian clock,[4] but nonphotic stimuli such as physical activity[5] and endogenous melatonin[6] also can alter the timing of circadian rhythms. In addition to its role in the timing and synchronization of biologic rhythms, the circadian pacemaker promotes alertness during the day and thus facilitates the consolidation of nocturnal sleep and daytime wakefulness across the 24-hour cycle.[7–11]

Significant changes in circadian regulation occur with aging and probably contribute to the higher prevalence of irregular sleep–wake rhythm disorder (ISWRD) in older adults. ISWRD is characterized by the relative absence of a circadian pattern in an individual's sleep–wake cycle. Common age-associated changes in circadian rhythm are the decreases in the amplitude of physiologic (eg, core body temperature) and hormonal circadian rhythms.[12–16] These age-related changes may be the result of degeneration or decreased neuronal activity of SCN neurons, decreased responsiveness of the circadian clock to entraining agents such as light, and decreased exposure to bright light and structured social and physical activity during the day.[17–20]

Alterations in the central regulation of circadian rhythms when combined with the decreased levels of light exposure and social/physical activity levels probably contribute to the increased prevalence of ISWRD in older adults. This tendency toward increased prevalence of ISWRD is often further exaggerated in older adults who have neurodegenerative disorders, such as Alzheimer's disease.[21]

CIRCADIAN RHYTHM SLEEP DISORDER, IRREGULAR SLEEP–WAKE RHYTHM TYPE (ALSO KNOWN AS IRREGULAR SLEEP–WAKE RHYTHM DISORDER)

Consolidation of nocturnal sleep and daytime alertness is achieved when the desired sleeping and waking times are synchronized with the timing of the endogenous propensity for a circadian rhythm of sleeping and waking. Although the primary pathophysiology of irregular sleep–wake rhythm (ISWR) is caused by a disruption of circadian timing, its actual clinical presentation also is influenced by a combination of behavioral and environmental factors.

Clinical Features and Diagnosis

ISWRD is characterized by the lack of a clearly defined circadian sleep–wake rhythm in which sleeping and waking periods are distributed in at

M.V.V. is supported by NIH Grants AG025515, AG031126, MH072736, NR001094, and CA116400. P.C.Z. is supported by NIH Grants AG11412, HL069988, and HL086461.
[a] Department of Neurology, Northwestern University Medical School, 710 N. Lake Shore, Suite 521, Chicago, IL 60611, USA
[b] Department of Psychiatry and Behavioral Sciences, University of Washington School of Medicine, 1959 NE Pacific St., Rm BB-1520D, Seattle, WA 98195, USA
* Corresponding author.
E-mail address: p-zee@northwestern.edu (P.C. Zee).

Sleep Med Clin 4 (2009) 213–218
doi:10.1016/j.jsmc.2009.01.009

least three short bouts (lasting 1–4 hours) throughout the 24 hours, but the total amount of sleep obtained over a 24-hour period is generally normal for the age of the patient (**Fig. 1**).[22] Although sleeping and waking periods are fragmented, the longest sleep period usually is between 2 and 6 AM.[23] Daytime sleep often is composed of multiple naps, whereas nighttime sleep is severely fragmented and shortened. Consequently the primary symptoms of ISWRD are chronic sleep-maintenance insomnia and excessive daytime sleepiness. Diagnosis is made by the clinical history of fragmented sleeping and waking periods along with chronic complaints, usually of sleep-maintenance insomnia and excessive daytime sleepiness. In addition, a sleep diary and/or actigraphy for at least 7 days should be undertaken and show at least three irregular intervals of sleeping and waking periods within a 24-hour period.[22]

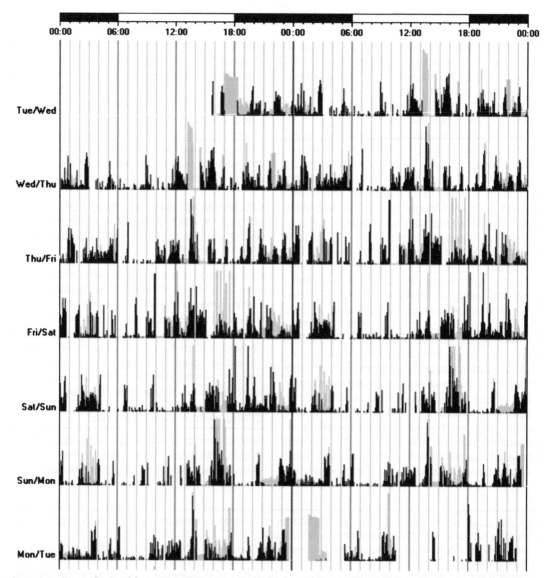

Fig. 1. Actogram obtained by actigraphy over a 7-day period from an older adult patient who has ISWRD. The yellow bars indicate timing and level of ambient light exposure, and the black bars indicate activity levels recorded at the nondominant wrist. Note the lack of a discernible circadian sleep–wake rhythm. Sleep is characterized by nocturnal fragmentation and multiple short periods of sleeping and waking across the entire 24-hour day.

Epidemiology

Although the prevalence of ISWRD increases in later life, age itself is not an independent risk factor for ISWRD. Rather, the age-associated increases in medical, neurologic, and psychiatric disorders have been shown to be the greatest contributors to the development of ISWRD.[24] The disorder is seen more commonly in institutionalized older adults and most commonly in patients who have Alzheimer's disease.[24] Other disorders of the central nervous system, including traumatic brain injury and mental retardation, also can lead to an ISWR pattern.[23,25–27]

Pathophysiology

It has been postulated that both dysfunction of the central processes responsible for the generation of the circadian rhythm and decreased exposure to external synchronizing agents termed "zeitgebers", such as light and social activities, play a role in the development and maintenance of ISWR. The findings of age-related loss of neurons and functional changes within the SCN[17] and a further decrease in the number of neurons within the SCN in patients who have Alzheimer's disease[28,29] suggest that neurodegeneration of the SCN may contribute to the development of ISWRD in older adults.

Older adults, especially those who have chronic medical and neurologic disorders, often are exposed to lower levels of daytime light than their younger counterparts.[30,31] This reduction may be exacerbated by age-related visual disorders, such as cataracts, which can further attenuate the effect of ambient light on the SCN. The impact of diminished exposure to circadian synchronizing agents such as light and activity is most pronounced in patients who have Alzheimer's disease. Low light levels and lack of structured social and physical activities in long-term care facilities may decrease further the amplitude of circadian rhythms. In fact, lower daytime light levels are associated with an increase in nighttime awakenings, even after controlling for the level of dementia.[32]

Finally, although there is no direct evidence for a genetic basis for ISWRD, several lines of evidence suggest that the sleep disturbance seen in Alzheimer's disease is at least partially based on genetic factors. Actigraphic studies of patients who have Alzheimer's disease have demonstrated longitudinal deterioration of sleep quality,[33,34] and most of this longitudinal variance in sleep seems to be related to an inherent trait of the individual patient. This evidence suggests that genetic factors may help determine the ultimate course and level of sleep deterioration seen in a given patient who has Alzheimer's disease,[35,36] a hypothesis consistent with considerable research suggesting that much of the circadian variation in many physiologic systems is controlled by a limited number of similar genes across species.[37] Further studies are needed to determine if certain mutations or polymorphisms of circadian clock genes play a role in the development of ISWR.

Treatment

The primary goals of treatment of an ISWR are to consolidate sleep during the night and wakefulness during the day. To this end, measures aimed at restoring or enhancing exposure to the various SCN time cues or zeitgebers are critical. Patients should be exposed to bright light during the day, and bright light should be avoided in the evening and at night.[38,39] Daytime physical and social activities also should be strongly encouraged.[40–43] A multicomponent approach using a variety of behavioral treatment options is recommended.

Light

The overall approach to light therapy for the treatment of the ISWR type is to increase both the duration and intensity of light exposure throughout the daytime and to avoid exposure to bright light in the evening. Bright light exposure delivered for 2 hours in the morning at 3000 to 5000 lux over the course of 4 weeks has been found to decrease daytime napping and increase nighttime sleep in demented subjects.[44] Light may help further consolidate nighttime sleep, decrease agitated behavior, and result in stronger amplitudes of the circadian rhythm.[38,39,44]

Melatonin

When compared with the effects of bright light, studies evaluating the use of melatonin in ISWRD have yielded less consistent results.[24] Serfaty and colleagues[45] randomly assigned 44 participants who had a *Diagnostic and Statistical Manual-IV* diagnosis of dementia and comorbid sleep disturbance to a 7-week double-blind crossover trial of 2 weeks of slow-release melatonin (6 mg) versus placebo. It should be noted that only 25 of the 44 patients completed the trial. Melatonin had no effect on actigraphically measured total sleep time, number of awakenings, or sleep efficiency. Another large scale trial of 157 patients who had Alzheimer's disease found no statistically significant differences in actigraphy-derived sleep measures between a control group and those taking 2.5 mg melatonin,[46] although a trend toward improvement was seen with 10 mg melatonin. Overall, the efficacy of melatonin treatment for circadian and sleep disorders remains undetermined (for review, see Brzezinski and colleagues[47]).

Some success, however, has been shown in small studies in using melatonin to treat sleep disturbances in children who have psychomotor retardation and presumed ISWR.[48] Significant, although incomplete, benefit also was reported in an open-label trial of melatonin, 2 to 20 mg, given at bedtime to children who had varied neurologic disabilities and chronic sleep–wake cycle disorders.[49,50] Furthermore, a more recent study indicates that a controlled-release melatonin formulation may be more effective for sleep maintenance than the immediate-release formulation in a similar population.

Other therapeutic approaches

Structured physical activity and social activity may help provide temporal cues to increase the regularity of the sleep–wake schedule. Allowing for a favorable sleep environment by reducing nighttime light and noise and improving incontinence care can reduce awakenings in nursing home residents.[51] Furthermore, Alessi and colleagues[52] documented that elderly subjects reported decreased daytime sleep and increased participation in social and physical activities and social conversation by following a regimen of reduced time in bed during the day, a structured bedtime routine at night, 30 minutes or more of sunlight exposure a day, and increased physical activity.

The use of a multimodal nonpharmacologic approach including an increase in sunlight exposure and social activity during the day and a decrease in daytime in-bed time and nighttime noise may be particularly effective. A recent randomized, controlled trial testing such an approach was conducted recently in a group of community-dwelling patients who had Alzheimer's disease with inferred ISWRD diagnoses.[53] Thirty-six community-dwelling patients who had Alzheimer's disease and their family caregivers participated. All participants received written materials describing age- and dementia-related changes in sleep and standard principles of good sleep hygiene. Caregivers in active treatment received specific recommendations about setting up and implementing a sleep hygiene program for the dementia patients and training in behavior management skills. Patients in active treatment also were instructed to walk daily and to increase daytime light exposure with the use of a light box. Control subjects received general dementia education and caregiver support. Sleep was measured actigraphically. Patients in the active-treatment arm showed significant reductions in number of nighttime awakenings and total time awake at night compared with control subjects. At 6-month follow-up, treatment gains were maintained, and additional significant improvements in the duration of night awakenings and circadian organization of sleep emerged.

The most effective ISWRD treatments seem to require a combination of structured social and physical activity, exposure to light during the day, and minimizing nighttime light and noise.[39,51,54,55] A more recent study, however, showed that light alone did not improve nocturnal sleep, but that a combination of light and melatonin (5 mg) increased daytime waking time and activity levels and also strengthened the rest–activity rhythm in patients who had Alzheimer's disease.[56] Riemersma-van der Lek and colleagues[57] found that exposure to bright light during the day had a modest benefit in improving cognitive function and mood, whereas 2.5 mg of melatonin taken in the evening shortened sleep latency and increased sleep duration but adversely affected mood in elderly residents of group-care facilities. Therefore, the authors concluded that melatonin should be used only in combination with light. In this same study, a combined treatment with light and melatonin decreased aggressive behavior and modestly improved sleep efficiency and decreased nocturnal restlessness.

SUMMARY

Individuals who have ISWRD often present with symptoms of sleep-maintenance insomnia and excessive daytime sleepiness. ISWR always should be considered in the differential diagnosis of sleep disturbances in older adults and in children who have neurologic impairments. It is commonly accepted that a combination of dysfunction of the circadian clock (SCN) and decreased exposure to circadian zeitgebers, such as timed bright light and structured physical or social activities, have important roles in the development and maintenance of the characteristic irregular low-amplitude circadian sleep–wake rhythm of ISWRD. Studies of the effectiveness of pharmacologic treatments for ISWRD generally have yielded negative or inconsistent results. One exception may be in children who have psychomotor retardation, in which melatonin has been shown to improve the sleep–wake pattern. Furthermore, the safety of pharmacologic agents has not been well studied, particularly in the elderly, who are more likely to suffer from ISWRD. Therefore, a mixed-modality behavioral approach to consolidate nocturnal sleep (improved sleep hygiene; decreased nocturnal light and noise levels) and enhance daytime alertness (increased daytime light exposure; increased social and physical activity) is the mainstay treatment for ISWRD. The success of treatment for this condition is highly variable and requires tailoring to individual needs. It is expected that rapid advances in the understanding of the genetic regulation of circadian rhythms will define better the genetic vulnerability for ISWRD and should lead to prevention and improved treatment of this circadian-based disorder.

REFERENCES

1. Moore RY, Eichler VB. Loss of a circadian adrenal corticosterone rhythm following suprachiasmatic lesions in the rat. Brain Res 1972;42(1):201–6.
2. Pittendrigh CS. Circadian oscillations in cells and the circadian organization of multicellular systems. In: Schmitt FC, Worden FG, editors. The neurosciences third study program. Cambridge (MA): MIT Press; 1974. p. 437–58.
3. Mouret J, Coindet J, Debilly G, et al. Suprachiasmatic nuclei lesions in the rat: alterations in sleep circadian rhythms. Electroencephalogr Clin Neurophysiol 1978;45(3):402–8.
4. Czeisler CA, Allan JS, Strogatz SH, et al. Bright light resets the human circadian pacemaker independent of the timing of the sleep-wake cycle. Science 1986; 233(4764):667–71.
5. Buxton OM, Lee CW, L'Hermite-Baleriaux M, et al. Exercise elicits phase shifts and acute alterations of melatonin that vary with circadian phase. Am J Physiol Regul Integr Comp Physiol 2003;284(3):R714–24.
6. Lewy AJ, Ahmed S, Jackson JM, et al. Melatonin shifts human circadian rhythms according to a phase-response curve. Chronobiol Int 1992;9(5): 380–92.
7. Akerstedt T, Gillberg M. The circadian variation of experimentally displaced sleep. Sleep 1981;4(2): 159–69.
8. Czeisler CA, Duffy JF, Shanahan TL, et al. Stability, precision, and near-24-hour period of the human circadian pacemaker. Science 1999;284(5423):2177–81.
9. Dijk DJ, Czeisler CA. Paradoxical timing of the circadian rhythm of sleep propensity serves to consolidate sleep and wakefulness in humans. Neurosci Lett 1994;166(1):63–8.
10. Wever RA. Influence of physical workload on free running circadian rhythms of man. Pflugers Arch 1979;381(2):119–26.
11. Zulley J, Wever R, Aschoff J. The dependence of onset and duration of sleep on the circadian rhythm of rectal temperature. Pflugers Arch 1981;391(4): 314–8.
12. Skene DJ, Swaab DF. Melatonin rhythmicity: effect of age and Alzheimer's disease. Exp Gerontol 2003; 38(1–2):199–206.
13. Touitou Y, Reinberg A, Bogdan A, et al. Age-related changes in both circadian and seasonal rhythms of rectal temperature with special reference to senile dementia of Alzheimer type. Gerontology 1986; 32(2):110–8.
14. Van Cauter E, Leproult R, Kupfer DJ. Effects of gender and age on the levels and circadian rhythmicity of plasma cortisol. J Clin Endocrinol Metab 1996;81(7):2468–73.
15. van Coevorden A, Mockel J, Laurent E, et al. Neuroendocrine rhythms and sleep in aging men. American Journal of Physiology 1991;260(4 Pt 1): E651–61.
16. Vitiello MV, Smallwood RG, Avery DH, et al. Circadian temperature rhythms in young adult and aged men. Neurobiol Aging 1986;7(2):97–100.
17. Swaab DF, Fliers E, Partiman TS. The suprachiasmatic nucleus of the human brain in relation to sex, age and senile dementia. Brain Res 1985;342(1): 37–44.
18. Swaab DF, VAn Someren EJ, Zhou JN, et al. Biological rhythms in the human life cycle and their relationship to functional changes in the suprachiasmatic nucleus. Prog Brain Res 1996; 111:349–68.
19. Hofman MA. The human circadian clock and aging. Chronobiol Int 2000;17(3):245–59.
20. Hofman MA, Swaab DF. Alterations in circadian rhythmicity of the vasopressin-producing neurons of the human suprachiasmatic nucleus (SCN) with aging. Brain Res 1994;651(1–2):134–42.
21. Reid KJ, Chang AM, Zee PC. Circadian rhythm sleep disorders. Med Clin North Am 2004;88(3): 631–51, viii.
22. Hauri PJ. AAOS Medicine. ICSD-2. The International Classification of Sleep Disorders: Diagnostic and Coding Manual. 2nd edition. Westchester(IL): American Academy of Sleep Medicine; 2005.
23. Wagner DR. Disorders of the circadian sleep-wake cycle. Neurol Clin 1996;14(3):651–70.
24. Sack RL, Auckley D, Auger RR, et al. Circadian rhythm sleep disorders: part II, advanced sleep phase disorder, delayed sleep phase disorder, free-running disorder, and irregular sleep-wake rhythm. An American Academy of Sleep Medicine review. Sleep 2007;30(11):1484–501.
25. Hoogendijk WJ, Van Someren EJ, Mirmiran M, et al. Circadian rhythm-related behavioral disturbances and structural hypothalamic changes in Alzheimer's disease. Int Psychogeriatr 1996;8(Suppl 3):245–52, discussion: 269–72.
26. Wagner DR. Circadian rhythm sleep disorders. Curr Treat Options Neurol 1999;1(4):299–308.
27. Witting W, Kwa IH, Eikelenboom P, et al. Alterations in the circadian rest-activity rhythm in aging and Alzheimer's disease. Biol Psychiatry 1990;27(6): 563–72.

28. Swaab DF. Ageing of the human hypothalamus. Horm Res 1995;43(1–3):8–11.

29. Zhou JN, Hofman MA, Swaab DF. VIP neurons in the human SCN in relation to sex, age, and Alzheimer's disease. Neurobiol Aging 1995;16(4):571–6.

30. Van Someren EJ, Kessler A, Mirmiran M, et al. Indirect bright light improves circadian rest-activity rhythm disturbances in demented patients. Biol Psychiatry 1997;41(9):955–63.

31. Van Someren EJ. Circadian rhythms and sleep in human aging. Chronobiol Int 2000;17(3):233–43.

32. Ancoli-Israel S, Klauber MR, Jones DW, et al. Variations in circadian rhythms of activity, sleep, and light exposure related to dementia in nursing-home patients. Sleep 1997;20(1):18–23.

33. Werth E, Savaskan E, Knoblauch V, et al. Decline in long-term circadian rest-activity cycle organization in a patient with dementia. J Geriatr Psychiatry Neurol 2002;15(1):55–9.

34. Yesavage JA, Friedman L, Kraemer HC, et al. A follow-up study of actigraphic measures in home-residing Alzheimer's disease patients. J Geriatr Psychiatry Neurol 1998;11(1):7–10.

35. Yesavage JA, Friedman L, Ancoli-Israel S, et al. Development of diagnostic criteria for defining sleep disturbance in Alzheimer's disease. J Geriatr Psychiatry Neurol 2003;16(3):131–9.

36. Yesavage JA, Taylor JL, Kraemer H, et al. Sleep/wake cycle disturbance in Alzheimer's disease: how much is due to an inherent trait? Int Psychogeriatr 2002;14(1):73–81.

37. Clayton JD, Kyriacou CP, Reppert SM. Keeping time with the human genome. Nature 2001;409(6822):829–31.

38. Ancoli-Israel S, Gehrman P, Martin JL, et al. Increased light exposure consolidates sleep and strengthens circadian rhythms in severe Alzheimer's disease patients. Behav Sleep Med 2003;1(1):22–36.

39. Ancoli-Israel S, Martin JL, Kripke DF, et al. Effect of light treatment on sleep and circadian rhythms in demented nursing home patients. J Am Geriatr Soc 2002;50(2):282–9.

40. Naylor E, Penev PD, Orbeta L, et al. Daily social and physical activity increases slow-wave sleep and daytime neuropsychological performance in the elderly. Sleep 2000;23(1):87–95.

41. Benloucif S, Orbeta L, Ortiz R, et al. Morning or evening activity improves neuropsychological performance and subjective sleep quality in older adults. Sleep 2004;27(8):1542–51.

42. Niggemyer KA, Begley A, Monk T, et al. Circadian and homeostatic modulation of sleep in older adults during a 90-minute day study. Sleep 2004;27(8):1535–41.

43. Vitiello MV, Prinz PN, Schwartz RS. Slow wave sleep but not overall sleep quality of healthy older men and women is improved by increased aerobic fitness. Sleep Res 1994;23:149.

44. Mishima K, Okawa M, Hishikawa Y, et al. Morning bright light therapy for sleep and behavior disorders in elderly patients with dementia. Acta Psychiatr Scand 1994;89(1):1–7.

45. Serfaty M, Kennell-Webb S, Warner J, et al. Double blind randomised placebo controlled trial of low dose melatonin for sleep disorders in dementia. Int J Geriatr Psychiatry 2002;17(12):1120–7.

46. Singer C, Tractenberg RE, Kaye J, et al. A multi-center, placebo-controlled trial of melatonin for sleep disturbance in Alzheimer's disease. Sleep 2003;26(7):893–901.

47. Brzezinski A, Vangel MG, Wurtman RJ, et al. Effects of exogenous melatonin on sleep: a meta-analysis. Sleep Med Rev 2005;9(1):41–50.

48. Pillar G, Shahar E, Peled N, et al. Melatonin improves sleep-wake patterns in psychomotor retarded children. Pediatr Neurol 2000;23(3):225–8.

49. Jan JE, Abroms IF, Freeman RD, et al. Rapid cycling in severely multidisabled children: a form of bipolar affective disorder? Pediatr Neurol 1994;10(1):34–9.

50. Jan JE, Freeman RD, Fast DK. Melatonin treatment of sleep-wake cycle disorders in children and adolescents. Dev Med Child Neurol 1999;41(7):491–500.

51. Schnelle JF, Alessi CA, Al-Samarrai NR, et al. The nursing home at night: effects of an intervention on noise, light, and sleep. J Am Geriatr Soc 1999;47(4):430–8.

52. Alessi CA, Martin JL, Webber AP, et al. Randomized, controlled trial of a nonpharmacological intervention to improve abnormal sleep/wake patterns in nursing home residents. J Am Geriatr Soc 2005;53(5):803–10.

53. McCurry SM, Gibbons LE, Logsdon RG, et al. Nighttime insomnia treatment and education for Alzheimer's disease: a randomized, controlled trial. J Am Geriatr Soc 2005;53(5):793–802.

54. Schnelle JF, Cruise PA, Alessi CA, et al. Sleep hygiene in physically dependent nursing home residents: behavioral and environmental intervention implications. Sleep 1998;21(5):515–23.

55. Yamadera H, Takahashi K, Okawa M. A multicenter study of sleep-wake rhythm disorders: therapeutic effects of vitamin B_{12}, bright light therapy, chronotherapy and hypnotics. Psychiatry Clin Neurosci 1996;50(4):203–9.

56. Dowling GA, Burr RL, Van Someren EJ, et al. Melatonin and bright-light treatment for rest-activity disruption in institutionalized patients with Alzheimer's disease. J Am Geriatr Soc 2008;56(2):239–46.

57. Riemersma-van der Lek RF, Swaab DF, Twisk J, et al. Effect of bright light and melatonin on cognitive and noncognitive function in elderly residents of group care facilities: a randomized controlled trial. JAMA 2008;299(22):2642–55.

Advance-Related Sleep Complaints and Advanced Sleep Phase Disorder

R. Robert Auger, MD[a,b,c,*]

KEYWORDS

- Circadian • Melatonin • Insomnia • Phototherapy
- Advanced • Treatment

Other articles from this issue review pertinent aspects of sleep and circadian physiology (see the articles by Gillette and Abbott, Dijk and Archer, Duffy and Czeisler, Rajaratnam, and Cohen and Rogers). Misalignment between endogenous circadian rhythms and the light/dark cycle can result in pathologic disturbances in the form of erratic sleep timing (irregular sleep-wake rhythm), complete dissociation from the light/dark cycle (circadian rhythm sleep disorder, free-running type), delayed sleep timing (delayed sleep phase disorder), or advanced sleep timing (advanced sleep phase disorder [ASPD]). This review focuses on the latter phenomenon, with an emphasis on epidemiology, diagnosis and assessment, etiologic underpinnings, and treatment options.

EPIDEMIOLOGY

ASPD is the sole entity within the International Classification of Sleep Disorders (ICSD) that specifically addresses "advance-related" sleep complaints (ie, difficulties remaining awake until bedtime, awakening earlier than desired, or both).[1] As can be seen in **Table 1**, the diagnosis requires the simultaneous presence of nighttime and morning complaints. Although not included among the actual criteria, the ICSD also states that sleep onset is "typically" advanced to

between 18:00 and 21:00 and wake times to between 02:00 and 05:00. In one large survey study that approximated this stringent definition (among a cohort aged 40 to 64 years), the population prevalence was estimated at 1%, although it is unclear what proportion of these subjects would deem their schedule to be significantly troublesome so as to warrant clinical attention, a requirement when invoking the disorder terminology.[2]

The existing literature and the author's personal experience suggest that clinicians are unlikely to encounter patients with ICSD-defined ASPD, as until the recent identification of familial cohorts, only four cases were described,[3–6] one of which was confounded by concomitant sleep-disordered breathing.[5] Select treatment trials[7,8] also support this contention, with objective demonstration of rather orthodox sleep and wake times despite eligibility for study entry based on subjective assessments. Fulfillment of ASPD criteria is made particularly difficult by the requirement of early evening sleep onset, as this can be more readily voluntarily modified than wake time[9] and is likely to be more actively resisted due to its propensity to conflict with social or familial obligations.

Based on the rarity of discrete ASPD in the clinical setting, knowledge of the epidemiology of the broader "advance-related" sleep complaint is

[a] Department of Psychiatry and Psychology and Psychology, Mayo Clinic College of Medicine, Rochester, MN 55905, USA
[b] Department of Medicine, Mayo Clinic College of Medicine, Rochester, MN 55905, USA
[c] Mayo Center for Sleep Medicine, Gonda Building 17W, 200 First Street SW, Rochester, MN 55905, USA
* Mayo Center for Sleep Medicine, Gonda Building 17W, 200 First Street SW, Rochester, MN 55905.
E-mail address: auger.raymond1@mayo.edu

Sleep Med Clin 4 (2009) 219–227
doi:10.1016/j.jsmc.2009.01.012

Table 1
Advanced sleep phase disorder diagnostic criteria

Diagnostic Criteria	Description
A	There is an advance in the phase of the major sleep period in relation to the desired sleep and wake-up time, as evidenced by a chronic or recurrent complaint of inability to stay awake until the desired conventional clock time, together with an inability to remain asleep until the desired and socially acceptable time for awakening.
B	When patients are allowed to choose their preferred schedule, sleep quality and duration are normal for age with an advanced, but stable, phase of entrainment to the 24-hour sleep-wake pattern.
C	Sleep logs or actigraphy monitoring (including sleep diaries) for at least 7 days demonstrate a stable advance in the timing of the habitual sleep period.
D	The sleep disturbance is not better explained by another current sleep disorder, medical or neurologic disorder, mental disorder, medication use, or substance use disorder.

From American Academy of Sleep Medicine. International classification of sleep disorders. Diagnostic and coding manual. 2nd edition. Westchester (IL): American Academy of Sleep Medicine; 2005; with permission.

required. For the purposes of discussion herein, such a description applies to sleep disturbances that are presumed to be primarily due to a pathologic phase advance (ie, ASPD, early morning awakenings, or maintenance insomnia) and therefore responsive to circadian-based interventions. Elderly status appears to be a risk factor, as advanced age (among a cohort aged 20 to 59 years) is associated with increased morningness (as assessed by the Horne-Ostberg or morningness-eveningness questionnaire [MEQ]), and this trait has been found to be a significant mediator of numerous age-sleep relationships.[10] A large survey study (involving a cohort aged 40 to 64 years) more directly supported a relationship with advance-related complaints, finding that the concomitant endorsement of both nighttime and morning aspects was twice as common ($\sim$7% of respondents) when compared with "delay-related" complaints.[11]

DIAGNOSIS AND ASSESSMENT

The attribution of a sleep complaint to a pathologic phase advance needs to be contemplated thoroughly, particularly when a discrete diagnosis of ASPD is not apparent. Exclusionary criteria for ASPD mandate that other psychiatric, medical, or substance-induced conditions not contribute primarily (see **Table 1**) and, as the condition is classically related to an aberration in the timing (but not quality) of sleep, the characterization of a disorder is invoked only if the schedule interferes significantly with social or occupational functioning. These same criteria are logically applied to patients who have presumed advance-related sleep complaints, which serve to optimize the likelihood that a circadian dysrhythmia is implicated, and that the condition will be responsive to circadian-based treatment interventions.

Important specific considerations within the differential diagnosis include depression, which often manifests with sleep complaints.[12] Poor sleep hygiene practices, particularly evening napping (reviewed later), and irregularity of the sleep/wake schedule, need also to be explored. The possibility of a "free-running" circadian rhythm is also worthy of contemplation (ie, a sleep/wake schedule that occurs independent of the light/dark cycle), but patients with this condition are most commonly blind and report only periodic complaints of insomnia depending on the relative relationship between their internal rhythm and that of the light/dark cycle.[1] As with any sleep disturbance that persists over time, a conditioned insomnia can develop secondarily. The presence of more than one contributing variable seems to be the norm, and each entity needs to be treated accordingly.

Much can be ruled in or out solely with a careful clinical history (preferably with collateral informants). Emblematic of the success of careful subjective screening, Lack and colleagues[13] recruited patients for a treatment study with the intent of selecting those that experienced early morning awakenings primarily as a result of phase-advanced circadian rhythms. Upon entering the active phase of the protocol, patients were found to have markedly advanced core body temperature minima (CBT) on the order of 02:00 or earlier. Typically, the CBT occurs several hours before habitual sleep offset, ranging between 04:00 and 06:00,[14] highlighting the fruitful efforts of these investigators.

Various assessment tools can also assist in establishing a diagnosis of an advance-related sleep complaint, particularly when its origins are multifactorial. Sleep logs or actigraphy (included in the ASPD ICSD diagnostic criteria, see **Table 1**) are essential to demonstrate stability of the sleep/wake schedule. Actigraphs are compact "motion detectors," the output of which allows longitudinal assessment of various sleep/wake parameters.[15] Studies that have compared data obtained in this fashion with those of polysomnography (gold standard) have shown excellent correlations,[16] and the device has been specifically endorsed as a means of assessing circadian rhythm sleep disorders.[15] Although either method is acceptable, recent studies support greater reliability of the data produced by these devices in comparison with sleep logs.[17,18] An idealized example of the utility of visual inspection of actigraphy is depicted in **Fig. 1**A and B. Although both patients presented with complaints of early-morning awakenings, one can readily see the stability of the phase advance depicted in **Fig. 1**A compared with the erratic sleep/wake schedule depicted in **Fig. 1**B, in which the influence of non-circadian (or multifactorial) variables seems more apparent.

Morningness tendencies of patients can be further verified with the MEQ.[19] This questionnaire contains 19 items aimed at determining when the respondent's natural propensity to be active lies during the daily temporal span. The sum score gives a value ranging from 16 to 86 (higher and lower values correspond to morning and evening types, respectively) and is thought to be a fair predictor of the endogenous circadian period or phase.[20] Select studies involving ASPD patients (that did not use an MEQ score as an entry criterion) support its use in narrowing the differential diagnosis for sleep maintenance complaints and also appear to highlight its ability to detect an innate circadian preference. In a study by Jones and colleagues[21] involving patients with familial advanced sleep phase disorder (FASPD), affected subjects scored remarkably high on the MEQ when compared with controls and, interestingly, unaffected blood relatives scored significantly higher than a non-sanguineous comparison group. More germane to typical clinical practice, a study involving patients with advance-related sleep complaints (ie, subjects did not meet ICSD-defined ASPD criteria) demonstrated morningness MEQ scores among 91% of participants.[8]

Physiologic circadian phase assessments (such as those obtained by salivary melatonin immunoassays) appear to have potential utility but are not yet routinely used clinically.[20,22] The necessity to develop normative values is exemplified by comparing phase markers obtained from FASPD

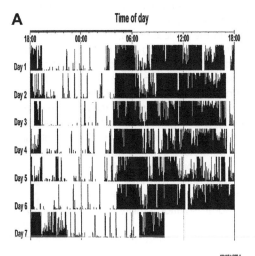
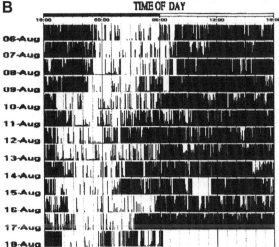

Fig. 1. (A) Actigraph recording from a patient with advance-related sleep complaints. (B) Actigraph recording from a separate patient with advance-related sleep complaints. Data represent sleep-wakefulness activity levels across sequential 24-hour periods as determined by an accelerometer typically worn on the nondominant wrist. The x-axis of each figure depicts clock times in 24-hour blocks, and the data are continuously plotted in subsequent rows until the device is removed (associated dates are depicted on the y-axis). Black "tick marks" represent periods of signal activity (or motion) detected by the device. Periods of time with comparatively less signal activity are representative of inactivity or sleep episodes; therefore, the tracing serves as a useful surrogate measure of the patient's longitudinal sleep/wake schedule (see the article by Wirz-Justice, Bromundt, and Cajochen elsewhere in this issue for a more detailed discussion of the clinical use of actigraphy).

patients with those from patients with non-familial ASPD or patients with advance-related sleep complaints. To preface, the dim light melatonin onset (DLMO) typically begins 14 hours after habitual sleep offset (or about 2 hours before sleep onset),[23] and the CBT occurs approximately 7 hours thereafter[24] or several hours before natural awakening.[14] A case-control comparison of FASPD patients (representative of the extreme phenotype) demonstrated markedly advanced DLMO (17:31 ± 1:49 versus 21:21 ± 0:28, $P<.0005$) and CBT values (23:22 ± 2:55 versus 03:35 ± 1:33, $P = .002$).[21] A review of CBT values obtained from nonfamilial ASPD patients (DLMO values not available for comparison) and those with advance-related complaints reveals a wider range of values (ranging from approximately 01:30 to 04:00),[7,13,25] with the latter range approaching those expected in unaffected populations. Taking into account that changes in circadian rhythms can be produced by voluntary manipulation of the sleep/wake schedule alone,[26] a physiologic assay would be useful in clinical practice only if extremes in values could be readily identified, prompting providers to search for further clinical correlation if the results fell into a "gray zone." Such an approach is familiar to those who interpret multiple sleep latency testing values on a regular basis.[27]

POTENTIAL MECHANISMS

In an individual normally entrained to the light/dark cycle, evening bright light (≥ 2500 lux) exposure (ie, light exposure before the CBT) delays circadian rhythms, and morning bright light exposure (ie, light exposure after the CBT) advances rhythms[7,13,28,29] (see the article by Duffy and Czeisler elsewhere in this issue). These opposing effects allow the majority of the population to be properly attuned to the light-dark cycle, such that sleep and wakefulness occur at a conventional schedule. Patients with pathologic advance-related sleep complaints live at a circadian phase that appears resistant to delays and is incompatible with their personal and social obligations.

Mechanistic postulations regarding this entity assume that numerous contributing variables have been evaluated and ruled out. Possible etiologies include an alteration in the ability of the clock to phase delay, a dominant phase advance region of the light phase response curve (PRC) to entraining agents, altered strength of zeitgebers to the pertinent portions of the light PRC (voluntarily or involuntarily induced), or a shortened endogenous circadian period of the pacemaker. Among these proposed mechanisms, only the latter has been

definitively demonstrated and is discussed herein.[21]

A patient's ability to sleep at an abnormal circadian phase ("phase tolerance") also impacts the degree to which adverse symptoms are experienced, and this adaptability varies among individuals.[30,31] In a simulated jet lag study (requiring a 6-hour phase advance), middle-aged subjects (37–52 years) experienced a greater degree of polysomnographically recorded fragmented sleep than their younger counterparts (18–25 years) and also exhibited greater impairments in daytime alertness, suggesting that advanced age reduces phase tolerance.[31] Conflicting results were obtained from two field studies (involving both eastward and westward travel), which suggested that age may actually be protective with respect to adaptation to circadian dyssynchrony[32,33] (reviewed in reference[20]). Methodological differences preclude direct comparisons of the investigations, as do wide variances in the age groups studied.

Familial Advanced Sleep Phase Disorder

The completion of the Human Genome Project has facilitated the discovery of genes responsible for complex behaviors. Recent descriptions of FASPD cohorts have spurred investigations of human clock genes in relation to circadian rhythm sleep disorders.[21,34] In contrast to the precautionary statements regarding rigid adherence to ICSD criteria in the clinical arena, stringent selection of patients in this setting has enabled researchers to study relatively homogenous populations with extreme phenotypes[9,21,34–36] (see Table 1). In the most productive research to date, three kindreds with FASPD were identified (Northern European descent) with highly penetrant autosomal dominant trait transmission.[21] In comparison with unaffected controls, markedly advanced sleep onset/offset (polysomnographically measured), CBT, and melatonin rhythms were demonstrated (Table 2). One of these subjects was admitted to a temporal isolation facility for a subsequent 18 days, during which time a significant shortening of the circadian period was demonstrated at 23.3 hours.

This dramatic phenotype was further exploited with genetic analyses, which revealed a missense mutation in a casein kinase ($CK1\epsilon$) binding region of a Period gene (hPer2), culminating in hypophosphorylation by $CK1\epsilon$ in vitro.[35] The importance of this finding can be demonstrated when considering the molecular mechanisms of the mammalian circadian clock (see the article by Gillette and Abbott elsewhere in this issue). Summarized

Table 2
Phase markers of familial advanced sleep phase disorder subjects versus unaffected controls

Phase Marker	Control (n = 6) (Mean ± SD)	FASPD (n = 6) (Mean ± SD)	Difference (Hours: Minutes)	P Value
Sleep onset	23:10 ± 0:40	19:25 ± 1:44	3:45	<.0005
Sleep offset[a]	07:44 ± 1:13	04:18 ± 2:00	3:26	<.0005
DLMO	21:21 ± 0:28	17:31 ± 1:49	3:50	<.0005
CBT[b]	03:35 ± 1:33	23:22 ± 2:55	4:13	.002

All values reported as 24-hour clock times.
Abbreviations: CBT, core body temperature minimum; DLMO, dim light melatonin onset; FASPD, familial advanced sleep phase disorder.
[a] n = 5 for FASPD only.
[b] n = 5 for controls and FASPD. Data include both nights of study.
Data from Jones C, Campbell S, Zone S, et al. Familial advanced sleep phase syndrome: a short-period circadian rhythm variant in humans. Nat Med 1999;5(9):1062–5.

briefly, *CK1ε* phosphorylation of the Period (*PER*) protein promotes *PER* degradation, which prevents the protein from dimerizing with the *Cryptochrome* (*Cry*) protein, translocating into the nucleus, and inhibiting its own transcription.[37] Hypophosphorylation of the *PER* protein results in promotion of its transcription and, ultimately, a decrease in the period length of the clock.

Although the importance of this finding cannot be overstated, genetic heterogeneity of FASPD is also apparent as demonstrated by the fact that other FASPD cohorts from this study[35] and another study (involving patients of Japanese descent)[9] did not reveal mutations in *hPer2*. A separate report of a Japanese FASPD cohort described a missense mutation in a different casein kinase gene (*CKIδ*), which also resulted in decreased enzymatic activity in vitro.[36]

TREATMENTS
Phototherapy

A variety of studies have employed evening phototherapy as a treatment for advance-related sleep complaints according to underlying knowledge of the human light PRC (see the article by Duffy and Czeisler elsewhere in this issue). In the two positive studies to date, compliance with treatment was systematically monitored, and physiologic circadian markers were employed.[7,13] In the first study, bright light (4000 lux) was administered for 2 hours between 20:00 and 23:00 for 12 consecutive nights in subjects' homes.[7] Significant phase delays were observed in the active treatment group (when compared with the sham intervention group), on the order of 3 hours, in association with an average delay in bedtime of nearly 30 minutes, an approximately 13% increase in sleep efficiency,

and a related decrease in wakefulness after sleep onset. The control group demonstrated no significant changes in sleep or circadian parameters. In the more recent study, similar magnitudes of phase delays were achieved using a lower intensity of light (2500 lux) and a shorter overall duration of treatment (two nights), but with administration at a later clock time (20:00–01:00) and with a greater length of exposure (4 hours).[13]

In an attempt to develop a protocol that was better tolerated and more practically implemented in the clinical setting, a separate group of investigators explored the efficacy of "enhanced evening light" (approximately 265 lux) as administered by an apparatus resembling a floor lamp.[8] The treatment was provided in subjects' homes for 2 to 3 hours at earlier clock times than described previously (19:00–22:00) for a duration of 4 weeks. Although overall compliance was monitored during the protocol, the placement of the lighting device in relation to the participant was unsupervised, and no objective benefits were demonstrated when compared with the placebo intervention. The importance of monitoring patient compliance and proper device use is further highlighted by two additional studies that more closely approximated the protocols of the aforementioned positive investigations,[38,39] including one with an otherwise identical protocol[39] to that described previously.[7]

A "bright light mask" that delivers the stimulus through closed eyelids (during sleep) presents a potential means of negating these issues and was reported as well tolerated in one study, with little sleep disturbance among subjects receiving the treatment for delayed sleep phase disorder.[40] This apparatus is not yet commercially available. Widely obtainable blue light boxes may also influence treatment factors; they have been reported to exhibit at least equivalent efficacy to bright light devices but with markedly decreased light intensity and fewer associated adverse effects.[41] This contention is reported by a company that markets the devices however, and there are no published reports to date of their efficacy among patients with advance-related sleep complaints. Despite these and other limitations, subjective benefits of light therapy in the reviewed studies were uniformly observed, and there is little risk in implementing a trial of treatment (**Fig. 2**). Caution should be taken in prescribing this therapy to patients using photosensitizing drugs or those with ocular or retinal pathology.[20]

Light and Darkness Exposure

In an interesting study using a constant routine protocol, evidence was provided for a darkness PRC such that exposure (with or without sleep) during the hours of 19:00 to 01:00 resulted in phase advances.[42] In a more naturalistic study of older subjects, those who took evening naps showed earlier sleep-offset times and a more advanced acrophase of the melatonin rhythm than subjects who refrained from napping.[43] Because both behaviors (ie, evening naps and early awakenings) could theoretically result in phase advances, the avoidance of evening naps and protection from morning light exposure are rational recommendations to provide to the patient (see **Fig. 2**). With respect to the latter intervention, the use of protective eyewear (approximately 15% visual light transmission with <3% blue light transmission) was shown to be effective in decreasing light exposure (and undesired phase advances)

in studies involving subjects exposed to simulated shift work.[44] Commercial products are also available that specifically inhibit the transmission of blue light (www.lowbluelights.com), but they have not been specifically studied in patients with advance-related sleep complaints.

Oral Melatonin

There are no systematic reports of melatonin administration for persons with advance-related sleep complaints,[22,45] but consideration of the melatonin PRC (nearly a mirror image of the light PRC) provides a rationale for low-dose administration after early morning awakenings or upon final arising in the morning (see **Fig. 2**, and article by Eastman and Burgess elsewhere in this issue for further details regarding the melatonin PRC).[46] Legitimate safety concerns arise when recommending a potentially sleep-promoting agent during morning hours, and appropriate precautions are required if treatment is initiated.[47]

Melatonin is not regulated by the US Food and Drug Administration and is available over-the-counter as a nutritional supplement. Verification of purity of the product is difficult. With regard to safety concerns, a comprehensive review by the National Academy of Sciences stated that, given available data, short-term use of melatonin in total daily doses of 10 mg or less in healthy adults appears to be safe, but caution should be heeded when administering this agent to children or women of reproductive age. Adverse effects have been reported at higher doses and even at lower doses in those with preexisting central nervous system, cardiovascular, gastrointestinal,

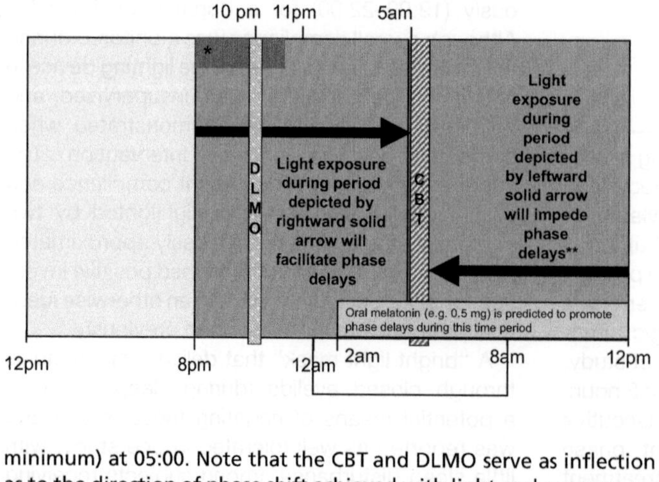

Fig. 2. Summary of circadian-based treatments for advance-related sleep complaints based upon human phase response curves. *Area denoted by *rightward solid arrow* represents recommended time period for evening phototherapy and specific avoidance of naps or darkness. **Area denoted by *leftward solid arrow* denotes times during which patients with advance-related sleep complaints should avoid or protect themselves from light exposure. The rectangle underneath the x-axis represents the nocturnal sleep period, occurring from midnight to 08:00. The DLMO (dim light melatonin onset) occurs at 22:00 and the CBT (core body temperature minimum) at 05:00. Note that the CBT and DLMO serve as inflection points (the former more so than the latter) as to the direction of phase shift achieved with light and exogenous melatonin, respectively. The times and phase relationships depicted are idealized and assume that the circadian clock is entrained to a 24-hour day. The local time axis would require adjustment in those with advanced or delayed circadian rhythms (see the articles by Duffy and Czeisler and Eastman and Burgess elsewhere in this issue for further details regarding the light and melatonin phase response curves, respectively). (*Courtesy of* J.K. Wyatt, PhD, Chicago, IL).

or dermatologic conditions.[48] Doses recommended for circadian-based interventions are typically physiologic in nature (ie, 0.5 mg or less),[46] which may serve to mitigate these concerns.

Chronotherapy

Chronotherapy is a treatment whereby patients are prescribed a sleep schedule that is delayed or advanced for several hours incrementally until sleep is aligned to a target bedtime. After this goal is reached, the individual is advised to rigorously maintain a regular sleep/wake schedule, repeating the process as necessary. There is one case report of successful use of this modality in a patient with presumed ASPD (an advance of 3 hours every 2 days for a 2-week period), with successful maintenance of the desired phase at 5-month follow-up assessment.[5] Further research is required regarding the efficacy and practicality of this intervention in the clinical setting.

Hypnotics

A discussion of the use of hypnotics for persons with maintenance or terminal insomnia is beyond the scope of this review and contrary to its chronobiologic focus. Adjunctive use of medications is sometimes required due to failure or impracticality of non-pharmacologic treatments. Practitioners are frequently reluctant prescribers owing to reports linking their use with exacerbation of sleep-disordered breathing and cognitive impairment,[49] as well as concerns regarding an increased risk of falls.[50,51] The latter concern must be balanced against the results of recent studies suggesting that sleep complaints are better predictors of falls in community-dwelling and institutionalized elderly adults when compared with medications, and that medications may simply be a proxy for the underlying sleep disturbance.[52-54] Bolstering this theory, the presence of untreated insomnia predicted more falls than insomnia despite the use of hypnotics, and subjects who took hypnotics but had no insomnia complaints had no significantly greater risk for falls.[54]

Although multiple hypnotics have demonstrated short-term efficacy, there are few long-term data (with the exception of studies on eszopiclone), and only select studies have specifically addressed the elderly population. Nightly administration of longer-acting agents (eg, eszopiclone) or intermittent dosing of shorter-acting agents (eg, zaleplon) seems most rational for patients with advance-related sleep complaints. Eszopiclone (1-2 mg) has shown favorable safety and efficacy in a large randomized controlled study of medically stable elderly individuals with primary insomnia (mean age 72.3 years) for a period of up to 2 weeks.[55] A similar short-term study investigating the use of zaleplon (5-10 mg) in elderly individuals with primary insomnia (mean age 72.5 years) was extended to a single-blinded, open-label phase with favorable results up to 12 months.[56]

Stimulants

Intermittent administration of a stimulant medication to promote evening alertness in patients who have discrete ASPD could be clinically justified, but there are no data addressing this practice. Clinical experience suggests that evening complaints are much less common than morning complaints among this patient population, but individuals occasionally present with reports of evening sleepiness that is socially embarrassing or detrimental to personal relationships.

Behavioral

In all instances, external contributors to advance-related sleep complaints should be pursued and addressed, including avoidance of evening naps.[42,43] As can occur in anyone with chronic sleep maintenance complaints, patients may have a concomitant conditioned insomnia that is often responsive to evidence-based behavioral treatments.[57]

Longitudinal Care

Regardless of which interventions are employed, the patient should be seen in follow-up in approximately 2 months (a sufficient length of time to ascertain benefit and compliance with the prescribed treatments), with the opportunity to contact the provider if questions or concerns arise before that time. A review of accompanying sleep logs or actigraph recordings is essential during this visit so that the timing or nature of interventions can be properly adjusted. Because there are no established guidelines for the longitudinal therapy of this condition, cessation of treatment occurs on a trial and error basis with resumption if symptoms recur. Alternatively, once a desired sleep/wake schedule is established, it can often be maintained with continued adherence to the measures initially employed.

SUMMARY

A thorough assessment of patients with advance-related sleep complaints can facilitate proper diagnostic assignation of a circadian dysrhythmia, which subsequently leads to rational therapy. Although stringent research protocols have demonstrated success of evening light in alleviating complaints, comparable achievements have not been realized in settings that more closely approximate the clinical realm in which patient selection and compliance monitoring are not rigorously observed. Nevertheless, subjective benefits are routinely reported by patients, and the treatment poses few risks. Future research will assist in the determination of optimal light intensity and duration of therapy. Other lesser-studied treatment options include exogenous melatonin, chronotherapy, and hypnotic medications. Stimulant medications may be justified for persons with predominant complaints of evening sleepiness. Proper recommendations regarding avoidance and receipt of light should be provided in all instances. Although the knowledge base surrounding circadian rhythm sleep disorders pales in comparison with that of the circadian biologic sciences, ongoing collaboration between the two arenas will likely yield further important mechanistic insights, ultimately enabling more sophisticated circadian-based treatment interventions.

REFERENCES

1. American Academy of Sleep Medicine. International classification of sleep disorders. Diagnostic and coding manual. 2nd edition. Westchester (IL): American Academy of Sleep Medicine; 2005.

2. Ando K, Kripke DF, Ancoli-Israel S. Estimated prevalence of delayed and advanced sleep phase syndromes [abstract]. J Sleep Res 1995;24:509.

3. Billiard M, Verge M, Aldaz C, et al. A case of advanced-sleep phase syndrome [abstract]. Sleep Research 1993;22:109.

4. Kamei R, Hughes L, Miles L, et al. Advanced-sleep phase syndrome studied in a time isolation facility. Chronobiologia 1979;6:115.

5. Moldofsky H, Musisi S, Phillipson EA. Treatment of a case of advanced sleep phase syndrome by phase advance chronotherapy. Sleep 1986;9(1):61–5.

6. Singer CM, Lewy AJ. Case report: use of the dim light melatonin onset in the treatment of ASPS with bright light [abstract]. Sleep Research 1989;18:445.

7. Campbell SS, Dawson D, Anderson MW. Alleviation of sleep maintenance insomnia with timed exposure to bright light. J Am Geriatr Soc 1993;41(8):829–36.

8. Palmer CR, Kripke DF, Savage HC Jr, et al. Efficacy of enhanced evening light for advanced sleep phase syndrome. Behav Sleep Med 2003;1(4):213–26.

9. Satoh K, Mishima K, Inoue Y, et al. Two pedigrees of familial advanced sleep phase syndrome in Japan. Sleep 2003;26(4):416–7.

10. Carrier J, Monk TH, Buysse DJ, et al. Sleep and morningness-eveningness in the 'middle' years of life (20–59 y). J Sleep Res 1997;6(4):230–7.

11. Ando K, Kripke DF, Ancoli-Israel S. Delayed and advanced sleep phase symptoms. Isr J Psychiatry Relat Sci 2002;39(1):11–8.

12. Ohayon M. Prevalence of DSM-IV diagnostic criteria of insomnia: distinguishing insomnia related to mental disorders from sleep disorders. J Psychiatr Res 1997;31(3):333–46.

13. Lack L, Wright H, Kemp K, et al. The treatment of early-morning awakening insomnia with 2 evenings of bright light. Sleep 2005;28(5):616–23.

14. Cagnacci A, Elliott JA, Yen SS. Melatonin: a major regulator of the circadian rhythm of core temperature in humans. J Clin Endocrinol Metab 1992; 75(2):447–52.

15. Morgenthaler TI, Alessi C, Friedman L, et al. Practice parameters for the use of actigraphy in the assessment of sleep and sleep disorders: an update for 2007. Sleep 2007;30(4):519–29.

16. Sadeh A, Hauri P, Kripke D, et al. The role of actigraphy in the evaluation of sleep disorders. Sleep 1995;18(4):288–302.

17. Bradshaw DA, Yanagi MA, Pak ES, et al. Nightly sleep duration in the 2-week period preceding multiple sleep latency testing. J Clin Sleep Med 2007;3(6):613–9.

18. Varghese R, Slocumb NL, Silber MH, et al. Comparative value of actigraphy versus sleep logs [abstract]. Sleep 2008;31(Abstract Supplement): A334–5.

19. Horne JA, Ostberg O. A self-assessment questionnaire to determine morningness-eveningness in human circadian rhythms. Int J Chronobiol 1976; 4(2):97–110.

20. Sack RL, Auckley D, Auger RR, et al. Circadian rhythm sleep disorders. Part I. Basic principles, shift work and jet lag disorders: an American Academy of Sleep Medicine review. Sleep 2007;30(11):1460–83.

21. Jones C, Campbell S, Zone S, et al. Familial advanced sleep phase syndrome: a short-period circadian rhythm variant in humans. Nat Med 1999; 5(9):1062–5.

22. Sack RL, Auckley D, Auger RR, et al. Circadian rhythm sleep disorders. Part II. Advanced sleep phase disorder, delayed sleep phase disorder, free-running disorder, and irregular sleep-wake rhythm: an American Academy of Sleep Medicine review. Sleep 2007;30(11):1484–501.

23. Burgess HJ, Eastman CI. The dim light melatonin onset following fixed and free sleep schedules. J Sleep Res 2005;14(3):229–37.

24. Lee C, Smith MR, Eastman CI. A compromise phase position for permanent night shift workers: circadian phase after two night shifts with scheduled sleep and light/dark exposure. Chronobiol Int 2006;23(4): 859–75.

25. Lack L, Wright H. The effect of evening bright light in delaying the circadian rhythms and lengthening the

sleep of early morning awakening insomniacs. Sleep 1993;16(5):436–43.

26. Wyatt JK. Delayed sleep phase syndrome: pathophysiology and treatment options. Sleep 2004; 27(6):1195–203.

27. Arand D, Bonnet M, Hurwitz T, et al. The clinical use of the MSLT and MWT. Sleep 2005;28(1):123–44.

28. Khalsa SB, Jewett ME, Cajochen C, et al. A phase response curve to single bright light pulses in human subjects. J Physiol 2003;549(Pt 3):945–52.

29. Rosenthal NE, Joseph-Vanderpool JR, Levendosky AA, et al. Phase-shifting effects of bright morning light as treatment for delayed sleep phase syndrome. Sleep 1990;13(4):354–61.

30. Dawson D, Campbell SS. Timed exposure to bright light improves sleep and alertness during simulated night shifts. Sleep 1991;14(6):511–6.

31. Moline ML, Pollak CP, Monk TH, et al. Age-related differences in recovery from simulated jet lag. Sleep 1992;15(1):28–40.

32. Waterhouse J, Edwards B, Nevill A, et al. Identifying some determinants of "jet lag" and its symptoms: a study of athletes and other travellers. Br J Sports Med 2002;36(1):54–60.

33. Tresguerres JA, Ariznavarreta C, Granados B, et al. Circadian urinary 6-sulphatoxymelatonin, cortisol excretion and locomotor activity in airline pilots during transmeridian flights. J Pineal Res 2001;31(1):16–22.

34. Reid KJ, Chang AM, Dubocovich ML, et al. Familial advanced sleep phase syndrome. Arch Neurol 2001;58(7):1089–94.

35. Toh K, Jones C, He Y, et al. An hPer2 phosphorylation site mutation in familial advanced sleep phase syndrome. Science 2001;291(5506):1040–3.

36. Xu Y, Padiath QS, Shapiro RE, et al. Functional consequences of a CKIdelta mutation causing familial advanced sleep phase syndrome. Nature 2005;434(7033):640–4.

37. Piggins HD. Human clock genes. Ann Med 2002; 34(5):394–400.

38. Pallesen S, Nordhus IH, Skelton SH, et al. Bright light treatment has limited effect in subjects over 55 years with mild early morning awakening. Percept Mot Skills 2005;101(3):759–70.

39. Suhner AG, Murphy PJ, Campbell SS. Failure of timed bright light exposure to alleviate age-related sleep maintenance insomnia. J Am Geriatr Soc 2002;50(4):617–23.

40. Cole R, Smith J, Alcala Y, et al. Bright-light mask treatment of delayed sleep phase syndrome. J Biol Rhythms 2002;17(1):89–101.

41. Apollo Health. BLUEWAVE Technology. Available at: http://www.apollohealth.com/bluewave_light_therapy.html; 2008. Accessed July 8, 2008.

42. Buxton O, L'Hermite-Baleriaux M, Turek F, et al. Daytime naps in darkness phase shift the human circadian rhythms of melatonin and thyrotropin

secretion. Am J Physiol Regul Integr Comp Physiol 2000;278(2):R373–82.

43. Yoon I, Kripke D, Elliott J, et al. Age-related changes of circadian rhythms and sleep-wake cycles. J Am Geriatr Soc 2003;51(8):1085–91.

44. Crowley SJ, Lee C, Tseng CY, et al. Combinations of bright light, scheduled dark, sunglasses, and melatonin to facilitate circadian entrainment to night shift work. J Biol Rhythms 2003;18(6):513–23.

45. Morgenthaler TI, Lee-Chiong T, Alessi C, et al. Response to Zee P, melatonin for the treatment of advanced sleep phase disorder. Sleep 2008;31(7): 925.

46. Lewy AJ. Clinical applications of melatonin in circadian disorders. Dialogues Clin Neurosci 2003;5:399–413.

47. Zee PC. Melatonin for the treatment of advanced sleep phase disorder [letter to the editor]. Sleep 2008;31(7):923.

48. Committee on the Framework for Evaluating the Safety of Dietary Supplements FaNB, Board on Life Sciences, Institute of Medicine and National Research Council of the National Academies. Dietary supplements: a framework for evaluating safety. Washington (DC): The National Academies Press; 2005.

49. Reynolds CF 3rd, Kupfer DJ, Hoch CC, et al. Sleeping pills for the elderly: are they ever justified? J Clin Psychiatry 1985;46(2 Pt 2):9–12.

50. Tinetti M, Speechley M, Ginter S. Risk factors for falls among elderly persons living in the community. N Engl J Med 1988;319(26):1701–7.

51. Wang P, Bohn R, Glynn R, et al. Zolpidem use and hip fractures in older people. J Am Geriatr Soc 2001;49(12):1685–90.

52. Koski K, Luukinen H, Laippala P, et al. Risk factors for major injurious falls among the home-dwelling elderly by functional abilities: a prospective population-based study. Gerontology 1998;44(4):232–8.

53. Brassington G, King A, Bliwise D. Sleep problems as a risk factor for falls in a sample of community-dwelling adults aged 64–99 years. J Am Geriatr Soc 2000;48(10):1234–40.

54. Avidan A, Fries B, James M, et al. Insomnia and hypnotic use, recorded in the minimum data set, as predictors of falls and hip fractures in Michigan nursing homes. J Am Geriatr Soc 2005;53(6):955–62.

55. Scharf M, Erman M, Rosenberg R, et al. A 2-week efficacy and safety study of eszopiclone in elderly patients with primary insomnia. Sleep 2005;28(6): 720–7.

56. Ancoli-Israel S, Richardson G, Mangano R, et al. Long-term use of sedative hypnotics in older patients with insomnia. Sleep Med 2005;6(2):107–13.

57. Morgenthaler T, Kramer M, Alessi C, et al. Practice parameters for the psychological and behavioral treatment of insomnia: an update. An American Academy of Sleep Medicine report. Sleep 2006; 29(11):1415–9.

Delayed Sleep-Phase Disorder

Leon C. Lack, PhD[a],*, Helen R. Wright, PhD[a],
Richard R. Bootzin, PhD[b]

KEYWORDS

- Circadian rhythms • Bright light • Melatonin
- Delayed sleep phase • Period length • Insomnia

Weitzman and colleagues[1,2] first defined delayed sleep-phase syndrome as a syndrome characterized by a delay of the usual sleep period by as much as 2 to 6 hours. According to the most recent *International Classification of Sleep Disorders (ICSD-2)*,[3] the terminology has been altered slightly to delayed sleep-phase disorder (DSPD). Individuals with DSPD have difficulty falling asleep at their desired bedtime and an inability to wake spontaneously at the desired time in the morning. For example, individuals with DSPD may wish to sleep between midnight and 8 AM to meet social or employment obligations. However, if they do go to bed at midnight, they experience sleep-onset insomnia and, if they must awaken at 8 AM, their total sleep time is curtailed. Repeated reduction of total sleep time results in an accumulated sleep debt and daytime sleepiness (especially in the mornings), irritability, and a lack of concentration, all of which can subsequently impair safety, performance at work, and family life.

PREVALENCE AND ETIOLOGY

Estimated prevalence rates for DSPD have ranged from 0.2% to 10% of the population.[1,2,4–6] The apparently large range of these prevalence estimates may be due to variation of the severity criteria for the delayed sleep period. Less severe cases of DSPD (eg, 2 AM to 10 AM sleep period) are likely to be more prevalent than the more extreme delayed cases (eg, 5 AM to 2 PM sleep period). A recent study found the habitual sleep-onset times of patients diagnosed with DSPD varied between about 11:30 PM and 5:15 AM with a majority before 2 AM.[7]

DSPD is associated with delayed endogenous circadian rhythms.[8–14] This includes delayed sleep-timing parameters, melatonin circadian rhythms, and core body temperature rhythms.[11,13,15–17] When core body temperature rhythms and melatonin circadian rhythms are delayed, then the "wake maintenance zone" (WMZ), which occurs about 6 PM and 9 PM in a normally entrained person, is also delayed.[18] For example, if the temperature minimum (CTmin) is delayed until 8 AM to 9 AM, the WMZ will occur from 10 PM to 2 AM, resulting in significant difficulty falling asleep until after 2 AM.[19] In such cases, a person attempting to awaken early for work or other obligations, at 8 AM for example, would be trying to arise around CTmin, the most sleepy circadian time. For this person, waking up would be especially difficult.

Researchers have speculated at the cause of this circadian rhythm phase delay. Putative circadian mechanisms include (1) a diminished response of phase advance to morning light stimulation, (2) enhanced phase-delay response to evening light stimulation, and (3) a longer than normal circadian period length (the time to complete one circadian cycle).[20] Just recently, Campbell and Murphy[21] explored the third possibility in a time-free isolation experiment with one DSPD participant in comparison with three normal control healthy sleepers. The DSPD person showed a consistent circadian period length of about 25.4 hours, 1 hour longer than the average for the three controls. This suggests that DSPD may arise from an inherently longer circadian

[a] School of Psychology, Flinders University, GPO Box 2100, Adelaide, SA 5001 Australia
[b] Department of Psychology, University of Arizona, Tucson, AZ 85721-0068, USA
* Corresponding author.
E-mail address: leon.lack@flinders.edu.au (L.C. Lack).

Sleep Med Clin 4 (2009) 229–239
doi:10.1016/j.jsmc.2009.01.006

period length, resulting in an unrelenting tendency to phase delay in our 24-hour world. This would imply that the DSPD patient is required to phase advance by 1 to 1.5 hours every day to remain synchronized with the 24-hour world. The fact that this seems to be possible most of the time for DSPD patients is somewhat surprising. It perhaps can be explained by the likelihood that their awakenings are usually later in the morning in the presence of generally stronger phase-advancing ambient light and the likelihood that the timing of this exposure to light is when it is most effective for phase-advancing their rhythms (eg, very soon after their temperature minimums). The possible genetic basis for this inherent tendency is being investigated.[22]

Although circadian rhythm phase delay is seen as the major contributor to DSPD, some behavioral and psychological factors are also likely to be important contributors, which should also be addressed to improve treatment effectiveness. The circadian phase delayed individual is likely to feel better in the evenings than in the mornings as indicated by their preference for doing things in the evening according to their responses in the Morning/Evening questionnaire.[23] They may want to prolong this period by staying up later. In addition, they are likely to engage in activities that interfere with sleep onset and sleep quality, including late-night socializing, computer use, and mobile phone use.[24–28] However, later bedtimes also tend to delay morning awakenings. "Sleeping in" leads to further delays of the circadian rhythm, which thus exacerbate the DSPD.[29–31] Because of this vicious cycle of circadian rhythm phase delay leading to behavior that further magnifies the circadian rhythm phase delay, therapies must address both behavior and circadian rhythm phase delay to be most effective.

When anticipating a necessary early awakening (eg, 8 AM), the DSPD sufferer is likely to attempt an earlier bedtime (eg, midnight would be "early" for them) in the hopes of obtaining sufficient sleep. However, because this bedtime is still within the circadian wake-maintenance or alert zone, DSPD sufferer will take a long time to fall asleep and the experience is likely to be frustrating or worrying. This frustration or worry may activate the "fight or flight" response and heightened arousal, which further inhibits sleep onset. Repetition of this experience over many nights can lead to more persistent conditioned or psychophysiologic insomnia. Even when DSPD sufferers sleep at their most preferred sleep time, they show evidence of having some sleep-onset insomnia. At these preferred later bedtimes, they had sleep-onset latencies that were still significantly

and clinically lengthened to 32 minutes versus 10 minutes for controls in one study[14] and to 38 minutes versus 17 minutes for controls in another study.[21] Therefore, in addition to a delayed circadian rhythm, DSPD sufferers are likely to have persistent sleep-onset insomnia.

In DSPD, behavioral or psychological factors, as well as the delayed circadian rhythm, may contribute to difficulty awakening in the morning. On those occasions when the DSPD sufferer is forced to awaken close to the circadian nadir (which is probably quite common), they experience lethargy, reduced motivation, irritability, or even mild depression. Falling back to sleep avoids these aversive experiences. Thus, the resumption of sleep rewards the sufferer by providing a way to avoid the morning period. Seeking this reward, the DSPD person could fall into a pattern of persistent conditioned sleep resumption. This possible conditioned sleep resumption also needs to be addressed in therapy. Furthermore, individuals with DSPD who must awaken for school or work may be more likely to use stimulants (eg, caffeine, nicotine) to stay awake. This may lead to a vicious cycle in which the use of stimulants delays sleep onset and produces further phase delays.[32] Therefore, the clinician should be alert to the possibility of multiple factors playing a role in DSPD and be willing to use therapies addressing those factors in addition to therapies dealing with circadian factors.[33]

CLINICAL DIAGNOSIS AND ASSESSMENT

It is suggested that virtually all DSPD patients score as extreme evening types although not all evening types report the distress required for a diagnosis of DSPD. Perhaps many of these non-distressed extreme evening types have adapted their lifestyles to accommodate delayed circadian rhythms.[34]

Diagnosis of a delayed sleep-wake schedule is made from a 1- to 2-week sleep-wake diary and actigraphy if available.[35] Sleep parameters documented on the diaries include bedtime and lights-out time, sleep-onset latency (SOL), time spent awake during the night after sleep onset (wake after sleep onset [WASO]), final wake-up time (including whether or not an alarm (AI) was needed), and estimated total sleep time (TST). Time of food, caffeine, and alcohol intake during the day is also entered on the diary each evening. Any change of sleep pattern between weekdays and weekends should be noted. **Fig. 1** is the 1-week sleep-wake diary of a 19-year-old university student with DSPD. The diary illustrates a delayed sleep pattern and sleep-onset difficulty. Despite bedtimes around midnight, his average

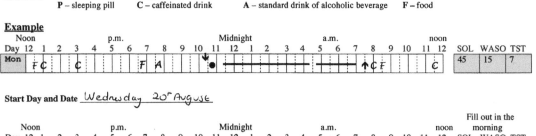

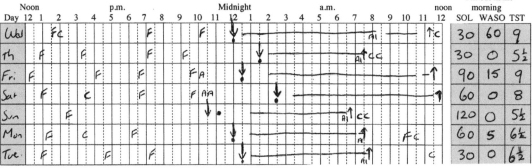

Fig. 1. A 1-week sleep-wake diary from a 19-year-old client indicating a delayed bedtime and wake-up time when an alarm did not result in an awakening. Explanations for symbols used appear at the top of the diary. Each line graph reflects a 24-hour day from 9 AM. Sleep-onset latency (SOL), time spent awake during the night (WASO) and total sleep time (TST) are estimated in the morning. Food, caffeine, alcohol, bedtime, and lights-out time are completed in the evening. (*Courtesy of* Dr. Michael Gradisar, Flinders University.)

sleep-onset time was between 1 AM and 2 AM. On one weekday morning, he slept through the alarm and woke spontaneously at 10:30 AM. On the weekend, he was able to sleep in until 11:30 AM. His total sleep time during the week averaged about 6 hours per night and on weekends 8 to 9 hours per night. Caffeine and alcohol intake were not excessive and meals appeared to be eaten at regular times, although his first meal was not until 10 AM to 11 AM each day. Typically, clients with DSPD have a decreased appetite in the early morning.

Fig. 2 shows the wrist actigraphy recording corresponding with the same 1-week sleep-wake diary above. At lights-out time and final wake-up time, he was instructed to move his hand for 2 minutes, resulting in the spikes on the actigram.

Chronotype questionnaires may be helpful in assessing the degree of "eveningness" and thus the probable degree of phase delay.[23,36] Self-assessment of "eveningness" is associated with a delayed sleep pattern,[37–39] a delayed temperature rhythm,[40] and a delayed melatonin rhythm.[41]

THERAPIES FOR DELAYED SLEEP-PHASE DISORDER

Treatments that change the circadian rhythm phase or timing, such as morning bright light, exogenous melatonin, and chronotherapy, have

been effective in treating delayed circadian rhythm sleep disorders.

Because of the very strong tendency for those with DSPD to phase delay, treatments to phase advance take longer and are more difficult than phase delaying the same degree of phase change or number of hours to achieve the target sleep period. For example, in a DSPD case with an unconstrained sleep period from 6 AM to 3 PM and target sleep period of midnight to 8 AM, a 6-hour phase advance may be more difficult and time consuming to achieve than an 18-hour delay to reach the target sleep period. A decision needs to be made as to whether it would be more efficacious, practical, and preferable for the client with DSPD to attempt the phase-advance therapy (morning bright light and evening melatonin) or the phase-delay therapy (chronotherapy). Individuals with less extreme phase delays (eg, less than 4 hours) would be advised to use a phase-advancing therapy and those with more extreme delays (eg, more than 6 hours) would be advised to use a phase-delay therapy, such as chronotherapy. The decision to use an advance or delay treatment schedule for those DSPD clients with a delay of about 5 hours from their target sleep period (4–6 hours) may depend more on convenience and palatability of the therapy rather than the precise amount of estimated delay.

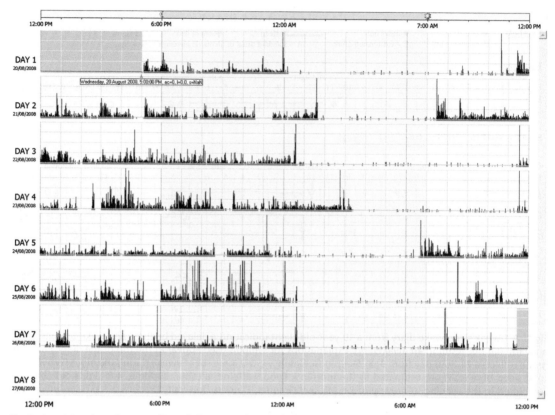

Fig. 2. A wrist actigraphy recording of the same client reflecting the sleep-wake diary. Vertical lines indicate the amount of activity in 1-minute epochs. (*Courtesy of* Dr. Michael Gradisar, Flinders University.)

MORNING BRIGHT-LIGHT THERAPY

Bright light is an effective intervention for phase advancing the circadian rhythm. The timing and duration of the light stimulus as well as the brightness and wavelength of light affect the magnitude of phase shift. The human phase response curve to light suggests a phase advance of the circadian rhythm is achieved when the light stimulus is presented immediately after the time at which core body temperature reaches CTmin, its endogenous minimum.[42–45]

Measuring CTmin or dim-light melatonin onset (DLMO) is expensive and time consuming. In good sleepers, an estimation of circadian timing has been derived from sleep-wake diaries with wake-up time able to predict DLMO within about 1 hour.[46–48] However, we found these correlations to be only moderate in those with a delayed circadian phase.[49] This finding is consistent with studies that have shown an altered phase relationship between CTmin or melatonin and the sleep-wake cycle in patients with DSPD.[11,15,17,21,50] However, to have an approximation of these parameters is valuable for determining treatment options. For good sleepers, CTmin is

approximately 2 hours before the spontaneous final wake-up time.[51] For predicting circadian timing, days of unconstrained sleep periods are more useful than days of forced awakening times.[46] For that reason phase estimation in those with DSPD should be made from the average ad lib sleep of preferably 2 weekends.

A few studies have used bright-light stimulation to advance the endogenous rhythm of people with DSPD.[12,42,52,53] Rosenthal and colleagues[12] evaluated the effects of 2 weeks of bright light (2500 lux) administered for 2 hours between 6 AM and 9 AM. Investigators found that CTmin advanced by 1 hour and 25 minutes and participants reported earlier sleep-onset times and increased morning alertness. In a study involving participants with sleep-onset insomnia and some DSPD, both DLMO and sleep-onset time advanced by about 1 hour following 1 week of 1-hour morning white light of 2500 lux.[52] In another study, the DLMO of participants with DSPD was advanced by over 2.5 hours after 1 week of 2-hour doses of 1000-lux blue light.[53]

Outdoor bright light is usually the most effective form of light. During the darker winter months, artificial lighting may be preferable or essential.

Generally, artificial broad-spectrum white light has been used to phase shift circadian rhythms. However, more recently, a maximal chronobiotic effect has been found for wavelengths in the blue end (420–500 nm) of the visible spectrum.[54–57]

LIFESTYLE CONSIDERATIONS

Before commencing light therapy, the clients' sleep and wake-up time goals need to be determined realistically, taking into account motivation to change their current sleep-wake schedule, difficulties with compliance to the treatment, and the amount of phase change required. If clients have significant early-morning obligations, then the motivation to comply with therapy instructions should be sufficient. On the other hand, simply the desire to achieve a more "normal" wake-up time without any morning obligations is unlikely to be sufficient motivation for adequate treatment compliance and long-term therapeutic success.

An expected outcome of a successful phase advance is that individuals will experience evening sleepiness rather than evening alertness. We advocate that during and after therapy any stimulating or obligatory activities now be pursued in the morning rather than the evening. The evenings should be time of relaxation under dim lighting. Such changes to lifestyle habits and attitude need to be discussed to ensure compliance and satisfaction with the therapy. Work, leisure, and family commitments need to be considered before commencing the therapy, and clients are encouraged to seek support from family members. The therapist and client need to work out the best time to commence therapy to ensure the least disturbance between the therapy schedule and the work/social schedule.

APPLICATION OF MORNING BRIGHT-LIGHT THERAPY

After estimating the CTmin from the sleep-wake diaries, a schedule for light exposure can be established, taking into account the client's practical obligations. Ideally, this schedule involves slowly advancing morning light exposure by 30 minutes each morning or alternate mornings until the target wake-up time is reached. Light exposure for at least 1 to 2 hours commencing about 1hour after the estimated CTmin is recommended. However, if the client's sleep-wake pattern is quite variable and the therapist is not confident of the estimated CTmin, it is prudent to commence light therapy at the time of spontaneous awakening from an unconstrained ad lib sleep period. In our example (see **Figs. 1** and **2**), the client wished to sleep between the hours of 11 PM and 7 AM. From his ad lib sleep episodes over the weekend, his estimated CTmin was about 9:30 AM and would thus require at least a 3.5-hour phase advance to 6 AM to achieve a more normal circadian and sleep-period phase relationship. **Fig. 3** shows a suggested bright-light protocol for this client. Bright-light therapy for at least 1 hour would begin just after 10:30 AM on the first morning and

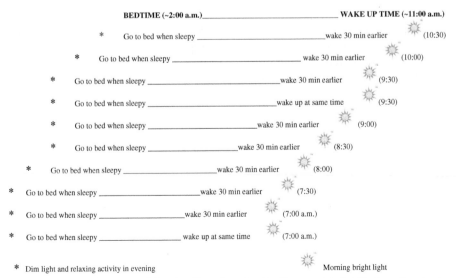

Fig. 3. A suggested bright-light protocol for the client described in **Figs. 1** and **2**. Ad lib sleep time is about 2 AM to 11 AM and target sleep time is between 11 PM and 7 AM. Asterisks denote dim light and quiet activity in the evening. The sun symbol denotes bright light (sunlight or artificial light source). Clients are reminded to go to bed only when feeling sleepy.

advance by about 30 minutes each day along with wake time (or perhaps advance 30 minutes every 2 days) until the target wake-up time has been reached. At that point, we recommend the continuation of light therapy, starting at the target wake-up time for at least another 7 mornings, including a weekend.[53]

To avoid a "reverse effect" (phase delay), it is important to precede the timed bright-light exposure with darkness or very dim light and to follow the bright-light exposure period with continued light exposure for preferably 2 to 3 hours, as intense as practicable. Therefore, it is usually best for clients to commence light therapy on a weekend when they usually have no work commitments. The client should not retreat to darkness or dim light following the bright-light pulse. If, during the therapy period, the client has early work/study commitments that require him or her to be outside before the start of the scheduled light pulse, then sunglasses need to be worn before that time. For example, if the client needs to leave for work at 7:30 AM but light exposure is not recommended until 8:30 AM for that morning, then dark glasses need to be worn on the way to work until 8:30 AM. Although neutral-density dark glasses are helpful, blue-blocking glasses that filter out more of the short-wavelength light may be more effective while allowing adequate visual intensity.

Since outdoor morning bright light is usually the most effective form of lighting following treatment, clients are encouraged to regularly eat breakfast outside or in a room exposed to bright morning light. They are asked not to wear sunglasses when they leave for work or school.

In winter, artificial light sources, such as commercially available light devices, may be necessary. Clients are encouraged to eat breakfast, read, work on a computer, or watch television, as long as they continue to gaze in the direction of the light if using a fixed-position light source. Some portable light-therapy devices now available have a light source that moves with the direction of the gaze, thus accommodating client mobility and enhancing compliance. We suggest that clients follow the instructions of the light device for method of use (eg, distance from light source). The brighter the light source (eg, the closer it is) and the longer its use, the greater will be the effect in phase changing the circadian rhythm. However, if side effects, such as eye irritations, headaches, or nausea, are experienced, then brightness and duration should be reduced,[58] but number of administrations increased.

We suggest that the client engage in relaxing and pleasant activities in the evening, especially 1 hour before bedtime and preferably in dim light. Studies have shown that using computers and playing computer games not only increase sleep latency,[25] but also can suppress nocturnal melatonin.[59] Similarly, adolescents who watch late-night television or receive or send text messages after lights are out are more likely to delay and disrupt their sleep.[24,26–28] Because evening is the time when individuals with DSPD habitually study, socialize, and are generally active, these lifestyle habits need to be changed. This can be a difficult part of the therapy because change in lifestyle requires some adjustment, discussion, and planning alternative activities to ensure success. In addition, caffeine, nicotine, and other stimulants should be avoided in the latter part of the day.

Following the advance in wake-up time, there will be a gradual phase advance in the time at which the individual starts to feel sleepy and is able to initiate sleep in the evening. However, this will probably not occur as quickly as the advance of wake-up time. For example, although Mundey and colleagues[7] found a phase advance of about 100 minutes in circadian rhythm, the 27-minute phase advance of sleep-onset time was not significant. Thus, during the initial treatment period, until sleep onset is advanced as much as wake-up time, the client may experience some sleep restriction and daytime sleepiness. However, it is not advisable to have a long nap during the day as this will reduce homeostatic sleep drive and inhibit an early sleep onset. On the other hand, napping research has shown that a brief 10-minute nap can alleviate sleepiness in the short term (up to 3 hours) without longer-term effects on nocturnal sleep.[60]

To prevent a relapse, we recommend that sleeping in, even after a late night, should be avoided or at least minimized. If a phase delay occurs after a sleep-in, then phase advancing using morning bright-light exposure is again recommended. The client should also continue exposure to morning bright light and avoid wearing sunglasses in the morning if possible. If, however, the client is walking or driving into the sun in the morning and needs protection, then blue-tinted sunglasses are appropriate for the capacity to diminish glare without decreasing the effective phase-advancing properties of shorter-wavelength light.[56] Booster administrations of morning bright light will be required if the sleep pattern again starts delaying.

MELATONIN

Exogenous melatonin administration is also capable of shifting the circadian rhythm to a more desired time.[61] Phase response curves for melatonin administration show that melatonin in the early evening phase advances the rhythm. The maximum advance occurs when multiple 3-mg doses are administered approximately 5 hours before the original DLMO or smaller doses (0.5 mg) are administered approximately 3 hours before the estimated DLMO.[62–64] For good sleepers, DLMO occurs approximately 2 hours before sleep onset.[7] Although this time interval may vary in people with DSPD,[15] one study found no difference between those with DSPD and a control group in the timing of melatonin onset relative to sleep onset.[13]

Various studies have evaluated the effect of exogenous melatonin on patients with DSPD. Varying doses, times, and number of doses make it difficult to compare studies. Nevertheless, early evening melatonin administration has resulted in phase advances,[7,9,65] improved physical and social functioning and mental health,[66] less daytime sleepiness and fatigue,[67] and overall sleep improvement.[68] A recent study[64] showed that the addition of evening melatonin treatment to morning bright-light therapy produced a significantly greater phase advance than that from morning bright light alone, suggesting that the effects of evening melatonin administration and morning bright light are additive. Melatonin doses of 0.3 or 0.5 mg can be administered 2 hours before estimated DLMO or 4 hours before estimated sleep-onset time.[61] In our example (see **Fig. 1**) melatonin would be administered about 10 PM on the first evening, and this time advanced by 30 minutes along with the advance of morning bright-light exposure and wake-up time as suggested by Lockley.[69] The final melatonin administration time would then be about 7 PM for the target bedtime of 11 PM.

Although exogenous melatonin appears safe with short-term use (less than 3 months), little information is available on its long-term administration.[70] The chronobiotic effects of lower doses (0.3–0.5 mg) appear to be as great as those for higher doses without requiring excessive supraphysiologic levels.[64] Some adverse side effects that have been reported following melatonin administration include headaches, dizziness, nausea, and drowsiness.[70]

Melatonin receptor agonists also have been shown to have chronobiotic effects on the circadian phase of healthy adults[71–73] and can also decrease sleep-onset latency in those with insomnia.[74–78] However, while melatonin receptor agonists might be expected to be effective in patients with DSPD, the use of melatonin receptor agonists in such an application has not been evaluated.

CHRONOTHERAPY

Chronotherapy involves progressively delaying bedtime each day until the desired bedtime for the individual has been reached.[2,79] The treatment shifts the individual's light-dark cycle as well as sleep period, and exposes the individual to light before the scheduled bedtime in the phase-delay portion of the phase-response curve, consequently facilitating the delay of the circadian rhythm.[80] Contributing to the phase delay is the endogenous tendency in most individuals for phase delaying relative to the 24-hour clock. Thus, free of 24-hour entraining cues (eg, a fixed 24 hour light-dark cycle), it would be expected that individuals with DSPD should also naturally phase delay each day by as much as 1.5 hours.[21,81]

Although an effective long-term treatment, chronotherapy can be difficult to implement because it can take from 8 to 10 days to complete. It is essential to draw up the phase-delaying protocol so that any necessary social and work activities can be planned around the programmed sleep and wake schedule.

We recommend 2-hour delays of the sleep period until the target bedtime and wake time have been reached. The original recommendations for more rapid 3-hour delays of bedtime could result, after a few days' administration, in inadvertent bright-light exposure following CTmin. This could inhibit the delay of circadian phase and result in an unsuccessful outcome following this arduous procedure. Two-hour delays ensure that the planned sleep-onset time and thus light exposure always occur before the CTmin and thus facilitate the delay process. Light before the sleep period (preferably outdoor sunlight or bright indoor light) and dim light (or blue-blocking glasses to filter out blue/green wavelengths) after the sleep period will enhance a phase delay.

When the target bed period is achieved, it is necessary to switch the timing of light relative to sleep to ensure bright-light exposure is in the morning and dim light is in the evening. Following chronotherapy, the client is advised to maintain a consistent sleep-wake schedule and to refrain from sleeping in.

BEHAVIORAL STRATEGIES

The conditioned activation response associated with sleep-onset insomnia can be ameliorated with the application of behavior therapy, such as stimulus control therapy.[82,83] For clients undergoing morning bright-light therapy, the time at which they are able to initiate sleep may advance slower than their bedtime if they advance their bedtime at the same pace as their wake-up time. This can produce lengthened sleep latencies and lead to the development or worsening of psychophysiologic insomnia. To prevent this problem, we ask clients to follow stimulus control therapy instructions.[82,84] They are encouraged in particular to go to bed only when feelings of sleepiness are apparent, as indicated in **Fig. 3**. If not asleep within 10 to 15 minutes, they should get out of bed and return to bed later when feeling sleepy again. Other activities, such as reading, watching television, talking on the phone, using computers, and eating are not to be performed in the bed or the bedroom.

In addition to problems with sleep, individuals who have the most delayed circadian sleep times have increased comorbid emotional and substance-abuse problems.[32,85] Consequently, simultaneous treatments to enhance social and emotional functioning, along with treatments for sleep, are likely to be beneficial.

SUMMARY

DSPD can range from mild to severe and affects not only an individual's sleep but also daytime functioning. A comprehensive assessment is necessary to reliably estimate the degree of circadian phase delay and thus determine the most effective treatment (morning bright light or chronotherapy). For phase advancing the circadian rhythms and sleep-wake cycle, the recommendation is a schedule of incremental advances of wake-up time and morning bright light as well as low-dose early-evening melatonin administration. It is also important to treat any psychophysiological insomnia with cognitive/behavior therapy. For the more extremely delayed DSPD individual, chronotherapy involving delays of scheduled sleep period in increments of 2 hours is recommended. Following either therapy, maintenance of consistent wake times, exposure to morning light, changes in lifestyle, and improvement of attitudes about morning times are also recommended to help prevent relapse.

Therefore, the treatment of DSPD needs to employ methods that focus on all the potential contributing factors, such as circadian phase delay, psychophysiological insomnia, and lifestyle issues.

REFERENCES

1. Weitzman ED, Czeisler CA, Coleman R, et al. Delayed sleep phase syndrome: a biological rhythm disorder. Sleep Res 1979;8:221.
2. Weitzman ED, Czeisler CA, Coleman RM, et al. Delayed sleep phase syndrome: a chronobiological disorder with sleep-onset insomnia. Arch Gen Psychiatry 1981;38:137–46.
3. American Academy of Sleep Medicine. International classification of sleep disorders. In: Diagnostic and coding manual. 2nd edition. Westchester (OL): American Academy of Sleep Medicine; 2005.
4. Lack LC. Delayed sleep and sleep loss in university students. J Am Coll Health 1986;35:105–10.
5. Pelayo RP, Thorpy MJ, Glovinsky P. Prevalence of delayed sleep phase syndrome among adolescents. J Sleep Res 1988;17:392.
6. Schrader H, Bovim G, Sand T. The prevalence of delayed and advanced sleep phase syndromes. J Sleep Res 1993;2:51–5.
7. Mundey K, Benloucif S, Harsanyi K, et al. Phase-dependent treatment of delayed sleep phase syndrome with melatonin. Sleep 2005;28:1271–8.
8. Kerkhof G, Van Vianen B. Circadian phase estimation of chronic insomniacs relates to their sleep characteristics. Arch Physiol Biochem 1999;107:383–92.
9. Nagtegaal JE, Kerkhof GA, Smits MG, et al. Delayed sleep phase syndrome: a placebo-controlled cross-over study on the effects of melatonin administered five hours before the individual dim light melatonin onset. J Sleep Res 1998;7:135–43.
10. Oren DA, Turner EH, Wehr TA. Abnormal circadian rhythms of plasma melatonin and body temperature in the delayed sleep phase syndrome. J Neurol Neurosurg Psychiatr 1995;58:379.
11. Ozaki S, Uchiyama M, Shirakawa S, et al. Prolonged interval from body temperature nadir to sleep offset in patients with delayed sleep phase syndrome. Sleep 1996;19:36–40.
12. Rosenthal NE, Joseph-Vanderpool JR, Levendosky AA, et al. Phase-shifting effects of bright morning light as treatment for delayed sleep phase syndrome. Sleep 1990;13:354–61.
13. Shibui K, Uchiyama M, Okawa M. Melatonin rhythms in delayed sleep phase syndrome. J Biol Rhythms 1999;14:72–6.
14. Wagner DR, Moline ML, Pollack CP, et al. Entrained sleep and temperature rhythms in delayed sleep phase syndrome. Sleep Res 1986;15:179.
15. Rodenbeck A, Huether G, Rüther E, et al. Altered circadian melatonin secretion patterns in relation to sleep in patients with chronic sleep-wake rhythm disorders. J Pineal Res 1998;25:201–10.
16. Shibu K, Uchiuama M, Kim K, et al. Melatonin, cortisol and thyroid-stimulating hormone rhythms are delayed in patients with delayed sleep phase syndrome. Sleep Biol Rhythms 2003;1:209–14.
17. Watanabe T, Kajimura N, Kato M, et al. Sleep and circadian rhythm disturbances in patients with delayed sleep phase syndrome. Sleep 2003;26:657–61.
18. Strogatz SH, Kronauer RE. Circadian wake maintenance zones and insomnia in man. Sleep Res 1985;14:219.

19. Morris M, Lack L, Dawson D. Sleep-onset insomniacs have delayed temperature rhythms. Sleep 1990;13:1–14.

20. Reid KJ, Burgess HJ. Circadian rhythm sleep disorders. Prim Care 2005;32:449–73.

21. Campbell SS, Murphy PJ. Delayed sleep phase disorder in temporal isolation. Sleep 2007;30:1225–8.

22. Archer SN, Robilliard DL, Skene DJ, et al. A length polymorphism in the circadian clock gene Per3 is linked to delayed sleep phase syndrome and extreme diurnal preference. Sleep 2003;26(4):413–5.

23. Horne JA, Östberg O. A self-assessment questionnaire to determine morningness-eveningness in human circadian rhythms. Int J Chronobiol 1976;4:97–110.

24. Dworak M, Schierl T, Bruns T, et al. Impact of singular excessive computer game and television exposure on sleep patterns and memory performance of school-aged children. Pediatrics 2007;120:978–85.

25. Higuchi S, Motohashi Y, Liu Y, et al. Effects of playing a computer game using a bright display on presleep physiological variables, sleep latency, slow wave sleep and REM sleep. J Sleep Res 2005;14:267–73.

26. Li S, Jin X, Wu S, et al. The impact of media use on sleep patterns and sleep disorders among school-aged children in China. Sleep 2007;30:361–7.

27. Suganuma N, Kikuchi T, Yanagi K, et al. Using electronic media before sleep can curtail sleep time and result in self-perceived insufficient sleep. Sleep Biol Rhythms 2007;5:204–14.

28. Van den Bulck J. Adolescent use of mobile phones for calling and for sending text messages after lights out: results from a prospective cohort study with a one-year follow-up. Sleep 2007;30:1220–3.

29. Yang C-M, Spielman A, D'Ambrosio P, et al. A single dose of melatonin prevents the phase delay associated with delayed weekend sleep pattern. Sleep 2001;24:272–81.

30. Burgess HJ, Eastman CI. A late wake time phase delays the human dim light melatonin rhythm. Neurosci Lett 2006;395:191–5.

31. Taylor A, Lack L, Wright H. Sleeping-in on the weekend delays circadian phase and increases sleepiness the following week. Sleep Biol Rhythms 2008;6:172–9.

32. Wittmann M, Dinich J, Merrow M, et al. Social jetlag: misalignment of biological and social time. Chronobiol Int 2006;23:497–509.

33. Campbell SS. Intrinsic disruption of normal sleep and circadian patterns. In: Turek FW, Zee PC, editors. Regulation of sleep and circadian rhythms. New York: Marcel Dekker; 1999. p. 465–8.

34. Zee PC. Delayed sleep phase disorder: psychiatric disturbances. J Sleep Res 2008;17(Supp 1):S45.

35. Littner M, Kushida CA, Anderson WM. Practice parameters for the role of actigraphy in the study of sleep and circadian rhythms: an update for 2002. Sleep 2003;26:337–41.

36. Roenneberg T, Wirz-Justice A, Merrow M. Life between clocks: daily temporal patterns of human chronotypes. J Biol Rhythms 2003;18:80–90.

37. Lack L, Bailey M. Endogenous circadian rhythms of evening and morning types. Sleep Res 1994;23:501.

38. Mongrain V, Lavoie S, Selmaoui B, et al. Phase relationships between sleep-wake cycle and underlying circadian rhythms in morningness-eveningness. J Biol Rhythms 2004;19:248–57.

39. Taillard J, Philip P, Chastang JF, et al. Validation of Horne and Ostberg morningness-eveningness questionnaire in a middle-aged population of French workers. J Biol Rhythms 2004;19:76–86.

40. Kerkhof GA, Van Dongen HP. Morning-type and evening-type individuals differ in the phase position of their endogenous circadian oscillator. Neurosci Lett 1996;218:153–6.

41. Gibertini M, Graham C, Cook MR. Self-report of circadian type reflects the phase of the melatonin rhythm. Biol Psychol 1999;50:19–33.

42. Czeisler CA, Kronauer RE, Allan JS, et al. Bright light induction of strong (type 0) resetting of the human circadian pacemaker. Science 1989;244(4910):1328–33.

43. Dawson D, Lack L, Morris M. Phase resetting of the human circadian pacemaker with use of a single pulse of bright light. Chronobiol Int 1993;10:94–102.

44. Lewy A, Sack R, Fredrickson R, et al. The use of bright light in the treatment of chronobiologic sleep and mood disorders: the phase-response curve. Psychopharmacol Bull 1983;19:523–5.

45. Minors DS, Waterhouse JM, Wirz-Justice A. A human phase-response curve to light. Neurosci Lett 1991;133:36–40.

46. Burgess HJ, Eastman CI. The dim light melatonin onset following fixed and free sleep schedules. J Sleep Res 2005;14:229–37.

47. Burgess HJ, Savic N, Sletten T, et al. The relationship between the dim light melatonin onset and sleep on a regular schedule in young healthy adults. Behav Sleep Med 2003;1:102–14.

48. Martin SK, Eastman CI. Sleep logs of young adults with self-selected sleep times predict the dim light melatonin onset. Chronobiol Int 2002;19:695–707.

49. Wright H, Lack L, Bootzin R. Relationship between dim light melatonin onset and the timing of sleep in sleep in sleep onset insomniacs. Sleep Biol Rhythms 2006;4:78–80.

50. Uchiyama M, Okawa M, Shibui K, et al. Altered phase relation between sleep timing and core body temperature in delayed sleep phase syndrome and non-24-hour sleep-wake syndrome in humans. Neurosci Lett 2000;294:101–4.

51. Dijk D-J, Lockley SW. Integration of human sleep-wake regulation and circadian rhythmicity. J Appl Phys 2002;92:852–62.

52. Lack L, Wright H, Paynter D. The treatment of sleep onset insomnia with morning b light. Sleep Biol Rhythms 2007;5:173–9.

53. Lack L, Bramwell T, Wright H. Morning bright blue light can advance the melatonin rhythm in mild delayed sleep phase syndrome. Sleep Biol Rhythms 2007;5:78–80.

54. Brainard GC, Hanifin JP, Greeson JM, et al. Action spectrum for melatonin regulation in humans: evidence for a novel circadian photoreceptor. J Neurosci 2001;21:6405–12.

55. Wright HR, Lack LC. Effect of wavelength on suppression and phase delay of the melatonin rhythm. Chronobiol Int 2001;18:801–8.

56. Wright HR, Lack LC, Kennaway DJ. Differential effects of light wavelength in phase advancing the melatonin rhythm. J Pineal Res 2004;35:1–5.

57. Warman VL, Dijk D-J, Warman GR, et al. Phase advancing human circadian rhythms with short wavelength light. Neurosci Lett 2003;342:37–40.

58. Chesson AL, Littner M, Davila D, et al. Practice parameters for the use of light therapy in the treatment of sleep disorders. Sleep 1999;22:641–60.

59. Higuchi S, Motohashi Y, Liu Y, et al. Effect of VDT tasks with a bright display at night on melatonin, core temperature, heart rate, and sleepiness. J Appl Physiol 2003;94:1773–6.

60. Brooks A, Lack LC. A brief afternoon nap following nocturnal sleep restriction: which nap duration is most recuperative? Sleep 2006;29:831–40.

61. Sack R, Lewy A, Hughes R. Use of melatonin for sleep and circadian rhythm disorders. Annu Mediaev 1998;30:115–21.

62. Burgess HJ, Revell VL, Eastman CI. A three pulse phase response curve to three milligrams of melatonin in humans. J Physiol 2008;586(2):639–47.

63. Lewy AJ, Bauer VK, Ahmed S, et al. The human phase response curve (PRC) to melatonin is about 12 hours out of phase with the PRC to light. Chronobiol Int 1998;15:71–83.

64. Revell VL, Burgess HJ, Gazda CJ, et al. Advancing human circadian rhythms with afternoon melatonin and morning intermittent bright light. J Clin Endocrinol Metab 2006;91:54–9.

65. Dahlitz M, Alvarez B, Vignau J, et al. Delayed sleep phase syndrome response to melatonin. Lancet 1991;337:1121–4.

66. Nagtegaal JE, Laurant MW, Kerkhof GA, et al. Effects of melatonin on the quality of life in patients with delayed sleep phase syndrome. J Psychosom Res 2000;48:45–50.

67. Kayamov L, Brown G, Jindal R, et al. A randomised, double-blind, placebo-controlled crossover study of the effect of exogenous melatonin on delayed sleep phase syndrome. Psychosom Med 2001;63:40–8.

68. Dagan Y, Yovel I, Hallis D, et al. Evaluating the role of melatonin in the long-term treatment of delayed sleep phase syndrome (DSPS). Chronobiol Int 1998;15:181–90.

69. Lockley SW. Timed melatonin treatment for delayed sleep phase syndrome: the importance of knowing circadian phase. Sleep 2005;28:1214–6.

70. Buscemi N, Vandermeer B, Hooton N, et al. The efficacy and safety of exogenous melatonin for primary sleep disorders a meta-analysis. J Gen Intern Med 2005;20:1151–8.

71. Kräuchi K, Cajochen C, Möri D, et al. Early evening melatonin and S-20098 advance circadian phase and nocturnal regulation of core body temperature. Am J Phys 1997;272:R1178–88.

72. Leproult R, Van Onderbergen A, L'Hermite-Balériaux M, et al. Phase-shifts of 24-h rhythms of hormonal release and body temperature following early evening administration of the melatonin agonist agomelatine in healthy older men. Clin Endocrinol (Oxf) 2005;63:298–304.

73. Nickelsen T, Samel A, Vejvoda M, et al. Chronobiotic effects of the melatonin agonist LY 156735 following a simulated 9h time shift: results of a placebo-controlled trial. Chronobiol Int 2002;19:915–36.

74. Mini L, Wang-Weigand S, Zhang J. Ramelton 8mg/d versus placebo in patients with chronic insomnia: post hoc analysis of a 5-week trial using 50% or greater reduction in latency to persistent sleep as a measure of treatment effect. Clin Ther 2008;30:1316–23.

75. Simpson D, Curran MP. Ramelteon: a review of its use in insomnia. Drugs 2008;68:1901–19.

76. Roth T, Seiden D, Sainati S, et al. Effects of ramelteon on patient-reported sleep latency in older adults with chronic insomnia. Sleep Med 2006;7:312–8.

77. Zammit G, Erman M, Wang-Weigand S, et al. Evaluation of the efficacy and safety of ramelteon in subjects with chronic insomnia. J Clin Sleep Med 2007;3:495–504.

78. Zemlan FP, Mulchahey J, Scharf MB, et al. The efficacy and safety of the melatonin agonist ß-methyl-6-chloromelatonin in primary insomnia: a randomized, placebo-controlled crossover clinical trial. J Clin Psychiatry 2005;66:384–90.

79. Czeisler CA, Richardson GS, Coleman RM, et al. Chronotherapy: resetting the circadian clocks of patients with delayed sleep phase insomnia. Sleep 1981;4:1–21.

80. Hughes R, Lewy A. Light and melatonin treatment of circadian phase sleep disorders. In: Lam R, editor. Seasonal affective disorder and beyond. Washington, DC: American Psychiatric Press Inc; 1998. p. 221–51.

81. Duffy JF, Rimmer DW, Ceisler CA. Association of intrinsic circadian period morningness-eveningness,

usual wake time and circadian phase. Behav Neurosci 2001;115:895–9.

82. Bootzin RR. A stimulus control treatment for insomnia. Proc Am Psychol Assoc 1972;7:395–6.

83. Bootzin RR, Nicassio P. Behavioral treatments for insomnia. In: Hersen M, Eisler RM, Miller PM, editors, Progress in behavior modification. vol. 6. New York: Academic Press; 1978. p. 1–45.

84. Bootzin RR, Epstein D, Wood JM. Stimulus control instructions. In: Hauri P, editor. Case studies in insomnia. New York: Plenum Press; 1991. p. 19–28.

85. Hasler BP, Bootzin RR, Cousins JC. Circadian phase in sleep-disturbed adolescents with a history of substance abuse: a pilot study. Behav Sleep Med 2008;6:55–73.

How to Travel the World Without Jet Lag

Charmane I. Eastman, PhD[a,b,*], Helen J. Burgess, PhD[a,b]

KEYWORDS
- Jet lag • Phase response curves • Melatonin
- Bright light • Sleep • Circadian rhythms

Several reviews on jet lag written by the authors[1,2] and others[3,4] have recently been published. The focus of this article is on describing in detail how melatonin, bright light, and sleep schedules can be used in conjunction with currently available flight times to reduce or eliminate jet lag. Our aim is to educate circadian rhythm researchers and sleep clinicians about the principles involved so that they can make similar jet travel schedules customized for individuals traveling in any direction across multiple time zones.

SYMPTOMS, HEALTH, AND SAFETY CONSEQUENCES OF JET LAG

Jet travel across multiple time zones produces jet lag, which includes difficulty initiating or maintaining nighttime sleep, daytime sleepiness, decreased alertness, loss of concentration, impaired performance, fatigue, irritability, disorientation, depressed mood, and gastrointestinal disturbances.[5–8] Jet lag is not just the bane of tourists; it can impair the judgment of business people and politicians, compromise the performance of athletes,[5,6] and pose a threat to public safety as it affects diplomats and the military.[9,10] In 2007, over 31 million US residents flew overseas, with about 12 million traveling to Europe and 7 million to Asia.[11] This census does not include military or government flights. Persons traveling for business and conventions took an average of 4.5 trips in the year.[11]

Frequent jet travel has long-term health risks. Cognitive deficits,[12] temporal lobe atrophy as determined by MRI scans,[13] and disturbances in the menstrual cycle[14] can all occur with frequent jet travel. Following transmeridian travel, it is likely that meals will be eaten at inappropriate circadian phases, and repeated occurrence of this could increase the risk of cardiovascular disease and type II diabetes.[15] There is an increased risk of cancer in flight attendants who frequently fly across many time zones.[16–18] Work in mice has shown that chronic jet lag accelerates the development of malignant tumors and reduces survival times.[19] Old mice subjected to weekly 6-hour phase shifts in the light-dark (LD) cycle died sooner when the LD cycle was advanced (equivalent to trips east across six time zones) than when it was delayed (trips west), and both groups died sooner than controls who were not shifted.[20] The effects of jet lag, both short and long term, are a public health issue that need to be addressed, and there is a need to prevent or at least minimize jet lag.

DURATION OF JET LAG AND WHY THERE IS MORE JET LAG AFTER FLYING EAST

Jet lag is caused by a temporary misalignment between the endogenous circadian clock,

This work was supported by grants R01 NR07677 and R01 HL086934 from the National Institutes of Health and by grant R01 OH003954 from the National Institute of Occupational Safety and Health (NIOSH) and the Centers for Disease Control and Prevention (CDC). The content is solely the responsibility of the authors and does not necessarily represent the official views of the National Institute of Nursing Research, the National Heart, Lung, and Blood Institute, the National Institutes of Health, the NIOSH, or the CDC.
[a] Behavioral Sciences Department, Rush University Medical Center, Chicago, IL, USA
[b] Biological Rhythms Research Laboratory, Rush University Medical Center, 1645 W. Jackson Boulevard, Suite 425, Chicago, IL 60612, USA
* Corresponding author. Biological Rhythms Research Laboratory, Rush University Medical Center, 1645 W. Jackson Boulevard, Suite 425, Chicago, IL 60612.
E-mail address: ceastman@rush.edu (C.I. Eastman).

Sleep Med Clin 4 (2009) 241–255
doi:10.1016/j.jsmc.2009.02.006

specifically the dorsomedial region of the supra-chiasmatic nucleus,[21] which controls the body's circadian rhythms and the destination time zone and sleep/wake schedule. The symptoms of jet lag dissipate as the circadian clock is gradually reset (gradually phase shifts) to realign (re-entrain) to the time cues (zeitgebers) of the new time zone, primarily the LD cycle. Flying east requires a phase advance of the circadian clock, whereas flying west requires a phase delay. For example, when it is early in the day in the United States, it may already be approaching nighttime in Europe. Common language for persons living in the United States is to say that Europe is ahead of us, and that when you arrive there, you must set your wrist-watch ahead by moving the hands later; however, your circadian clock has to be reset earlier, and the technical term is a *phase advance*. For example, if you flew east seven time zones (eg, Chicago to Paris) and expect to go to sleep at midnight in Paris, you are really trying to go to sleep at 5:00 PM according to the time of your circadian clock, which is still on Chicago time. You are trying to go to sleep earlier, to advance the time of your sleep, and your internal circadian clock has to phase advance to realign with your advanced sleep schedule and the new local time.

It takes longer to reset or re-entrain the circadian clock following eastward than westward flight,[22,23] which can be explained, at least in part, by the fact that the average free-running period (tau) of the human circadian clock is slightly longer than 24 hours.[24–26] Thus, most humans already have a natural tendency to drift slighter later each day, and it is much more difficult to phase advance the human circadian clock than to phase delay it,[27–29] even in older people.[30] Early estimates from real jet travelers are that the circadian clock phase delays 92 minutes per day after westward flights and phase advances 57 minutes per day after eastward flights.[22] Laboratory studies with an abrupt shift of the sleep/wake schedule, which mimic what happens after jet travel, show that the circadian clock can phase shift faster when people are exposed to bright light at the appropriate time. For example, in a study in which the sleep schedule was shifted 12 hours,[31] which is the largest possible shift, circadian rhythms shifted 9.6 hours over the first 4 days when they phase de-layed (2.4 h/d or 144 min/d) and 6.2 hours when they phase advanced (1.6 h/d or 93 min/d, see Fig. 1 in the article by Eastman and Martin[28]). Previously we have developed jet travel plans assuming phase advances of 1.5 hours per day and phase delays of 2 hours per day, given appro-priately timed bright light after landing.[32] These numbers are estimates, and, as explained herein,

the exact magnitude of the phase shift will vary de-pending on the individual and the timing and inten-sity of bright light they receive at their destination. More research in real jet travelers is required to know the magnitude of the phase shifts that can be produced using schedules of bright light expo-sure and avoidance after landing.

The jet travel plans described later in this article do not include the large abrupt shifts of the sleep schedule typical after crossing many time zones, because this is what causes circadian misalign-ment. In the example with the 12-hour abrupt shift mentioned previously,[28] the circadian clock was still misaligned with the sleep schedule 8 days after the shift when the clock phase advanced and was just approaching complete re-entrain-ment 4 days after the shift when the clock phase delayed. Thus, for many days, jet lag symptoms would have been felt. This example also illustrates directional asymmetry, that is, the circadian clock phase delays faster than it phase advances. In the jet travel plans presented later, we use bright light to shift the circadian clock but we also gradually shift the sleep schedule to keep it aligned with the shifting circadian clock, avoiding circadian misalignment and jet lag. Before presenting these plans, we show what happens with an abrupt shift of the sleep schedule, which is what most people subject themselves to after flying across many time zones.

Fig. 1 shows what might happen to the circadian clock of a traveler, called Henry, marked by the time of his temperature minimum (Tmin) shown by the triangles. At home in San Francisco, Henry typically sleeps from 11:30 PM to 7:00 AM and remains on this sleep schedule in China, producing an abrupt 9-hour delay of his sleep schedule and an abrupt 9-hour advance after returning home. Under usual circumstances, the Tmin occurs about 3 to 4.5 hours before wake time with an 8-hour sleep episode.[33] While home, Henry usually only allows himself 7.5 hours of sleep. He cuts his sleep short by waking up earlier than would be natural (although he probably sleeps later on the weekends); therefore, we esti-mate his Tmin to be 3 hours before wake time at 4:00 AM. After the trip west from San Francisco to Beijing, his circadian clock phase delays 1.5 hours per day, and complete re-entrainment, with the Tmin in the same phase relationship to sleep (3 hours before waking), occurs 5 days after landing. In contrast, after the return flight east, his circadian clock may phase advance by 1 hour per day (shown by the filled triangles), and it takes much longer for complete re-entrainment to occur (9 days). However, it is possible that on his return flight his circadian clock will phase delay rather

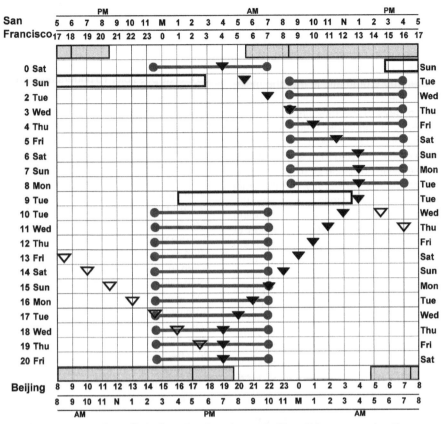

Fig. 1. Diagram showing a round trip flight from San Francisco to Beijing, China, across nine time zones. The rectangle on days 0 to 1 shows the time of the flight from San Francisco to Beijing (westward flight), and the rectangle on day 9 shows the return flight (eastward). The time lines on the top show the time in San Francisco (in daylight savings time), and the time lines on the bottom show the equivalent time in Beijing. The yellow horizontal bars show the maximum duration of the photoperiod (at the summer solstice), and the vertical lines within the bars show the minimum duration of the photoperiod (at the winter solstice). In-bed times (dark) are represented by the two circles connected by a line. This schedule shows what might happen to a traveler, called Henry, who usually sleeps from 11:30 PM to 7:00 AM and maintains that schedule while in Beijing. The triangle represents the temperature minimum (Tmin), a marker for the phase of the circadian clock, the sleepiest circadian time, and a rough marker for the crossover point from phase delays to phase advances in the light PRC. The Tmin phase delays by 1.5 hours per day after landing in Beijing until the original phase position of 4:00 AM is reached on day 6. After the return flight east (a phase advance of zeitgebers), two possibilities for re-entrainment are shown: (1) a phase delay of 1.5 hours per day (antidromic re-entrainment shown by the open triangles), and (2) a phase advance of 1 hour per day (orthodromic re-entrainment shown by the filled triangles). These daily phase shifts are the classic averages for phase shifts after flights as described by Aschoff and coworkers[22] but will be altered by the actual pattern of light and dark to which Henry is exposed. Because the Tmin quickly reaches the time for sleep after the trip west, Henry should have few days of jet lag. In contrast, after the return trip east, it takes a long time for the Tmin to reach sleep regardless of the direction of re-entrainment. The day of the week listed on the left and right sides changes at midnight, which is 9 hours later in the bottom time lines when compared with the top. On the days of the flights, it appears that Henry "gains" or "loses" a day (see the days of the week on the left and on the right), because he crosses the International Date Line twice. In reality, there are still 24 hours in a day. For the purposes of our descriptions, day numbers refer to the rows shown and do not change at midnight.

than phase advance (shown by the open triangles), and in this case complete re-entrainment will take 10 days. When the circadian clock phase shifts in the opposite direction to the shift in the LD cycle and sleep/wake schedule, this shift is considered re-entrainment in the "wrong" direction (antidromic re-entrainment).

Antidromic re-entrainment is common following eastward travel, especially when eight or more time zones are crossed.[23,34–37] For example, in one study[37] subjects flew eleven time zones east, and the circadian rhythm of endogenous melatonin was assessed before and after the flight. Seven of the eight subjects re-entrained by phase delaying instead of phase advancing. In another study with similar methodology,[35] six subjects flew eight time zones east but only four of them phase advanced. The melatonin rhythm of one subject phase delayed instead of phase advancing. Even more dramatic is that the melatonin rhythm of the sixth subject did not shift at all, even after 5 days in the new time zone (Los Angeles). Indeed, a previous study from the authors' laboratory has shown that phase advancing and phase delaying forces can conflict, resulting in essentially no phase shift.[27]

Jet lag symptoms are the worst when the Tmin occurs during the waking period, because the traveler will be sleepy in the hours surrounding the Tmin and will also have difficulty sleeping at times that are far from the Tmin. Even if adequate sleep is obtained (eg, because one uses hypnotics, because there is a lot of previous sleep deprivation, or because the individual is "phase tolerant"[38] and able to sleep at the wrong circadian phase), daytime activities will be impaired, especially near the Tmin. With age we become less phase tolerant,[39–41] and it follows that we will suffer more from the circadian misalignment of jet lag. Jet lag is not just due to loss of sleep on the day of travel. Such a sleep debt can be substantially "made up" the next night, but jet lag lingers due to circadian misalignment and the relatively slow moving circadian clock.

Henry (see **Fig. 1**) should start to feel good by day 3 after flying west to Beijing because his Tmin, which marks the sleepiest circadian time, will occur at the beginning of sleep, and it feels good to go to bed when you are very sleepy. This phase relationship is found in people living in temporal isolation who free-run with all of their rhythms synchronized (see Fig. 7 in the article by Eastman[42] and Fig. 17 in the article by Wever[24]). After the return trip east, if Henry's circadian clock phase advances (filled triangles), he should start to feel good by day 16, waking up slightly after the Tmin. We have previously stated that the goal for circadian adaptation to jet lag and to night shift work is to at least get the Tmin within the sleep episode.[28,43] However, when the Tmin is phase advancing into the sleep episode, it may be better to phase advance it 1 or 2 hours into sleep, because waking up at the sleepiest time is unpleasant. Eastman and Martin[28] have previously estimated that good sleep can be obtained for 6 hours before and 6 hours after the Tmin based on the results of several studies[44] and this interval may widen with increasing sleep debt. Henry should have the most difficulty maintaining sleep on day 2, and later on will have difficulty sleeping especially on days 11 to 14.

LIGHT AND MELATONIN PHASE RESPONSE CURVES

The most effective treatments for jet lag rely on shifting the circadian clock to the new time zone as fast as possible. To understand these schemes, one must understand phase response curves (PRCs). **Fig. 2** shows that bright light can help produce phase advances when applied late in the sleep episode and in the morning after the Tmin and can help produce phase delays when applied early in the sleep episode before the Tmin. Most human light PRCs show the crossover point from phase advances to phase delays around the time of the Tmin or a little later.[28,45–47] **Fig. 2** also shows that melatonin pills produce the greatest phase advances when taken in the afternoon and the greatest phase delays when taken in the morning. In the United States, melatonin pills are classified as a dietary supplement and are not approved by the Food and Drug Administration (FDA) for treating jet lag. Nevertheless, a wide body of research, including the melatonin PRC in **Fig. 2**, indicates that melatonin pills do effectively shift the circadian clock and are thus a useful tool for reducing jet lag. It is often said that the light and melatonin PRCs are 180 degrees out of phase, but **Fig. 2** shows this to be a bit of an oversimplification.

The light PRC can explain why Henry's circadian clock might phase delay rather than phase advance after the return flight east from China (ie, antidromic re-entrainment). In the first few days back home, days 10 to 12 in **Fig. 1**, if he spends more time outside before his Tmin than after, this light could push his circadian clock to phase delay (see Fig. 2 in the article by Eastman and Martin[28]) even though the zeitgebers and his sleep schedule advanced. We can also imagine that if he was exposed to enough phase advancing light on some days and phase delaying light on others, the net effect could be no phase shift at all. The authors have seen this occur in a laboratory study,[27] and it was observed in the traveler mentioned earlier who flew eight time zones east.[35] Travelers often develop superstitions about which procedures may help them overcome jet lag. It is probable that the time of landing combined with the light exposure during the first few days after landing explains most of the improvement commonly attributed to other factors such as diet or the amount of sleep obtained during the flight. Of course, sleep deprivation due to the flight will have its consequences, but, as mentioned earlier, one night of sleep deprivation can be mostly made up in a day, whereas jet lag can last much longer.

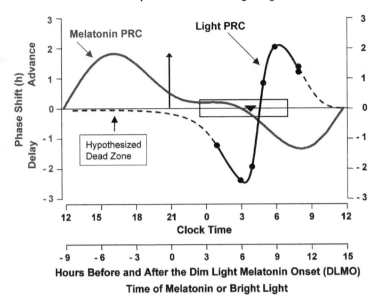

Human Phase Response Curves To Bright Light and Melatonin

Fig. 2. PRCs generated from subjects free-running through an ultradian LD cycle (LD, 2.5:1.5) for three 24-hour days. Melatonin pills (3.0 mg) or bright light pulses (2 hours of ~3500 lux) were given each day, with different subjects receiving the zeitgeber at different times of day. Phase shifts were derived from circadian phase assessments conducted before and after the 3 days of free-running. The x-axis shows the time the pill was given or the time the bright light pulse began relative to each subject's DLMO, represented by zero on the bottom time line and the upward arrow. For convenience, we added a clock time axis for a subject with a DLMO of 21:00, a rectangle showing a typical entrained sleep time (starting 2.5 hours after the DLMO and lasting for 7.5 hours), and a triangle 7 hours after the DLMO showing the typical time of the temperature minimum (Tmin). The melatonin PRC is a curve fit to 27 points (27 subjects); the data points can be seen in the article by Burgess and coworkers.[83] The bright light PRC should be considered preliminary because there were only 7 points (7 subjects). The dashed sections correspond to times with no data points. This preliminary light PRC can also be seen in the article by Revell and Eastman.[1] The 2.5-hour interval from the DLMO to sleep onset was based on averages from our laboratory studies.[84,85]

Fig. 2 shows roughly equivalent magnitudes of phase advances for two specific doses of melatonin and bright light. The melatonin dose of 3.0 mg is typically sold over the counter as a sleeping aid and produces pharmacologic levels of melatonin. The light level of 3500 lux is more intense than what is usually obtained indoors and is produced by bright light boxes. Outdoor sunlight is even more intense, ranging from about 10,000 to 100,000 lux. The roughly equivalent maximum phase advances in these two PRCs may be a surprise to many circadian rhythm researchers who consider bright light to be more powerful at phase shifting the clock. Part of this preconception comes from a comparison between previous light PRCs in which the sleep/dark episode was shifted many hours in a laboratory[48] and the melatonin PRC in which sleep was at home and was not shifted; therefore, the magnitude of the phase shift was constrained by entrainment to the 24-hour day.[49] In the authors' PRCs shown in **Fig. 2**, the subjects were free-running and free to phase shift without constraint. To more accurately compare PRCs for light and melatonin, they need to be generated using the same protocol. Thus far, only the authors' PRCs in **Fig. 2** are available for such a comparison; however, even the

comparison in **Fig. 2** is preliminary because the light PRC has so few points. The fact that there are roughly equivalent phase advances and a slightly larger phase delay with light given these two particular doses should be considered preliminary.

Fig. 2 shows that the light and melatonin PRCs have times of reduced sensitivity when the zeitgeber has very little phase shifting effect. These periods are often called "dead zones" and are a common feature of PRCs.[50] The dead zone in the light PRC in our figure is hypothetical because we do not yet have data in that region, but some other human light PRCs appear to have minimal phase shifts there in the middle of the day.[47] In contrast, the human bright light PRC does not have much of a dead zone when generated in protocols containing a sleep/dark episode that is shifted.[48,51] In these protocols, not only is bright light applied in the middle of the day, but the slight shift of sleep/dark permits dim light to impinge upon the sensitive portions of the PRC. This dim light could be responsible for the small phase shifts. In any case, humans are like other animals in that the timing of the circadian clock is not strongly affected by bright light in the middle of the day.

The dead zone in the 3-mg melatonin PRC shows that melatonin taken 1 or 2 hours before usual sleep onset and in the first half of the usual sleep episode will not greatly phase shift the clock. One explanation for this is that the dead zone begins when endogenous melatonin is first secreted from the pineal gland, marked by the dim light melatonin onset (DLMO), and ends several hours later on the falling limb of the melatonin profile after the pineal gland has shut off or greatly reduced its production of melatonin, a time often referred to as the SynOff.[52] Thus, exogenous melatonin has more of a phase shifting effect when there is less endogenous melatonin in the circulation, just like bright light has more of a phase shifting effect at night when bright light is ordinarily not present.

Fig. 3 shows that melatonin PRCs to different doses of melatonin have different shapes, just as light PRCs to different durations of light have different shapes.[53] The maximum of the phase advance portion of the 3-mg PRC is a few hours earlier than for the 0.5-mg PRC. Our working estimates for the best times to take these doses to help produce the largest phase advance are as follows: take the 3-mg dose 5 hours before the DLMO (7.5 hours before usual sleep onset or 12 hours before the Tmin), and take the 0.5-mg dose 2 hours before the DLMO (4.5 hours before

sleep onset or 9 hours before the Tmin). Our recommended times for the 0.5-mg dose are based on a PRC to which there is no curve fit;[49] therefore, our estimates of the optimal time to take the 0.5-mg dose vary slightly depending on what curve fitting procedures are used (see Fig. 1 in the article by Revell and Eastman[1]). A further caveat to directly comparing these two melatonin PRCs is that they were generated from different protocols. We are currently generating a 0.5-mg PRC using the same method used to generate the 3.0-mg PRC, with subjects free-running through an ultradian LD cycle, so that we will have a better comparison of the PRC shapes with these different doses of melatonin in the near future. The working estimates mentioned previously for giving these doses for maximum phase advances are more precise when using the numbers relative to the DLMO than those relative to sleep onset or the Tmin. Both of the melatonin PRCs were generated using the DLMO as a phase marker, whereas the times for sleep onset and the Tmin were derived from the DLMO based on averages from our studies and others.[54–56] Of course, we often do not know the time of an individual's DLMO unless we invest the time and money to measure it. Most often, the advice on when to take melatonin is referenced to the individual's typical sleep onset time. Despite these limitations, if the timing of the

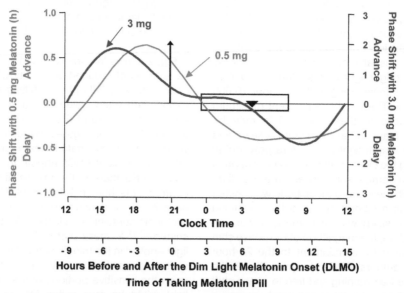

Human Phase Response Curves to Different Doses of Melatonin

Fig. 3. The melatonin PRC to 3.0 mg from **Fig. 2** and a melatonin PRC to 0.5 mg. The curve for 0.5 mg was fit to the data reported by Lewy and coworkers.[49] Note the different y-axes for the different doses. This difference is probably not due to the difference in dose but rather to the difference in protocols (ie, free-running subjects for 3.0 mg and entrained subjects for 0.5 mg). These PRCs show that the 3.0-mg dose needs to be taken earlier than the 0.5-mg dose to produce the maximum phase advance.

dose ends up being about 2 hours earlier or later than the ideal (relative to the DLMO), it will still fall within a high amplitude part of the advance portions of these melatonin PRCs and will help to phase advance the circadian clock (see **Fig. 3**).

Obviously there is a need to generate PRCs to different doses of melatonin besides 0.5 and 3 mg. Other doses are available over the counter and on the Internet in the United States. However, we have chosen to start with these two doses because the 0.5-mg dose is a low dose intended only for phase shifting the circadian clock and for which sleepiness is an unwanted side effect, and the 3.0-mg dose is a large pharmacologic dose marketed primarily for its soporific effects. Despite melatonin often being marketed as a sleep aid, it is not universally associated with sleep or increased sleepiness because, in nocturnal animals, melatonin is associated with waking activity. Instead, the release of melatonin appears to signal darkness.

HOW TO MINIMIZE OR AVOID JET LAG

Given the knowledge of when to apply bright light or give melatonin pills to get the largest phase shifts, how can we help Henry minimize or avoid jet lag? **Fig. 4** shows one possibility. Henry uses a bright light box in the 2 hours before sleep the two nights before the flight to China. Commercially available light boxes are usually advertised for the treatment of winter depression or seasonal affective disorder, but these boxes are also useful for helping to phase shift the circadian clock, and therefore minimize or avoid jet lag. In addition to using the light box, Henry goes to bed 2.5 hours later on day −1, which helps place the bright light exposure closer to the Tmin and into a higher amplitude part of the phase delay portion of the light PRC (see **Fig. 2**). He delays bedtime by 2 hours for the next two nights to keep up with the phase delaying circadian clock and its PRC, which is also phase delaying, so that the bright light will continue to coincide with the delay portion of the light PRC. The bright light on day −1 helps push the Tmin 2 hours later from 4:00 to 6:00 AM, and the bright light on day 0 helps phase delay the Tmin another 2 hours to 8:00 AM. Bright light is avoided after waking (indicated by the Ds) because it could coincide with the phase advance portion of the light PRC. During this time Henry would do well to wear dark sunglasses if he needed to go outside. For the same reason, it is necessary to sleep in a dark bedroom or, if that is not possible, to use an eye mask while in bed. An early study in which the sleep schedule was delayed 2 hours per day and bright light from light boxes (about 2000–4000 lux) was used in the 2 hours before bed showed that the Tmin of most subjects entrained to the 26-hour day (ie, they phase delayed by 2 h/d);[57] therefore, a phase delay of 2 hours per day is a reasonable estimate when a light box is used. After landing, the light exposure that Henry receives (days 1–3) is unpredictable and dependent on his activities, the weather, and the temperature in Beijing; therefore, we show his Tmin phase delaying by only 1 hour per day. Because a study of subjects kept in room light (70 lux) showed that the circadian clock phase delayed by about 1 hour per day with a sleep schedule delay of 2 hours per day,[58] we believe that a rate of 1 hour per day is a reasonable estimate for how Henry's circadian clock will phase delay after landing. If Henry happens to be exposed to enough bright light before bed, his circadian clock might phase delay even faster. The phase delays stop when complete re-entrainment is reached.

To phase advance his circadian clock back to San Francisco time, Henry uses bright light in the morning and melatonin in the afternoon (days 8–15). He also advances his sleep schedule by 1 hour per day. In a recent study, we showed that a 1 hour per day advance of the sleep schedule combined with intermittent bright light from light boxes (∼5000 lux) for the first 3.5 hours after waking and melatonin in the afternoon phase advanced the circadian clock by about 1 hour per day. Furthermore, this regimen did not produce jet lag type symptoms.[59] We found no difference in the magnitude of phase advance when a 0.5-mg dose was taken (on average 2.4 hours before the DLMO) and when a 3.0-mg dose was taken (on average 4.8 hours before the DLMO). These circadian times of administration coincide with the highest amplitude parts of the advance portions of the respective PRCs, close to our working estimates for optimal times of 2 hours and 5 hours before the DLMO. Although there was no significant difference in phase shift between the two doses, there was a slight difference in the sleepiness they produced. The 3.0-mg dose made our subjects slightly, although not significantly, more sleepy, whereas sleepiness after the 0.5-mg dose was almost identical to after placebo (see Fig. 6 in the article by Revell and coworkers[59]). To be safe and to avoid the mild soporific effects of melatonin, we have Henry use the 0.5-mg dose. On day 8, he takes it 4.5 hours before bedtime and 1 hour earlier each day. He could use a light box in the morning to help phase advance his circadian clock, but, because it is daylight in San Francisco, we recommend he go outside as much as possible because natural light

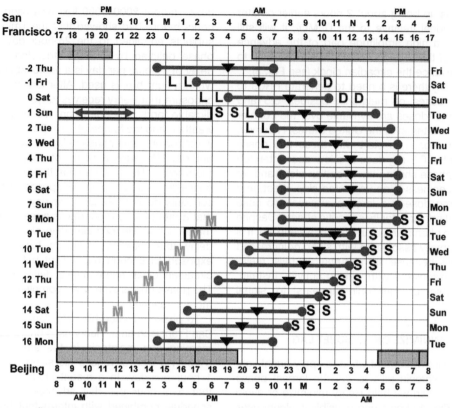

Fig. 4. The same flight schedule shown in **Fig. 1** but, in this case, Henry gradually changes the time of his sleep episodes (dark), controls light exposure, and takes melatonin to phase shift his circadian clock and avoid circadian misalignment and jet lag. Bright light can be obtained by going outside (S indicates sunlight exposure) or from a light box (L), but S is always preferable to L. Intermittent bright light exposure should be sufficient during the times indicated. A light box is needed for days −1 and 0; Henry can seek brightly lit places for the Ls during the next few days in Beijing. The Ms on days 8 to 15 indicate 0.5 mg of melatonin, timed to coincide with the maximum phase advance portion of the 0.5-mg melatonin PRC. This low dose should not make Henry sleepy. The Ds indicate the times to stay indoors and avoid bright light or, if it is necessary to go out, to wear very dark sunglasses. Note that Henry stays on a slightly earlier sleep schedule while in Beijing compared with when home. The 10:30 PM to 6:30 AM sleep schedule makes it quicker and easier to phase advance back to San Francisco time after the return flight home. The sleep line within the rectangle on day 1 shows that it is OK to sleep on the plane, and the best time for a nap (siesta time in the middle of the day) is indicated. It is good to nap whenever the sleep episodes are gradually delaying. The sleep line within the return flight rectangle on day 9 starts with an arrow indicating it is OK to go to sleep earlier, which is true whenever a schedule has gradually advancing sleep episodes.

is almost always more intense than the light from light boxes and should have a greater phase shifting effect. We also recommend that he gradually change the time of his meals to keep them aligned with his circadian clock. Henry's circadian clock represented by the Tmin and his sleep schedule remain aligned; therefore, he should be free of the physiologic symptoms of jet lag, the suppression of endogenous melatonin by light, and, we believe, from the health hazards of circadian misalignment.

There are individual differences in the magnitude of phase shifts produced by bright light even in strictly controlled laboratory studies.

What would happen to Henry if his circadian clock did not phase delay as much as 2 hours per day from days −2 to 0? There are two consequences: (1) it might take a few more days for complete re-entrainment, and (2) he might have trouble sleeping as late as planned (sleep maintenance insomnia) while the Tmin was very early within the sleep episode. Especially for early birds, who probably have shorter taus[60] and thus more trouble phase delaying, we recommend starting the light box treatment even before the sleep schedule is shifted, in this case on day −2, and/or delaying sleep by only 1 or 1.5 hours per day rather than 2 hours per day. The initial delay of bedtime on day −1 of 2.5 hours might be difficult for early birds, although it should be no trouble for night owls. If the traveler does not know whether he or she is an early bird or a night owl, most likely he or she is not either extreme. For most people, if scheduling permits, it would be even better to start the delaying schedule and light treatment a few days earlier than shown and to use a slow delay of the sleep schedule (ie, 1 h/d).

What would happen if Henry's clock did not phase advance as much as shown in **Fig. 4** (1 h/d) after the return flight east? His Tmin would gradually move later within the sleep episodes, and he might have difficulty falling asleep (sleep onset insomnia) and would feel sleepy upon waking. He would experience what extreme night owls or people with a delayed sleep phase live with every day when they try to conform to the 9 to 5 or 8 to 6 early bird world. This slight circadian misalignment is undesirable but is certainly not as bad as the massive circadian misalignment most travelers are subjected to when they abruptly shift the time of their sleep by several hours. We conducted a study in which the sleep schedule was advanced by 2 hours per day and intermittent bright light from light boxes was used upon waking in the morning in the hope of producing larger phase advances;[61] however, the circadian clock only phase advanced slightly more than when the sleep schedule was advanced by 1 hour per day, and the difference was not statistically significant. We deduced that circadian misalignment, with the Tmin occurring slightly after wake up time, occurred on average after the second advanced sleep episode; therefore, we do not recommend advancing the sleep schedule more than 1 hour per day. Furthermore, when scheduling permits, and especially for night owls who probably have longer taus, we recommend advancing by even less than 1 hour per day (eg, 0.5 h/d). Night owls might need more bright light in the morning to use a sleep schedule advance of 1 hour per day. Alternatively, they could choose to follow a delaying schedule for flying east.

We recognize that Henry might not be able to maintain the sleep schedule shown in **Fig. 4** upon his return to San Francisco or in the 2 days before the flight to China depending on his work and family commitments. However, given the increasing prevalence of flex time and working from home (telecommuting), he may be able to arrange it, especially with some advance notice. When people first hear about such sleep schedules and light treatments they sometimes develop the misconception that it will take too much time; however, after careful explanation, they understand that it only requires a rearrangement of

time. For some people the scheduling and planning required to rearrange meetings and activities can seem overwhelming. Our Henry is in charge of his own work schedule and has no objection to following the prescribed sleep schedule. If he chooses to use a light box in the morning on days 10 to 15 rather than go outside to get his bright light exposure, he can do many activities while sitting there, such as reading, writing, working on a computer, watching television, eating, or talking on the phone. The intermittent nature of the light treatment means that, with a little bit of planning, he can get up to shower, dress, or prepare breakfast without interfering with the treatment. He could also get some of his bright light exposure from natural outdoor light while commuting to work. Another alternative would be to have a second light box at work to start the bright light exposure at home and do the rest at work. This approach would work well for people with desk jobs. We envision a future in which companies keep light boxes on hand for this purpose. After all, it is in their best interests to have a highly functioning employee rather than one who is sleepy and jet lagged.

A large variety of commercial light boxes are marketed for jet lag and seasonal affective disorder. We recommend boxes with the largest illuminated area because they are easier to sit in front of without having the head move out of range and are usually less intense and less aversive. One advantage of the very small light boxes is that they could be taken to work or on the plane and used overseas (providing the box is battery powered or able to process any variations in voltage that may occur). Light boxes that are enriched with blue wavelengths or that produce only blue light are currently in vogue because the circadian system is most sensitive to blue light;[62,63] however, we have shown that the older light boxes with cool white fluorescent lamps produce the same magnitude of phase shifts as those observed with blue-enriched fluorescent light in protocols with gradually advancing or gradually delaying sleep schedules.[64,65]

The melatonin PRCs (see **Fig. 3**) show that melatonin could be taken in the morning to help Henry when he needs to phase delay his circadian clock. We did not include it in the jet travel plan (see **Fig. 4**) because we have no experimental evidence that it would increase the phase delay produced by the bright light before bed. A 2 hour per day phase delay may be the maximum one can delay the circadian clock while using a gradually delaying sleep schedule. Furthermore, the 3.0-mg dose could make him sleepy, and we will not know the optimal time to give the 0.5-mg dose to produce delays until we generate our own 0.5 mg PRC.

Let us now consider a traveler, called Susan, who flies from Chicago to Paris and does nothing to phase shift her circadian clock before the flight. **Fig. 5** shows what she can do to try to minimize jet lag, but this last minute approach has many problems. Obtaining outdoor light exposure and avoiding it at the appropriate times may be difficult due to weather or scheduled indoor or outdoor activities. If she happens to experience the wrong pattern of light exposure in the first few days in Paris (ie, a lot of bright light before her Tmin and none after), she could suffer from antidromic re-entrainment (her circadian clock could phase delay), or her clock might not shift at all. Furthermore, even under the best circumstances, several days are wasted because of extreme circadian misalignment and jet lag. Susan will not be back to normal until 5 days after the flight, when she is waking up slightly after the Tmin.

Several publications, commercial computer sites, and programs and devices are available to tell the traveler when to seek and when to avoid

outdoor light in the days after landing. For more discussion of several of these sources, the reader is referred to the article by Eastman and colleagues.[61] Although these schemes are based on the light PRC, they differ in ways which can result in completely opposite, and often incorrect, instructions for the traveler. For example, most expect the circadian clock to phase advance much faster than our 1 hour per day estimate. If the time scheduled for bright light exposure each day changes faster than the shifting of the circadian clock, the bright light could end up falling on the wrong side of the crossover point (other side of the Tmin) and hinder rather than help produce phase advances. With our preflight schedules, there is little danger of this because the bright light is applied far from the crossover point (Tmin), and knowing the exact time of the crossover point is not as crucial as it is when bright light exposure and avoidance are started after landing.

We recommend resetting the circadian clock at least partially toward the destination time zone before flying. **Fig. 6** shows an example for Susan's trip to Paris. Four days before the flight she takes

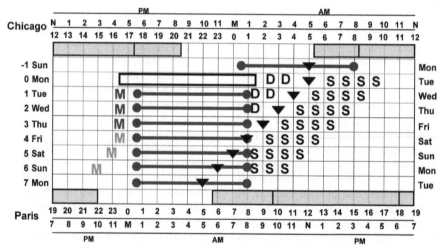

Fig. 5. Diagram showing a flight from Chicago to Paris, seven time zones east, with both time lines in daylight savings time. Other symbols are the same as in **Figs. 1** and **4**, with green Ms for 0.5 mg melatonin and red Ms for 3.0 mg melatonin. This schedule shows what might happen to a traveler, called Susan, who usually sleeps from 12:30 AM to 8:00 AM and does not do any preparation to avoid jet lag until after landing in Paris. On arrival, she is careful to get the ideal light exposure pattern to help phase advance her circadian clock to Paris time according to the light PRC; however, regardless of how much sleep she obtains at night, she will be sleepy during the day, especially in the hours around her Tmin (the triangles). Susan takes melatonin before bedtime on days 1 to 3, a large dose of 3.0 mg, to make her slightly sleepy and help her fall asleep so early (relative to home time). It will also help phase advance her clock according to the 3.0-mg melatonin PRC. On day 4 she switches to the smaller dose of melatonin, 0.5 mg, because her circadian clock has phase advanced so far that the 3.0-mg dose would no longer coincide with the times for maximum phase advances in the 3.0-mg PRC. She takes the 0.5-mg dose at the ideal times for maximum phase advances according to the 0.5-mg melatonin PRC. Susan's circadian clock phase advances by 1 hour per day. Her Tmin reaches the sleep episode by day 4, at which time her circadian misalignment and jet lag symptoms should start to subside. We do not think that this schedule is the best solution, because circadian misalignment is pronounced during the first few days after landing.

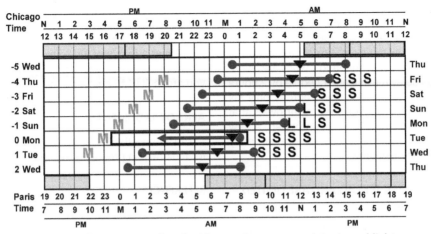

Fig. 6. Same flight schedule shown in **Fig. 5** but, in this case, Susan uses melatonin and light exposure to phase advance her circadian clock toward the destination time zone before the flight and avoids circadian misalignment and jet lag. She advances her sleep schedule by 1 hour per day. She exposes herself to bright light in the morning either by going outside (S), which is best, or by using a light box (L) when it is before sunrise or otherwise impractical. She takes 0.5 mg of melatonin in the afternoon timed to produce the maximum phase advance according to the 0.5-mg melatonin PRC. This low dose should not make her sleepy. The arrow within the flight indicates that this is a good time to sleep and that going to sleep earlier is encouraged, as it is whenever the sleep schedule is gradually advanced.

0.5 mg of melatonin 4.5 hours before her usual sleep onset. That night she goes to bed 1 hour earlier than usual and wakes up 1 hour earlier than usual. She gets intermittent bright light in the morning, preferably by going outside. The whole schedule is advanced by 1 hour per day. Depending on the time of year, at some point she will be waking up before sunrise and will need to use a light box (Ss change to Ls). After landing (day 0), all of the bright outdoor light she receives will help phase advance her circadian clock because none will occur before her Tmin. This approach will prevent antidromic re-entrainment. Her circadian clock and her sleep schedule remain aligned throughout, and she should have little or no jet lag. It may be difficult for her to fall asleep early on the first night (day −4), but if she thinks that will be a problem she can minimize it by starting the melatonin and bright light even before shifting her sleep schedule (on day −5). If she can fly business or first class, she may be able to sleep on the plane; it will be the ideal circadian time for her to sleep, and she should arrive with little sleep deprivation. If she has to fly coach, she may arrive slightly sleep deprived; however, one night of sleep deprivation can largely be made up in a day, whereas jet lag can last much longer.

Obviously, a schedule like this (see **Fig. 6**) can be made for flying east across different numbers of time zones, not just seven, and contain more or less days of phase advancing before the flight.

The more days of phase shifting before the flight, the less jet lag after landing and the quicker the remaining jet lag will dissipate. We have made personalized advancing schedules like these for ourselves, friends, and colleagues. They usually report little trouble falling asleep or waking up earlier following the sleep schedule before the flight, which makes sense because their circadian clocks are phase advancing. The most troubling inconvenience to them is missing out on evening social and family contacts because of the early bedtimes. The importance of a few nights of social contacts has to be balanced with that of optimal performance and alertness for several days after landing. A key point is that even just 1 or 2 days of a preflight shift will help reduce the subsequent jet lag.

As mentioned previously, it is easier for most people to phase delay than to phase advance; therefore, especially for night owls, if scheduling permits, it would be better to delay the sleep schedule before flying east rather than to advance it. Intermittent bright light should be used in the 2 hours before bed (see the first few days in **Fig. 4**). The decision of whether to try to phase advance the circadian clock or phase delay it before flying east depends on the number of time zones crossed, the sleep schedule desired at the destination, whether the individual is an extreme along the morningness-eveningness continuum, and the scheduling constraints of the individual. Even general guidelines, such as phase advance the circadian clock for crossing up to seven time zones east and phase delay the clock for crossing eight or more time zones east[1,32,66] may not always apply to all travelers. For example, one of the authors and her husband, who are night owls, always delay their sleep schedule by 2 hours per day before flying east, even across only six time zones. The advantage for a night owl is that the delaying schedule can be stopped a few days early, leaving the individual on an early schedule at the destination.

DRUGS ONLY MASK JET LAG AND ARE LIMITED IN THEIR EFFECTS

With no preparation before jet travel and random light exposure on arrival, the nighttime insomnia and daytime sleepiness often associated with jet lag can be treated with drugs and naps as a last resort. In this scenario, one treats the symptoms only, and the cause, the underlying circadian misalignment, will continue until the circadian clock finally re-entrains to the new time zone. Re-entrainment to the new time zone may take a week or more (see **Fig. 1**) or longer still if you are unfortunate enough to suffer from a clock that does not initially shift.[35] Pharmaceutical treatment of jet lag symptoms, such as with caffeine[67] and hypnotics[68–70] or large doses of melatonin at bedtime for its soporific effect[9,67,69,71,72] will not eliminate jet lag. Research indicates that although hypnotic medications can improve sleep quantity, sleepiness will still be felt around the Tmin when it occurs during waking hours.[73–75] Caffeine can be used during the day, but even moderate doses taken well before bedtime will impair sleep[76] (although this effect may be overridden by further uses of hypnotics). Furthermore, stimulants such as caffeine,[77] modafinil (Provigil),[78,79] and even bright light exposure[80] and prophylactic naps[77] can all improve alertness and performance but do not return them to normal levels while the underlying circadian misalignment persists. Modafinil is not yet FDA approved for treating jet lag related sleepiness. All drugs have some risks for abuse and dependence, some hypnotics may produce morning hang-over effects,[81] and short-acting benzodiazepines have been associated with transient global amnesia when taken for jet lag.[82]

SUMMARY

In this article we have explained the circadian principles behind how to phase shift the circadian clock with bright light and melatonin and have presented current light and melatonin PRCs that indicate the correct timing of these zeitgebers to produce the desired phase shifting effect. We have provided detailed examples of a few jet travel plans and hope that you are now equipped to devise your own. If you have difficulty doing this, you are invited to contact us for advice.

ACKNOWLEDGMENTS

The authors thank Heather Holly and Tom Molina for their help in preparing the figures.

REFERENCES

1. Revell VL, Eastman CI. How to trick mother nature into letting you fly around or stay up all night. J Biol Rhythms 2005;20:353–65.
2. Reid KJ, Burgess HJ. Circadian rhythm sleep disorders. Prim Care 2005;32:449–73.
3. Sack R, Auckley D, Auger R, et al. Circadian rhythm sleep disorders. Part 1. Basic principles, shift work and jet lag disorders. Sleep 2007;30:1460–83.
4. Waterhouse J, Reilly T, Atkinson G, et al. Jet lag: trends and coping strategies. Lancet 2007;369: 1117–29.
5. Waterhouse J, Edwards B, Nevill A, et al. Identifying some determinants of "jet lag" and its symptoms: a study of athletes and other travellers. Br J Sports Med 2002;36:54–60.
6. Lemmer B, Kern RI, Nold G, et al. Jet lag in athletes after eastward and westward time-zone transition. Chronobiol Int 2002;19:743–64.
7. Wright JE, Vogel JA, Sampson JB, et al. Effects of travel across time zones (jet-lag) on exercise capacity and performance. Aviat Space Environ Med 1983;54:132–7.
8. Rogers HL, Reilly SM. A survey of the health experiences of international business travelers. Part one: physiological aspects. AAOHN J 2002;50:449–59.
9. Comperatore CA, Lieberman HR, Kirby AW, et al. Melatonin efficacy in aviation missions requiring rapid deployment and night operations. Aviat Space Environ Med 1996;67:520–4.
10. Reynolds NC, Montgomery R. Using the Argonne diet in jet lag prevention: deployment of troops across nine times zones. Mil Med 2002;167:451–3.
11. US Department of Commerce, International Trade Administration. Profile of US resident travelers visiting overseas destinations. outbound. Available at: http://tinet.ita.doc.gov/outreachpages/download_data_table/2007_Outbound_Profile.pdf. Accessed March 16, 2009.
12. Cho K, Ennaceur A, Cole JC, et al. Chronic jet lag produces cognitive deficits. J Neurosci 2000;20:1–5.
13. Cho K. Chronic 'jet lag' produces temporal lobe atrophy and spatial cognitive deficits. Nat Neurosci 2001;4:567–8.

14. Iglesias R, Terres A, Chavarria A. Disorders of the menstrual cycle in airline stewardesses. Aviat Space Environ Med 1980;51:518–20.

15. Hampton SM, Morgan LM, Lawrence N, et al. Postprandial hormone and metabolic responses in simulated shift work. J Endocrinol 1996;151:259–67.

16. Rafnsson V, Tulinius H, Jonasson JG, et al. Risk of breast cancer in female flight attendants: a population-based study (Iceland). Cancer Causes Control 2001;12:95–101.

17. Reynolds P, Cone J, Layefsky M, et al. Cancer incidence in California flight attendants (United States). Cancer Causes Control 2002;13:317–24.

18. Pukkala E, Aspholm R, Auvinen A, et al. Incidence of cancer among Nordic airline pilots over five decades: occupational cohort study. BMJ 2002;325:567–71.

19. Filipski E, Delaunay F, King VM, et al. Effects of chronic jet lag on tumor progression in mice. Cancer Res 2004;64:7879–85.

20. Davidson AJ, Sellix MT, Daniel J, et al. Chronic jet lag increases mortality in aged mice. Curr Biol 2006;16:R914–6.

21. Nagano M, Adachi A, Nakahama K, et al. An abrupt shift in the day/night cycle causes desynchrony in the mammalian circadian center. J Neurosci 2003; 23:6141–51.

22. Aschoff J, Hoffmann K, Pohl H, et al. Re-entrainment of circadian rhythms after phase shifts of the zeitgeber. Chronobiologia 1975;2:23–78.

23. Boulos Z, Campbell SS, Lewy AJ, et al. Light treatment for sleep disorders: consensus report. VII. Jet lag. J Biol Rhythms 1995;10:167–76.

24. Wever RA. The circadian system of man. Heidelberg-Berlin. New York: Springer-Verlag; 1979.

25. Czeisler CA, Duffy JF, Shanahan TL, et al. Stability, precision, and near-24-hour period of the human circadian pacemaker. Science 1999;284:2177–81.

26. Burgess HJ, Eastman CI. Human tau in an ultradian light-dark cycle. J Biol Rhythms 2008;23:374–6.

27. Mitchell PJ, Hoese EK, Liu L, et al. Conflicting bright light exposure during night shifts impedes circadian adaptation. J Biol Rhythms 1997;12:5–15.

28. Eastman CI, Martin SK. How to use light and dark to produce circadian adaptation to night shift work. Ann Med 1999;31:87–98.

29. Shanahan TL, Kronauer RE, Duffy JF, et al. Melatonin rhythm observed throughout a three-cycle bright-light stimulus designed to reset the human circadian pacemaker. J Biol Rhythms 1999;14:237–53.

30. Monk TH, Buysse DJ, Carrier J, et al. Inducing jet lag in older people: directional asymmetry. J Sleep Res 2000;9:101–16.

31. Eastman CI. High intensity light for circadian adaptation to a 12-h shift of the sleep schedule. Am J Phys 1992;263:R428–36.

32. Burgess HJ, Eastman CI. Prevention of jet lag. Physicians' Information and Education Resource (PIER). American College of Physicians; 2003. Available at: http://Pier.acponline.org.

33. Baehr EK, Revelle W, Eastman CI. Individual differences in the phase and amplitude of the human circadian temperature rhythm: with an emphasis on morningness-eveningness. J Sleep Res 2000;9: 117–27.

34. Gundel A, Wegmann HM. Transition between advance and delay responses to eastbound transmeridian flights. Chronobiol Int 1989;6(2):147–56.

35. Takahashi T, Sasaki M, Itoh H, et al. Re-entrainment of circadian rhythm of plasma melatonin on an 8-h eastward flight. Psychiatry Clin Neurosci 1999;53:257–60.

36. Gundel A, Spencer MB. A circadian oscillator model based on empirical data. J Biol Rhythms 1999;14: 516–23.

37. Takahashi T, Sasaki M, Itoh H, et al. Re-entrainment of the circadian rhythms of plasma melatonin in an 11-h eastward bound flight. Psychiatry Clin Neurosci 2001;55:275–6.

38. Dawson D, Campbell SS. Timed exposure to bright light improves sleep and alertness during simulated night shifts. Sleep 1991;14:511–6.

39. Campbell SS. Effects of timed bright-light exposure on shift-work adaptation in middle-aged subjects. Sleep 1995;18:108–16.

40. Dijk DJ, Duffy JF, Riel E, et al. Ageing and the circadian and homeostatic regulation of human sleep during forced desynchrony of rest, melatonin and temperature rhythms. J Physiol 1999;516(2):611–27.

41. Moline ML, Pollak CP, Monk TH, et al. Age-related differences in recovery from simulated jet lag. Sleep 1992;15:28–40.

42. Eastman CI. Are separate temperature and activity oscillators necessary to explain the phenomena of human circadian rhythms? In: Moore-Ede MC, Czeisler CA, editors. Mathematical models of the circadian sleep-wake cycle. New York: Raven Press; 1984. p. 81–103.

43. Burgess HJ, Sharkey KM, Eastman CI. Bright light, dark and melatonin can promote circadian adaptation in night shift workers. Sleep Med Rev 2002;6:407–20.

44. Zulley J, Wever R, Aschoff J. The dependence of onset and duration of sleep on the circadian rhythm of rectal temperature. Pflugers Arch 1981;391: 314–8.

45. Jewett ME, Kronauer RE, Czeisler CA. Phase-amplitude resetting of the human circadian pacemaker via bright light: a further analysis. J Biol Rhythms 1994;9:295–314.

46. Dijk DJ, Lockley SW. Functional genomics of sleep and circadian rhythm. Invited review: integration of human sleep-wake regulation and circadian rhythmicity. J Appl Phys 2002;92:852–62.

47. Minors DS, Waterhouse JM, Wirz-Justice A. A human phase-response curve to light. Neurosci Lett 1991;133:36–40.

48. Czeisler CA, Kronauer RE, Allan JS, et al. Bright light induction of strong (type 0) resetting of the human circadian pacemaker. Science 1989;244:1328–33.

49. Lewy AJ, Bauer VK, Ahmed S, et al. The human phase response curve (PRC) to melatonin is about 12 hours out of phase with the PRC to light. Chronobiol Int 1998;15:71–83.

50. Johnson CH. Forty years of PRCs: what have we learned? Chronobiol Int 1999;16:711–43.

51. Khalsa SBS, Jewett ME, Cajochen C, et al. A phase response curve to single bright light pulses in human subjects. J Physiol 2003;549(3):945–52.

52. Lewy AJ, Cutler NL, Sack RL. The endogenous melatonin profile as a marker of circadian phase position. J Biol Rhythms 1999;14:227–36.

53. Comas M, Beersma DG, Spoelstra K, et al. Phase and period responses of the circadian system of mice (Mus musculus) to light stimuli of different duration. J Biol Rhythms 2006;21:362–72.

54. Eastman CI, Martin SK, Hebert M. Failure of extraocular light to facilitate circadian rhythm reentrainment in humans. Chronobiol Int 2000;17:807–26.

55. Griefahn B. The validity of the temporal parameters of the daily rhythm of melatonin levels as an indicator of morningness. Chronobiol Int 2002;19:561–77.

56. Benloucif S, Guico MJ, Reid KJ, et al. Stability of melatonin and temperature as circadian phase markers and their relation to sleep times in humans. J Biol Rhythms 2005;20:178–88.

57. Eastman CI, Miescke KJ. Entrainment of circadian rhythms with 26-hr bright light and sleep-wake schedules. Am J Phys 1990;259:R1189–97.

58. Monk TH, Buysse DJ, Billy BD, et al. Using nine 2-h delays to achieve a 6-h advance disrupts sleep, alertness, and circadian rhythm. Aviat Space Environ Med 2004;75:1049–57.

59. Revell VL, Burgess HJ, Gazda CJ, et al. Advancing human circadian rhythms with afternoon melatonin and morning intermittent bright light. J Clin Endocrinol Metab 2006;91:54–9.

60. Duffy JF, Rimmer DW, Czeisler CA. Association of intrinsic circadian period with morningness-eveningness, usual wake time, and circadian phase. Behav Neurosci 2001;115:895–9.

61. Eastman CI, Gazda CJ, Burgess HJ, et al. Advancing circadian rhythms before eastward flight: a strategy to prevent or reduce jet lag. Sleep 2005;28:33–44.

62. Lockley SW, Brainard GC, Czeisler CA. High sensitivity of the human circadian melatonin rhythm to resetting by short wavelength light. J Clin Endocrinol Metab 2003;88:4502–5.

63. Warman VL, Dijk DJ, Warman GR, et al. Phase advancing human circadian rhythms with short wavelength light. Neurosci Lett 2003;342:37–40.

64. Smith MR, Revell VL, Eastman CI, et al. Phase advancing the human circadian clock with blue-enriched polychromatic light. Sleep Med 2009;10:287–94.

65. Smith MR, Eastman CI, et al. Phase delaying the human circadian clock with blue-enriched polychromatic light. Chronobiology International 2009;28(4):709–25.

66. Burgess HJ, Crowley SJ, Gazda CJ, et al. Preflight adjustment to eastward travel: 3 days of advancing sleep with and without morning bright light. J Biol Rhythms 2003;18:318–28.

67. Beaumont M, Batejat D, Pierard C, et al. Caffeine or melatonin effects on sleep and sleepiness after rapid eastward transmeridian travel. J Appl Phys 2004;96:50–8.

68. Jamieson AO, Zammit GK, Rosenberg RS, et al. Zolpidem reduces the sleep disturbance of jet lag. Sleep Med 2001;2:423–30.

69. Suhner A, Schlagenhauf P, Hofer I, et al. Effectiveness and tolerability of melatonin and zolpidem for the alleviation of jet lag. Aviat Space Environ Med 2001;72:638–46.

70. Daurat A, Benoit O, Buguet A. Effects of zopiclone on the rest/activity rhythm after a westward flight across five time zones. Psychopharmacology (Berl) 2000;149:241–5.

71. Edwards BJ, Atkinson G, Waterhouse J, et al. Use of melatonin in recovery from jet lag following an eastward flight across 10 time-zones. Ergonomics 2000; 43(10):1501–13.

72. Nickelsen T, Lang A, Bergau L. The effect of 6-, 9- and 11-hour time shifts on circadian rhythms: adaptation of sleep parameters and hormonal patterns following the intake of melatonin or placebo. In: Arendt J, Pevet P, editors, Advances in pineal research, 5. London: John Libbey; 1991. p. 303–6.

73. Walsh JK, Muehlbach MJ, Schweitzer PK. Hypnotics and caffeine as countermeasures for shiftwork-related sleepiness and sleep disturbance. J Sleep Res 1995;4:80–3.

74. Schweitzer PK, Koshorek G, Muehlbach MJ, et al. Effects of estazolam and triazolam on transient insomnia associated with phase-shifted sleep. Hum Psychopharmacol 1991;6:99–107.

75. Paul MA, Brown G, Buguet A, et al. Melatonin and zopiclone as pharmacologic aids to facilitate crew rest. Aviat Space Environ Med 2001;72:974–84.

76. Landolt HP, Werth E, Borbely AA, et al. Caffeine intake (200 mg) in the morning affects human sleep and EEG power spectra at night. Brain Res 1995; 675:67–74.

77. Schweitzer PK, Randazzo AC, Stone K, et al. Laboratory and field studies of naps and caffeine as practical countermeasures for sleep-wake problems associated with night work. Sleep 2006;29: 39–50.

78. Walsh JK, Randazzo AC, Stone KL, et al. Modafinil improves alertness, vigilance, and executive function during simulated night shifts. Sleep 2004;27: 434–9.

79. Czeisler CA, Walsh JK, Roth T, et al. Modafinil for excessive sleepiness associated with shift-work sleep disorder. N Engl J Med 2005;353:476–86.

80. Campbell SS, Dijk DJ, Boulos Z, et al. Light treatment for sleep disorders: consensus report. III. Alerting and activating effects. J Biol Rhythms 1995;10:129–32.

81. Roehrs T, Roth T. Hypnotics: efficacy and adverse effects. In: Kryger MH, Roth T, Dement WC, editors. Principles and practice of sleep medicine. 3rd edition. Philadelphia: WB Saunders; 2000. p. 414–8.

82. Morris HH, Estes ML. Transient global amnesia secondary to triazolam. JAMA 1987;258:945–6.

83. Burgess HJ, Revell VL, Eastman CI. A three pulse phase response curve to three milligrams of melatonin in humans. J Physiol 2008;586(2):639–47.

84. Burgess HJ, Eastman CI. The dim light melatonin onset following fixed and free sleep schedules. J Sleep Res 2005;14:229–37.

85. Burgess H, Fogg L. Individual differences in the amount and timing of salivary melatonin secretion. PLoS ONE 2008;3:e3055.

Sleep Loss and Fatigue in Shift Work and Shift Work Disorder

Torbjörn Åkerstedt, PhD[a],*, Kenneth P. Wright, Jr, PhD[b]

KEYWORDS

• Sleep • Sleepiness • Shiftwork • Night • Work • Disorder

Work hours that displace sleep to the daytime and work to the nighttime will interfere with the circadian and homeostatic regulation of sleep. Such work hours will in several ways constitute a health problem with respect to sleep and fatigue, cardiovascular disease, accidents, and cancer[1] (see the article by Litinski, Scheer, and Shea elsewhere in this issue). Herein the focus will be on sleep and fatigue. The terminology with regard to work that extends outside the day hours is somewhat diffuse, and several attempts have been made to classify and bring order to the description of the types of schedules.[2] Normally, the term *shift work* is used to denote work schedules that divide the 24 hours into roughly similar sizes and that use three or more teams to provide full 24-hour coverage. The teams can alternate between early morning, afternoon (swing), and night shifts or may work a permanent shift. The latter is more common in the United States, whereas rotating shifts dominate in Europe. Shift work is mainly used in the production industry. "Roster work" or other terms are used to denote schedules that are more irregular but still cover all or most of the 24 hours. Roster work is more common in transport work and health care. Essentially, the same conflict occurs between circadian regulation and the sleep/work pattern, as is true with shift work. For simplicity, we will use the term *shift work* for both of these types. There are also varieties of shift work that do not infringe on the normal sleep hours. These types are not dealt with herein.

CIRCADIAN AND HOMEOSTATIC REGULATION OF SLEEP AND WAKEFULNESS

The quality of waking cognition and of sleep is determined to a large extent by circadian and sleep homeostatic brain processes. From a circadian perspective, cognition is optimal during the internal biologic day, whereas sleep is optimal during the internal biologic night. Homeostatic sleep drive increases with the duration of prior wakefulness, whether due to acute total sleep deprivation or chronic short sleep schedules. Higher homeostatic sleep drive results in impaired cognition, increased sleepiness, and increased propensity for sleep. Importantly, these circadian and homeostatic processes interact to influence the quality of waking cognition and of sleep. As discussed herein, shift work schedules often require work to occur during the biologic night when the circadian system is promoting sleep, and sleep to occur during the biologic day when the circadian system is promoting wakefulness. The resulting misalignment between internal circadian time and the required wakefulness-sleep, work-rest schedules leads to impaired wakefulness and disturbed sleep. The reader is referred to the article by Dijk and Archer elsewhere in this issue for further discussion of the circadian and homeostatic regulation of sleep and wakefulness.

Dr. Wright was funded by NIH grant HL081761 and by National Space Biomedical Research Institute Cooperative Agreement NCC 9-58-202 with NASA.
[a] Clinical Neuroscience, Karolinska Institutet, Box 230, 17177 Stockholm, Sweden
[b] Sleep and Chronobiology Laboratory, Department of Integrative Physiology, University of Colorado, Boulder, CO 80309, USA
* Corresponding author.
E-mail address: torbjorn.akerstedt@ipm.ki.se (T. Åkerstedt).

SHIFT WORK AND SLEEP

The dominating health problem reported by shift workers is disturbed sleep as acknowledged in early studies.[3–5] At least three fourths of the shift working population is affected.[6] Disturbed sleep seems to be the decisive factor with respect to the attitude to one's work hours.[7] Findings from several questionnaire studies[8] have shown sleep durations of around 5 to 6 hours in relation to the night shift. Objective assessment of sleep via electroencephalography (EEG) of rotating shift workers indicates that day sleep is 1 to 4 hours shorter than night sleep.[9–14] Lockely and colleagues have shown similar values for interns on call.[15]

Night shifts are reported to result in greater loss of total sleep time than evening and slow rotating shift schedules.[14,16,17] Although some have argued that permanent night work may have benefits in terms of circadian adjustment to shift work, there is little support for this argument.[18] Rapid shift rotations are reported to be associated with reduced total sleep duration when compared with slower rotations (eg, at least 3 weeks per shift schedule).[16] Rapid counterclockwise rotations appear to especially disrupt sleep immediately prior to the night shift.[19] These effects are thought to be less severe for workers experiencing a clockwise rotation because of the natural tendency of the circadian clock to delay to a later hour[20,21] and because of increased time between shifts.[22] Some individuals have circadian clock periods that are shorter than 24 hours, and these persons would be expected to adapt easier to counterclockwise shift rotations. Before a counterclockwise rotation, 80% to 90% of workers nap before the midnight shift, as opposed to 40% to 60% before a clockwise rotation, which may help to ameliorate some of the expected impairments in sleep and sleepiness during a counterclockwise rotation. This interpretation is also consistent with numerous studies demonstrating the beneficial effects of napping among shift workers.[23–27]

Sleep episodes during shift work are terminated after only 4 to 6 hours, with the individual being unable to return to sleep, presumably because the internal circadian clock is promoting wakefulness during the schedule-induced circadian misalignment. The sleep loss is primarily taken out of stage 2 sleep (the dominant sleep stage) and stage REM sleep (dream sleep). Stages 3 and 4 ("deep" sleep) do not seem to be affected. The latter changes in sleep architecture during shift work schedules are consistent with the sleep architecture changes observed during restricted sleep schedules.[28,29] Furthermore, the time taken to fall asleep (sleep latency) is usually shorter.

Night sleep before an early morning shift is also reduced, but the termination is through external means (ie, awakening with an alarm) and the awakening usually difficult and unpleasant.[30–33] In a rotating system, some of the sleep loss appears to be repaid in connection with working the afternoon shift, with sleep durations often extending beyond 8 hours.

Interestingly, day sleep does not seem to improve much across a series of night shifts;[34,35] however, night workers seem to sleep slightly better (longer) than rotating workers on the night shift.[36–38] The same lack of adjustment is seen in subjective sleep reports.[39] The assumed explanation for nonadjustment is the conflict with the external light-dark cycle.[39] Strict control over exposure to light and darkness can facilitate complete or partial circadian adaptation to permanent night work schedules.[40–42] Application of circadian principles to shift work has been demonstrated to adjust the sleep duration, as well as alertness, in real night shift operations on Norwegian oil production platforms.[43]

The long-term effects of shift work on sleep are poorly understood. Dumont and colleagues[44,45] found that the amount of sleep/wake and related disturbances in present day workers were positively related to their previous experience of night work. Guilleminault and colleagues[46] found an overrepresentation of former shift workers with different clinical sleep/wake disturbances appearing at a sleep clinic. Recently, the first author (TA) and colleagues have shown that, in pairs of twins discordant on night work exposure, the exposed twin reports somewhat deteriorated sleep quality and health after retirement.[47] Disturbed sleep is reported as a major problem in shift work, but it is not clear to what extent this actually constitutes a problem when compared with the effect of an extended time awake or work at the circadian trough. No study has attempted to dissect the relative contributions of these factors in shift work, but the findings from other types of studies show that the short sleep durations found in shift work (approximately 6 hours) may cause meaningful sleepiness or impaired performance in the average shift worker.[48–50] It is unknown whether extended sleep, after the night shift or during days off, compensates for prior loss during shift work operations.

In a recent representative health survey it was demonstrated that day and shift workers did not differ on most items of sleep quality on a questionnaire.[51] The only item that did differ significantly was "sufficient sleep." It was concluded that shift workers do not consider their sleep "disturbed" more than do day workers. Furthermore, diagnosed insomniacs, with whom the results were compared, scored much worse on most items. The lack of difference between shift workers and day workers could possibly be due to shift workers not seeing their sleep as disturbed because their sleep, although short, is consolidated, as documented in the polysomnographic studies listed previously. Shift workers also sleep well before an early morning shift, even if the awakening is difficult. They also sleep well after an evening shift. The observations suggest that shift workers in general do not fulfill the criteria for chronic insomnia despite frequent occurrence of reduced sleep duration.

PHYSIOLOGIC SLEEPINESS

Although short or otherwise impaired sleep may be the most common complaint in shift workers, the amount of sleepiness may determine the level of difficulty with shift work. If sleep would be impaired without consequences to alertness, it is doubtful that this would be seen as a problem.

In the sleep clinic, the Multiple Sleep Latency Test (MSLT) is considered the gold standard measure of physiologic sleepiness. The MSLT is a series of brief nap opportunities provided across the day, typically in 2-hour increments. The naps are ended after the patient falls asleep as determined by the EEG. The average latency to sleep across the day is then determined. Average latencies below 5 minutes are considered to represent a pathologic level of physiologic sleepiness[52] that is seen commonly in patients with sleep disorders such as sleep apnea and narcolepsy. An average latency to sleep of between 5 to 10 minutes is considered an intermediate level of sleepiness, and average latencies greater than 10 minutes are considered to represent low levels of physiologic sleepiness. No study has been performed to document the incidence of pathologic sleepiness in shift workers at night, but data from simulated shift work studies suggest that average MSLT sleep latencies are lower during the biologic night.[53,54]

Data from post–night shift bedtimes exist in field studies.[9–14] Essentially they indicate short (<5 minutes) latencies, attesting to excessive sleepiness according to clinical criteria.[52] Other indicators of physiologic sleepiness include EEG measures of alpha (8–12 Hz) and theta (4–8 Hz) activity,[55] slow eye movements,[56] or blink duration.[57] In general, alpha activity is an EEG pattern associated with relaxed wakefulness and increased sleepiness, and theta activity is a sleep EEG pattern. Slow eye movements are commonly seen during the transition from wakefulness to

sleep.[58] In laboratory studies, alpha and theta EEG activity, as well as slow eye movements and blink duration measures of physiologic sleepiness, have been shown to be increased when homeostatic sleep drive is high and when wakefulness occurs during the biologic night.[59]

Physiologic measures give strong support to the notion of night shift sleepiness. In an EEG study of night workers at work (train drivers), it was found that one fourth showed pronounced increases in alpha (8–12 Hz) and theta (4–8 Hz) activity as well as slow eye movements towards the early morning, but these changes were absent during day driving.[60] The correlations with ratings of sleepiness were high (r = .74). In some instances, obvious performance lapses such as driving against a red light occurred during bursts of slow eye movements and of alpha/theta activity. The pattern is very similar in truck drivers during long haul (8–10 hour) drives,[14,61] and similar results have been demonstrated for air crew during long haul flights (**Fig. 1**).[62]

Process operators were found to have not only sleepiness-related increases in alpha and theta activity but also full-fledged sleep during the night shift.[13] Such incidents of sleep proper occurred in approximately one fourth of the subjects. Usually, they occurred during the second half of the night shift and never in connection with any other shift. Importantly, sleep on the job was not condoned by the company, nor was there any official awareness that sleep would or could occur during work hours. Interestingly, the subjects were unaware of having slept but were aware of sleepiness.

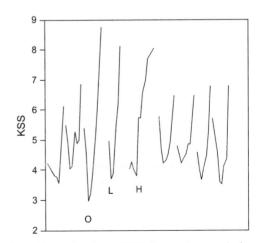

Fig. 1. Mean sleepiness (KSS) in an air crew before, during, and after a westward flight across nine time zones (Copenhagen to Los Angeles). O = outbound flight day; L = layover day in Los Angeles; H = homebound flight day. Ratings are made from awakening to bedtime.

Furthermore, hospital interns on call show "attentional failures" (defined as sleep intrusions in the EEG), particularly during early morning work.[63] The occurrence of sleep intrusions was reduced when continuous on-call duty across days was broken up to permit relatively normal amounts of sleep each day.

Increased alpha and theta activity in the waking EEG have also been demonstrated in truck drivers driving a truck simulator at night,[64] in power station operators during a night shift,[65] and in shift workers driving a simulator home after a normal night shift.[66] Findings from these studies also showed large increases in subjective sleepiness. In addition, findings from the driving simulator studies showed impaired performance in the form of increased variation in lateral position on the road. However, the use of simulated night shift operations is limited in that it is difficult to truly simulate real-world operational demands, interpersonal interactions, and challenges.

Findings from studies of physiologic sleepiness clearly show strong effects of night shifts. Nevertheless, it is possible that the degree of sleepiness is underestimated, because it appears that many individuals start counteracting sleepiness when they start to feel the symptoms. This reaction probably prevents sleepiness from appearing in many physiologic indicators, because EEG and electro-oculogram (EOG) signs of sleepiness only occur at higher levels of sleepiness when the individual is "fighting sleep" and has reached a maximum level of sleepiness.[56] Physiologic changes may occur only when no countermeasures are applied; however, this is an unsystematic impression by the primary author from natural observations in many studies. Findings from laboratory studies indicate that signs of physiologic sleepiness at night are still observed, even when using wakefulness-promoting countermeasures such as caffeine.[67,68]

SUBJECTIVE SLEEPINESS

Subjective sleepiness is obviously easier to measure than physiologic sleepiness; therefore, a wealth of results is available for inspection. Although it has sometimes been argued that subjective measures are less valid than other measures, it is mainly subjective complaints that make individuals seek medical attention. This observation is certainly true for insomnia or hypersomnia, the diagnosis of which is based on complaints of difficulties initiating and maintaining sleep, of nonrestorative sleep, or of excessive sleepiness.[69]

In this context one should also point out that "sleepiness" is not the same thing as "fatigue," at least not scientifically. It would lead too far to try to introduce strict definitions. Nevertheless, "sleepiness" refers to the tendency of falling asleep.[70] Fatigue may include sleepiness but also states such as physical and mental fatigue. Often, the two conepts are interconnected, but they need not be. The issue of the differential definition of sleepiness and fatigue has been subject to a constant debate.[71,72] One clinically useful distinction between fatigue and sleepiness is that cognitive and muscle fatigue symptoms may be reduced by sedentary activity or rest without sleeping, whereas subjective sleepiness and the propensity for sleep are often exacerbated by sedentary activity or rest.

A wealth of early questionnaire studies suggests that the overwhelming majority of shift workers experience sleepiness in connection with night shift work, whereas day work is associated with no, or marginal, sleepiness.[5,73,74] The studies by Verhaegen[74] and Paley[73] and colleagues report that fatigue increases on entering and decreases on leaving shift work. In many studies, a majority of shift workers admit to having experienced involuntary sleep on the night shift, whereas this is less common on day-oriented shifts.[75–77]

Between 10% and 20% of workers report falling asleep during night work. Although the popular Epworth scale has not been used frequently in relation to shift work, one recent study showed values of 9.2 in night workers, 8.6 in rotating shift workers, and 8.0 in day workers.[78] The differences are small, and the Epworth scale[79] in its present form may not be ideal for studying shift work because it contains questions which often refer to activities that may be difficult to relate to night-time work, such as falling asleep at a red light (while in the drivers seat of a car).

If one wants to obtain a detailed impression of subjective sleepiness in shift work, multiple measurements must be made across each shift and on days off, including during leisure time. When this has been done, the results indicate moderate-to-high sleepiness during the night shift and no sleepiness at all during the day shifts,[30,80,81] again providing evidence that shift work sleepiness is associated with the work schedule and cannot be considered a primary sleep disorder of excessive sleepiness that is always present. Data are presented herein to illustrate subjective sleepiness at night in the laboratory and during real shift work. We use these studies because the same self-rating scale of sleepiness has been used in all of them, allowing the possibility of making comparisons. The scale is the Karolinska Sleepiness Scale (KSS) which ranges from 1 to 9, with 1 = very alert, 3 = rather alert, 5 = nether alert nor sleepy, 7 = sleepy but no difficulty remaining awake, and 9 = very sleepy (fighting sleep, an effort to remain awake).[56] Physiologic intrusions of sleep in the EEG or EOG usually start at level 7 and dominate the recording at level 9. The KSS has been shown to be sensitive to sleepiness due to total sleep deprivation[82] and circadian phase (eg, **Fig. 2**), chronic sleep loss,[83] sleep disorders,[84,85] as well as treatment of sleepiness with wakefulness and sleep-promoting countermeasures.[85,86]

Findings from a shift work study (**Fig. 3**) show subjective sleepiness ratings in 60 workers in the paper industry working an extremely rapidly rotating shift system with very short rest between the shifts.[7] The schedule started with a night shift (2100–0600 hours) followed by 8 hours off, an afternoon shift (1400–2100 hours) with 8 hours

off, and a morning shift (0600–1400 hours). This "triad" was followed by 56 hours off and included two normal night sleeps. The triad pattern was repeated seven times, and the cycle ended with 8 days off. **Fig. 3** shows the last triad, together with the first 2 days off. Sleepiness rose to high levels during the first night shift (6.5), fell to intermediate levels (4–4.5) during the afternoon shift (after 5.4 hours of sleep), and reached high levels (5–5.5) again during the morning shift (after 4.5 hours of sleep). Sleepiness was back to normal levels (mostly <4) on the first recovery day.

The morning shift effect seems to be similar to that seen in the middle of the night shift but seems, on the other hand, to be present throughout the entire shift[80,87] and may reach very high levels[5,6] when the start time is earlier than 6 AM.[88] This sleepiness leads to an early afternoon nap in about

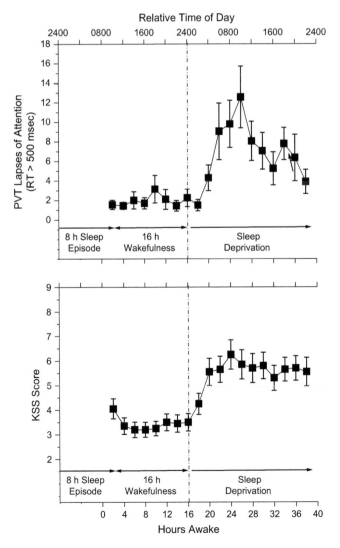

Fig. 2. Subjective sleepiness (KSS) and psychomotor vigilance test (PVT) performance scores (lapses of attention, reaction times >500 ms) across 40 hours of total sleep deprivation. Sleepiness and performance lapses are low during the habitual day across the first ∼16 hours of wakefulness, whereas, thereafter, sleepiness and PVT lapses of attention increase across the habitual night with peaks around 26 hours awake. PVT lapses, and to a lesser extent, KSS sleepiness then improve the next day because the circadian clock promotes wakefulness even though sleep did not occur. These data show what would likely happen to sleepiness and performance on the first night shift in a series if shift workers did not nap prior to the shift.

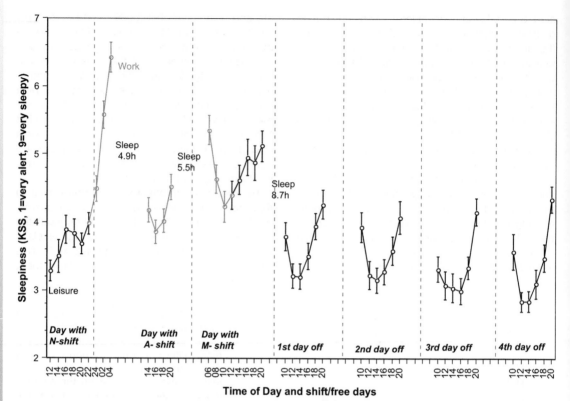

Fig. 3. Subjective sleepiness (KSS) in rapidly rotating shift workers (mean ± SE). Filled points (*grey*) indicate sleepiness during work hours.

one third of the workers.[89–91] Morning work seems to be increasing in many areas, particularly in transport work and in the media. One may also consider the effects of traffic congestion in large populated areas resulting in earlier commuting times in order for travelers to reduce travel time.

For comparison, burnout subjects (extreme exhaustion) show daytime values of 5 to 6, whereas controls show values of 3 to 4 and even lower values during days off.[92] Healthy subjects reach levels of 6 to 7 after 5 days of 4 hours of night sleep.[83]

The second shift work illustration (**Fig. 4**) concerns adjustment to night work under special circumstances. Adjustment to night shifts normally does not occur because shifts alternate, or because of the exposure to daylight when returning home from the night shift, which counteracts the expected delay of the circadian clock.[93] When light is not interfering, such as when night workers are provided with strong sunglasses for the morning commute home, partial adjustment can occur.[40,93] This adjustment may also be seen in situations when no daylight is present. **Fig. 4** shows the results from a study of seven workers on an oil production platform in the North Sea.[94] They worked 14 consecutive days between

1900 and 0700 hours. These days were followed by 3 weeks off. The workers were not exposed to outdoor light because the platform was a self-contained work place in which all aspects of life took place indoors. **Fig. 4** shows the sleepiness pattern across the working days and the first

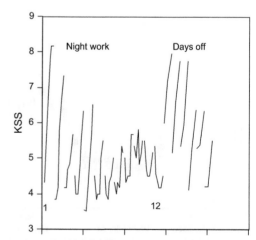

Fig. 4. Mean subjective sleepiness in oil platform workers on 12-night shifts and 6 days off (*dashed lines*).

6 days off. Sleepiness reached extremely high levels during the first days, but the pattern gradually changed. In about the middle, the pattern and levels become similar to day work patterns, although at a level of intermediate sleepiness. On return home, the pattern was strongly changed again, and sleepiness levels remained high for 4 to 5 days. In fact, daytime levels never seemed to reach normal day life levels. Because the study did not include further weeks off, it is unclear whether recovery may have proceeded further.

The daytime sleep data during the night work schedule showed that the bedtime gradually changed from 0800 hours to close to 1100 hours. Similarly, the time of awakening changed from 1700 hours to 1800 hours, yielding a sleep length of just below 8 hours. During the days off, a midnight bedtime was adopted throughout, but the time of awakening changed from 0600 hours to 0800 hours on day 6. Taken together, the results suggest that the circadian system adjusted strongly to night work, although not perfectly, and that the readjustment back to reasonably normal levels took around 6 days. Indeed, it is possible that even some days more would have been required to reach full recovery.

An important question is the implications of the rated sleepiness discussed previously, such as impaired performance. Is there a level of sleepiness that might be "acceptable" considering a putative right of individuals to lead their lives at reasonable levels of alertness? We have suggested that the KSS level of 5 to 6 characterizes subjects high on burnout[92] and patients with a burnout diagnosis at slightly higher levels.[95] One might also consider the level of sleepiness in individuals with a negative attitude to shift work in the study by Axelsson and colleagues.[7] That group reached a maximum of 7.2 on the night shift, 5.2 on the afternoon shift, and 5.9 on the morning shift. The corresponding values for workers with a positive attitude were 5.7, 3.9, and 4.8, respectively. Similarly, Czeisler and colleagues[85] showed that workers diagnosed with shift work disorder (SWD) had a mean KSS value of 7 out of 9 on the night shift. The comparisons attempted here suggest that night shift sleepiness for average shift workers is higher than acceptable, and that some shift workers have even higher levels of night shift sleepiness.

The effects of shift work on sleepiness are obviously profound, but an important question is whether it is related to the ability to function. This seems to be true,[82,96] although the relation between subjective sleepiness and many performance tasks appears to be moderate.[83,97–103] Yang and colleagues[104] have reported that if the self-rating is carried out after a minute of sitting quietly with closed eyes, the correlation is increased, although it is still moderate. In most studies, self-ratings are carried out without any control of the situation leading up to the rating, whereas performance tests are carried out under controlled conditions and with a task load that may unmask sleepiness.

PERFORMANCE AND ACCIDENTS AT WORK

As might be expected from the effects of shift work on sleepiness, performance and safety are also affected.[105] Road transport is the area where the link between safety and night work sleepiness is most pronounced. Harris[106] and Hamelin[107] and Langlois and colleagues[108] convincingly demonstrated that single-vehicle truck accidents have, by far, the greatest probability of occurring at night (early morning). Single-vehicle automobile highway accidents are also greatest at night.[109–111] Furthermore, the United States National Transportation Safety board (NTSB) found that 30% to 40% of all US truck accidents are fatigue related (and grossly underestimated in conventional reports). The latter investigation was extended to search for the immediate causes of fatigue-induced accidents.[112] The most important factor was the amount of sleep obtained during the preceding 24 hours and split-sleep patterns, whereas the length of time driven seemed to have a minor role.

The NTSB also concluded that the Exxon Valdez accident in 1989 was due to fatigue, caused by reduced sleep and extended work hours.[113] The extent of fatal, fatigue-related accidents is considered to be approximately 30%.[114] This rate is approximately the same level of incidence in the air traffic sector, whereas equivalent accidents at sea are estimated at slightly below 20%.

In industry, a classic study by Bjerner and colleagues[115] showed that errors in meter readings over a period of 20 years in a gas works had a pronounced peak on the night shift. There was also a secondary peak during the afternoon. Similarly, Brown[116] demonstrated that telephone operators connected calls considerably slower at night. Woyczak-Jaroszova found that the speed of spinning threads in a textile mill went down during the night.[117] From conventional industrial operations, less data are available[118,119] but indicate that overall accidents tend to occur, not surprisingly, when activity is at its peak. These values do not take account of exposure. Findings from some other studies show night shift dominance for accidents[120–122] but not all.

It is also believed that the (nighttime) nuclear plant meltdown at Chernobyl was due to human error related to work scheduling.[123] Similar observations have been made for the Three Mile Island reactor accident and the near miss incidents at the David Beese reactor in Ohio and at the Rancho Seco reactor in California. These observations are all anecdotal, and few additional data are available.

The most carefully executed study, from car manufacturing, indicates a 30% to 50% increase in accident risk on the night shift.[124] Åkerstedt and colleagues[125] showed that fatal occupational accidents were higher in shift workers in a prospective study (controlling for physical work load, stress, and other factors). Extended duration work shifts also increase the risk of automobile accidents.[126] A study of interns on call showed that improving rest conditions (maximum of 16 consecutive hours of work and 60 hours per week) greatly reduced many types of medical mistakes, of which several were serious.[15] The performance decrement during simulated[127] and actual shift work[128] has been compared with the effects of blood alcohol levels of 0.05% and greater.

Several studies have tried to evaluate the costs to society of alertness-related accidents and loss of performance (which does not reflect only the costs of shift work). One estimate from the 1990s exceeds $40 billion per year in the United States.[129]

SPECIAL CASES

With regard to shift scheduling, attempts have shown that clockwise shift changes should be less negative for performance than counterclockwise ones, but the results are not encouraging.[23,130,131] There has also been a continuous discussion of whether permanent shifts are better than rotating ones[16,132–134] This issue has not been resolved. One could also conceive of longer shifts because they would leave more days free for recuperation. This approach is probably not applicable to all occupations because of too high a work load, but in many studies shifts up to 12 hours have been shown not to affect performance negatively[80,135–137] and seem to be attractive to the employees. Findings from other studies indicate that shifts of 10 hour duration and greater increase sleepiness[138,139] and the risk of accidents.[126,137,140]

SHIFT WORK (SLEEP) DISORDER

The effects of shift work are relatively pronounced, such as a reduction of sleep by 1.5 to 2 hours when working the night shift schedule and considerable sleepiness (reaching 2–3 minutes on average for the MSLT and average subjective

sleepiness of 7 on the 1–9 level KSS scale). Clearly, some individuals appear to be more negatively affected by shift work than others. There is a diagnostic category called "shift work sleep disorder" (SWSD), also referred to as SWD or shift work type (DSM IV).[141] SWSD is defined as the "report of difficulty falling asleep, staying asleep, or non-restorative sleep for at least one month" associated with "a work period that occurs during the habitual sleep phase." The International Classification of Sleep Disorders (ICSD)[69] defines the diagnosis of SWD (the word "sleep" has been dropped) on four criteria: (1) a complaint of insomnia or excessive sleepiness temporally associated with a recurring work schedule that overlaps the usual time for sleep, (2) symptoms associated with the shift work schedule over the course of at least 1 month, (3) circadian and sleep-time misalignment as demonstrated by a sleep log or actigraphical monitoring for 7 days or more, and (4) the presence of a sleep disturbance not explainable by another sleep disorder, medical or neurologic disorder, mental disorder, medication use, or substance use disorder.

The prevalence of SWD is not clear because most studies have not used standardized diagnostic criteria;[142] however, one estimate arrives at 10% using the ICSD-2 criteria (sleep difficulties or sleepiness sometimes or often at a severity level of 6 on a 1–10 scale).[78] In another study, a figure of 8% was found when using "very negative or rather negative to present work hours" as a criterion.[7]

Czeisler and colleagues[85] used ICSD-2 SWD criteria, with MSLT values of less than 6 minutes during the night to objectively verify excessive nighttime sleepiness, and sleep efficiency of less than 87.5% during day sleep (8-hour time in bed) after a night shift to objectively verify daytime insomnia. The resulting group showed a mean MSLT during the night shift of less than 2 minutes, an average sleepiness rating of approximately 7 on the KSS,[56] and an average sleep duration of 6 hours. The MSLT and sleepiness ratings were clearly below what is usually found to be average in other studies, whereas the sleep duration was similar to that in most other studies. The controlled and soporific laboratory situation may not be representative of the real-life situation, at least not with respect to absolute levels of sleepiness.

COUNTERMEASURES

The most logical countermeasure for the sleep/wake problems in night work is to discontinue that activity. If that is not possible, several aspects of scheduling have been recommended as improvements.[7] Among them are clockwise rotation (the sequence of morning-night-afternoon shifts), but the empirical support is rather weak.[143] Some obvious adverse types of schedules should be avoided. One includes short rest periods between shifts. In many countries, 8 hours of rest frequently appear in between, for example, a night shift and a morning shift. This results in short sleep and sleepiness during work.[7,80]

One should probably also avoid several night shifts in succession, because sleepiness will 22accumulate, as will accidents.[144] Flexibility and influence on scheduling will have positive effects on sleep.[145] Strategic distribution of rest days will improve alertness.[136] Rest breaks seem to be efficient barriers to increased accident risk (and presumably sleepiness/fatigue) across the night shift.[146] Late changeovers seem preferable to early ones.[147]

Education of shift workers is needed regarding good sleep habits and environment, the need for protected time for sleep, as well as recognition of critical times of vulnerability. Among acute countermeasures for night shift fatigue/sleepiness, is are one possibility,[148] but few real-life shift work studies are available.[24,26,149,150] If naps are used as a countermeasure to shift work–induced sleepiness, evidence from laboratory studies suggests that prophylactic naps of 2 hours in duration before an overnight shift (eg, late afternoon) are more effective at reducing nighttime sleepiness than are 2-hour naps during the night shift.[151] The latter effect is likely due to the negative impact of sleep inertia[152] following long work shift naps, because such naps are likely to include deep slow wave sleep and sleep inertia is worst when awakening from deep sleep. If naps are used during shift work operations, very short naps of less than 10 minutes may be effective because there is less sleep inertia after short naps. Short 10-minute naps have been reported to reduce sleepiness during the daytime;[153] however, the effectiveness of short naps to reduce sleepiness has not been tested at night.

Sleepiness at night can also be reduced by wakefulness-promoting drugs. Caffeine is perhaps the most common self-selected countermeasure used by shift workers. No operational field studies have been performed with caffeine; however, findings from laboratory studies indicate that caffeine can reduce nighttime sleepiness and improve performance.[67,150,154] Prophylactic use of caffeine before the onset of sleepiness[67,154] appears to be more effective than use of caffeine to reverse sleepiness.[155] Recent work on alertness-enhancing drugs such as modafinil has shown improvement in nighttime sleepiness in patients with SWD, although clinically significant sleepiness is still present.[85] Treating otherwise healthy shift workers with pharmaceutical products is questionable, however, and the risks associated with treatment need to be weighed against the risks associated with no treatment or the effectiveness of alternate treatments. The case is probably the same with the "chronobiotic" melatonin.[156] Exogenous melatonin has been tried in an actual shift work situation but with moderate success.[157] Light treatment is a third possibility, but little applied field work has been carried out and with modest effects.[40–42,154,157–159]

With respect to driving, rolling down a window, turning on the radio, and stopping for exercise have been tried in simulator studies without success.[160] Interestingly, a recent study by Anund and colleagues[161] showed that hitting a so-called "rumble strip" due do sleepiness only brings back alertness (physiologic, behavioral) for 1 to 2 minutes. The sleepiness then returns to pre-hit levels.

Perhaps the most effective way of promoting wakefulness at night is through the use of combined countermeasures. In laboratory studies assessing nighttime performance, it has been demonstrated that combinations of bright light and caffeine, naps and caffeine, as well as naps and modafinil improve cognitive performance and alertness at night more than either treatment alone.[150,154,155,162]

SUMMARY

Shift work that includes the night will have pronounced negative effects on sleep, sleepiness, performance, and accident risk. Misalignment between internal circadian physiology and the required work schedule is thought to be a primary cause of shift work schedule–induced sleepiness and sleep disruption. Wakefulness and sleep-promoting countermeasures can provide some help to reduce sleepiness and improve sleep, but, currently, there are no effective treatments that can counteract all of the negative impact that shift work schedules have on human physiology and behavior. Additional research is necessary to determine why some individuals have particular vulnerability to nighttime sleepiness and daytime insomnia. In addition, more research is needed to develop effective countermeasures for both sleepiness and insomnia associated with shift work, because shift work is now an important and established component of local and world economies.

ACKNOWLEDGMENTS

The authors wish to acknowledge the many helpful discussions and research collaborations with Drs. Göran Kecklund and Charles A. Czeisler, which have influenced our thinking on shift work and shift work disorder.

REFERENCES

1. Knutsson A. Health disorders of shift workers. Occup Med (Lond) 2003;53(2):103–8.
2. Knauth P. Categories and parameters of shiftwork systems. In: Colquhoun WP, Costa G, Folkard S, et al, editors. Shiftwork: problems and solutions. Frankfurt am Main: Peter Lang GmbH; 1996. p. 17–28.
3. Aanonsen A. Shift work and health. Oslo: Universitetsforlaget; 1964.
4. Tune GS. A note on the sleep of shift workers. Ergonomics 1968;11(2):183–4.
5. Andersen JE. Three-shift work. Copenhagen: Socialforskningsinstituet; 1970.
6. Åkerstedt T. Sleepiness as a consequence of shift work. Sleep 1988;11:17–34.
7. Axelsson J, Akerstedt T, Kecklund G, et al. Tolerance to shift work: how does it relate to sleep and wakefulness? Int Arch Occup Environ Health 2004;77(2):121–9.
8. Pilcher JJ, Schoeling SE, Prosansky CM. Self-report sleep habits as predictors of subjective sleepiness. Behav Med 2000;25(4):161–8.
9. Foret J, Lantin G. The sleep of train drivers: an example of the effects of irregular work schedules on sleep. In: Colquhoun WP, editor. Aspects of human efficiency: diurnal rhythm and loss of sleep. London: The English Universities Press; 1972. p. 273–81.
10. Foret J, Benoit O. Structure du sommeil chez des travailleurs à horaires alternants [Sleep patterns of workers on rotating shifts]. Electroencephalogr Clin Neurophysiol 1974;37(4):377–444 [in French].
11. Matsumoto K. Sleep patterns in hospital nurses due to shift work: an EEG study. Waking Sleeping 1978;2:169–73.
12. Tilley A, Wilkinson RT, Drud M. Night and day shifts compared in terms of the quality and quantity of sleep recorded in the home and performance measures at work: a pilot study. Night and shift work: biological and social aspects. Oxford: Pergamon Press; 1981. p. 187–96.
13. Torsvall L, Akerstedt T, Gillander K, et al. Sleep on the night shift: 24-hour EEG monitoring of spontaneous sleep/wake behavior. Psychophysiol 1989; 26(3):352–8.
14. Mitler MM, Miller JC, Lipsitz JJ, et al. The sleep of long-haul truck drivers. N Engl J Med 1997; 337(11):755–61.
15. Lockley SW, Cronin JW, Evans EE, et al. Effect of reducing interns' weekly work hours on sleep and attentional failures. N Engl J Med 2004;351(18): 1829–37.
16. Pilcher JJ, Lambert BJ, Huffcutt AI. Differential effects of permanent and rotating shifts on self-report sleep length: a meta-analytic review. Sleep 2000;23(2):155–63.
17. Park YM, Matsumoto PK, Seo YJ, et al. Sleep-wake behavior of shift workers using wrist actigraph. Psychiatry Clin Neurosci 2000;54(3):359–60.
18. Folkard S. Do permanent night workers show circadian adjustment? A review based on the endogenous melatonin rhythm. Chronobiol Int 2008;25(2): 215–24.
19. Signal TL, Gander PH. Rapid counterclockwise shift rotation in air traffic control: effects on sleep and night work. Aviat Space Environ Med 2007; 78(9):878–85.
20. Czeisler CA, Duffy JF, Shanahan TL, et al. Stability, precision, and near-24-hour period of the human circadian pacemaker. Science 1999;284(5423): 2177–81.
21. Wright KP Jr, Hughes RJ, Kronauer RE, et al. Intrinsic near-24-hour pacemaker period determines limits of circadian entrainment to a weak synchronizer in humans. Proc Natl Acad Sci USA 2001;98(24):14027–32.
22. Czeisler CA, Mooreede MC, Coleman RM. Rotating shift work schedules that disrupt sleep are improved by applying circadian principles. Science 1982;217(4558):460–3.
23. Cruz C, Boquet A, Detwiler C, et al. Clockwise and counterclockwise rotating shifts: effects on vigilance and performance. Aviat Space Environ Med 2003;74(6 Pt 1):606–14.
24. Garbarino S, Mascialino B, Antonietta M, et al. Professional shift-work drivers adopting prophylactic naps can reduce the risk of car accidents during night work. Sleep 2004;27.
25. Rosekind MR, Smith RM, Miller DL, et al. Alertness management: strategic naps in operational settings. J Sleep Res 1995;4(S2):62–6.
26. Smith-Coggins R, Howard SK, Mac DT, et al. Improving alertness and performance in emergency department physicians and nurses: the use of planned naps. Ann Emerg Med 2006; 48(5):596–604.
27. Signal TL, Gander PH, Anderson H, et al. Scheduled napping as a countermeasure to sleepiness in air traffic controllers. J Sleep Res 2009;18(1):11–9.
28. Webb WB, Agnew HW Jr. Sleep: effects of a restricted regime. Science 1965;150:1745–7.
29. Akerstedt T, Gillberg M. A dose-response study of sleep loss and spontaneous sleep termination. Psychophysiol 1986;23(3):293–7.
30. Tilley AJ, Wilkinson RT, Warren PSG, et al. The sleep and performance of shift workers. Hum Factors 1982;24:629–41.

31. Dahlgren K. Adjustment of circadian rhythms and EEG sleep functions to day and night sleep among permanent nightworkers and rotating shiftworkers. Psychophysiol 1981;18(4):381–91.

32. Akerstedt T, Kecklund G, Knutsson A. Spectral analysis of sleep electroencephalography in rotating three-shift work. Scand J Work Environ Health 1991;17(5):330–6.

33. Kecklund G. Sleep and alertness: effects of shift work, early rising, and the sleep environment. Stress Research Report 1996;252:1–75.

34. Foret J, Benoit O. Shiftwork: the level of adjustment to schedule reversal by a sleep study. Waking and Sleeping 1978;2:107–12.

35. Dahlgren K. Long-term adjustment of circadian rhythms to a rotating shiftwork schedule. Scand J Work Environ Health 1981;7(2):141–51.

36. Kripke DF, Cook B, Lewis OF. Sleep of night workers: EEG recordings. Psychophysiol 1970; 7(3):377–84.

37. Bryden G, Holdstock TL. Effects of night duty on sleep patterns of nurses. Psychophysiol 1973; 10(1):36–42.

38. Tepas DI, Walsh JK, Moss PD, et al. Polysomnographic correlates of shift worker performance in the laboratory. In: Reinberg A, Vieux N, Andlauer P, editors. Night and shift work: biological and social aspects. Oxford: Pergamon Press; 1981. p. 179–86.

39. Akerstedt T. Adjustment of physiological circadian rhythms and the sleep-wake cycle to shiftwork. In: Folkard S, Monk TH, editors. Hours of work. London: John Wiley and Sons; 1985. p. 185–97.

40. Smith MR, Eastman CI. Night shift performance is improved by a compromise circadian phase position. Study 3. Circadian phase after 7 night shifts with an intervening weekend off. Sleep 2008; 31(12):1639–45.

41. Horowitz TS, Cade BE, Wolfe JM, et al. Efficacy of bright light and sleep/darkness scheduling in alleviating circadian maladaptation to night work. Am J Physiol Endocrinol Metab 2001;281(2):E384–91.

42. Boivin DB, James FO. Circadian adaptation to night-shift work by judicious light and darkness exposure. J Biol Rhythms 2002;17(6):556–67.

43. Bjorvatn B, Stangenes K, Oyane N, et al. Subjective and objective measures of adaptation and readaptation to night work on an oil rig in the North Sea. Sleep 2006;29(6):821–9.

44. Dumont M, Montplaisi J, Infante-Rivard C. Insomnia symptoms in nurses with former permanent night-work experience. In: Koella WP, Obal F, Schultz H, et al, editors. Sleep '86. Stuttgart: Gustav Fischer Verlag; 1988. p. 405–6.

45. Dumont M, Montplaisir J, Infante-Rivard C. Sleep quality of former night-shift workers. Int J Occup Environ Health 1997;3(Suppl 2):S10–4.

46. Guilleminault C, Czeisler S, Coleman R, et al. Circadian rhythm disturbances and sleep disorders in shift workers. In: Buser PA, Cobb WA, Okuma T, editors. Kyoto symposia. Amsterdam: Elsevier; 1982. p. 709–14.

47. Ingre M, Akerstedt T. Effect of accumulated night work during the working lifetime, on subjective health and sleep in monozygotic twins. J Sleep Res 2004;13(1):45–8.

48. Wilkinson RT, Edwards RS, Haines E. Performance following a night of reduced sleep. Psychon Sci 1966;5:471–2.

49. Roehrs T, Burduvali E, Bonahoom A, et al. Ethanol and sleep loss: a "dose" comparison of impairing effects. Sleep 2003;26(8):981–5.

50. Van Dongen HPA, Maislin G, Mullington JM, et al. The cumulative cost of additional wakefulness: dose-response effects on neurobehavioral functions and sleep physiology from chronic sleep restriction and total sleep deprivation. Sleep 2003;26(2):117–26.

51. Akerstedt T, Ingre M, Broman JE, et al. Disturbed sleep in shift workers, day workers, and insomniacs. Chronobiol Int 2008;25(2):333–48.

52. Roehrs T, Roth T. Multiple Sleep Latency Test: technical aspects and normal values. J Clin Neurophysiol 1992;9(1):63–7.

53. Porcu S, Bellatreccia A, Ferrara M, et al. Performance, ability to stay awake, and tendency to fall asleep during the night after a diurnal sleep with temazepam or placebo. Sleep 1997;20(7):535–41.

54. Muehlbach MJ, Walsh JK. The effects of caffeine on simulated night-shift work and subsequent daytime sleep. Sleep 1995;18(1):22–9.

55. Santamaria J, Chiappa KH. The EEG of drowsiness in normal adults. J Clin Neurophysiol 1987;4(4): 327–82.

56. Akerstedt T, Gillberg M. Subjective and objective sleepiness in the active individual. Int J Neurosci 1990;52(1–2):29–37.

57. Wierwille WW, Ellsworth LA. Evaluation of driver drowsiness by trained raters. Accid Anal Prev 1994;26(5):571–81.

58. Ogilvie RD, McDonagh DM, Stone SN, et al. Eye movements and the detection of sleep onset. Psychophysiol 1988;25(1):81–91.

59. Cajochen C, Khalsa SBS, Wyatt JK, et al. EEG and ocular correlates of circadian melatonin phase and human performance decrements during sleep loss. Am J Physiol 1999;277:R640–9.

60. Torsvall L, Akerstedt T. Sleepiness on the job: continuously measured EEG changes in train drivers. Electroencephalogr Clin Neurophysiol 1987;66(6):502–11.

61. Kecklund G, Akerstedt T. Sleepiness in long distance truck driving: an ambulatory EEG study of night driving. Ergonomics 1993;36(9):1007–17.

62. Rosekind MR, Graeber RC, Dinges DF, et al. Crew factors in flight operations. IX. Effects of planned cockpit rest on crew performance and alertness in long haul operations. Technical Memorandum No. A-94134. Moffett Field (CA): NASA Technical Memorandum; 1995.

63. Landrigan CP, Rothschild JW, Conin JW, et al. Effect of reducing interns' work hours on serious medical errors in intensive care units. N Engl J Med 2004;351(18):1838–48.

64. Gillberg M, Kecklund G, Akerstedt T. Sleepiness and performance of professional drivers in a truck simulator: comparisons between day and night driving. J Sleep Res 1996;5(1):12–5.

65. Gillberg M, Kecklund G, Goransson B, et al. Operator performance and signs of sleepiness during day and night work in a simulated thermal power plant. Int J Ind Ergon 2003;31(2):101–9.

66. Akerstedt T, Peters B, Anund A, et al. Impaired alertness and performance driving home from the night shift: a driving simulator study. J Sleep Res 2005;14(1):17–20.

67. Walsh JK, Muehlbach MJ, Schweitzer PK. Hypnotics and caffeine as countermeasures for shiftwork-related sleepiness and sleep disturbance. J Sleep Res 1995;4(S2):80–3.

68. Schweitzer PK, Muehlbach MJ, Walsh JK. Countermeasures for night work performance deficits: the effect of napping or caffeine on continuous performance at night. Work Stress 1992;6(4):355–65.

69. American Academy of Sleep Medicine. The International Classification of Sleep Disorders (ICSD). 2nd edition. Chicago: American Academy of Sleep Medicine; 2005.

70. Dement WC, Carskadon MA. Current perspectives on daytime sleepiness: the issues. Sleep 1982;5(Suppl 2):S56–66.

71. Dement WC, Hall J, Walsh JK. Tiredness versus sleepiness: semantics or a target for public education? Sleep 2003;26(4):485–6.

72. Horne T. The semantics of sleepiness. Sleep 2003;26(6):763.

73. Paley MJ, Tepas DI. Fatigue and the shiftworker: firefighters working on a rotating shift schedule. Hum Factors 1994;36(2):269–84.

74. Verhaegen P, Maasen A, Meers A. Health problems in shift workers: biological rhythms and shift work. New York: Spectrum; 1981. p. 271–82.

75. Prokop O, Prokop L. Ermüdung und einschlafen am steuer [fatigue and falling asleep in driving]. Zbl Verkehrsmed 1955;1:19–30 [in German].

76. Coleman RM, Dement WC. Falling asleep at work: a problem for continuous operations. Sleep Res 1986;15:265.

77. Luna TD, French J, Mitcha JL. A study of USAF air traffic controller shiftwork: sleep, fatigue, activity, and mood analyses. Aviat Space Environ Med 1997;68(1):18–23.

78. Drake CL, Roehrs T, Richardson G, et al. Shift work sleep disorder: prevalence and consequences beyond that of symptomatic day workers. Sleep 2004;27(8):1453–62.

79. Johns MW. A new method for measuring daytime sleepiness: the Epworth sleepiness scale. Sleep 1991;14(6):540–5.

80. Lowden A, Kecklund G, Axelsson J, et al. Change from an 8-hour shift to a 12-hour shift, attitudes, sleep, sleepiness and performance. Scand J Work Environ Health 1998;24(Suppl 3):69–75.

81. Harma M, Sallinen M, Ranta R, et al. The effect of an irregular shift system on sleepiness at work in train drivers and railway traffic controllers. J Sleep Res 2002;11(2):141–51.

82. Gillberg M, Kecklund G, Akerstedt T. Relations between performance and subjective ratings of sleepiness during a night awake. Sleep 1994;17(3):236–41.

83. Axelsson J, Kecklund G, Akerstedt T, et al. Sleepiness and performance in response to repeated sleep restriction and subsequent recovery during semi-laboratory conditions. Chronobiol Int 2008;25(2):297–308.

84. Greneche J, Krieger J, Erhardt C, et al. EEG spectral power and sleepiness during 24 h of sustained wakefulness in patients with obstructive sleep apnea syndrome. Clin Neurophysiol 2008;119(2):418–28.

85. Czeisler CA, Walsh JK, Roth T, et al. Modafinil for excessive sleepiness associated with shift-work sleep disorder. N Engl J Med 2005;353(5):476–86.

86. Suhner A, Schlagenhauf P, Johnson R, et al. Comparative study to determine the optimal melatonin dosage form for the alleviation of jet lag. Chronobiol Int 1998;15(6):655–66.

87. Kecklund G, Akerstedt T, Lowden A. Morning work: effects of early rising on sleep and alertness. Sleep 1997;20(3):215–23.

88. Strogatz SH, Kronauer RE, Czeisler CA. Circadian pacemaker interferes with sleep onset at specific times each day: role in insomnia. Am J Physiol 1987;253(1 Pt 2):R172–8.

89. Knauth P, Rutenfranz J. Duration of sleep related to the type of shift work. In: Reinberg A, Vieux N, Andlauer P, editors. Night and shift work: biological and social aspects. Oxford: Pergamon Press; 1981. p. 161–8.

90. Tepas DI. Shiftworker sleep strategies. J Hum Ergol (Tokyo) 1982;11(Suppl):325–36.

91. Harma M, Knauth P, Ilmarinen J. Daytime napping and its effects on alertness and short-term-memory performance in shiftworkers. Int Arch Occup Environ Health 1989;61(5):341–5.

92. Soderstrom M, Ekstedt M, Akerstedt T, et al. Sleep and sleepiness in young individuals with high burnout scores. Sleep 2004;27(7):1369–77.

93. Eastman CI, Stewart KT, Mahoney MP, et al. Shiftwork: dark goggles and bright light improve circadian rhythm adaptation to night-shift work. Sleep 1994;17(6):535–43.

94. Bjorvatn B, Kecklund G, Akerstedt T. Rapid adaptation to night work at an oil platform, but slow readaptation after returning home. J Occup Environ Med 1998;40(7):601–8.

95. Ekstedt M, Soderstrom M, Akerstedt T, et al. Disturbed sleep and fatigue in occupational burnout. Scand J Work Environ Health 2006;32(2): 121–31.

96. Hoddes E, Zarcone V, Smythe H, et al. Quantification of sleepiness: a new approach. Psychophysiol 1973;10(4):431–6.

97. Dorrian J, Lamond N, Holmes AL, et al. The ability to self-monitor performance during a week of simulated night shifts. Sleep 2003;26(7):871–7.

98. Dorrian J, Lamond N, Dawson D. The ability to self-monitor performance when fatigued. J Sleep Res 2000;9(2):137–44.

99. Ingre M, Akerstedt T, Peters B, et al. Subjective sleepiness, simulated driving performance and blink duration: examining individual differences. J Sleep Res 2006;15(1):47–53.

100. Johnson LC, Spinweber CL, Gomez SA, et al. Daytime sleepiness, performance, mood, nocturnal sleep: the effect of benzodiazepine and caffeine on their relationship. Sleep 1990;13(2):121–35.

101. Kaida K, Akerstedt T, Kecklund G, et al. Use of subjective and physiological indicators of sleepiness to predict performance during a vigilance task. Ind Health 2007;45(4):520–6.

102. Kaida K, Takahashi M, Akerstedt T, et al. Validation of the Karolinska Sleepiness Scale against performance and EEG variables. Clin Neurophysiol 2006;117(7):1574–81.

103. Rogers NL, Dinges DF. Subjective surrogates of performance during night work. Sleep 2003;26(7): 790–1.

104. Yang CM, Lin FW, Spielman AJ. A standard procedure enhances the correlation between subjective and objective measures of sleepiness. Sleep 2004;27(2):329–32.

105. Folkard S, Akerstedt T. Trends in the risk of accidents and injuries and their implications for models of fatigue and performance. Aviat Space Environ Med 2004;75(3 Suppl):A161–7.

106. Harris W. Fatigue, circadian rhythm and truck accidents. In: Mackie RR, editor. Vigilance. New York: Plenum Press; 1977. p. 133–46.

107. Hamelin P. Lorry driver's time habits in work and their involvement in traffic accidents. Ergonomics 1987;30(9):1323–33.

108. Langlois PH, Smolensky MH, Hsi BP, et al. Temporal patterns of reported single-vehicle car and truck accidents in Texas, U.S.A. during 1980-1983. Chronobiol Int 1985;2(2):131–40.

109. Horne JA, Reyner LA. Sleep related vehicle accidents. BMJ 1995;310(6979):565–7.

110. Pack AI, Pack AM, Rodgman E, et al. Characteristics of crashes attributed to the driver having fallen asleep. Accid Anal Prev 1995;27(6):769–75.

111. Akerstedt T, Kecklund G, Horte LG. Night driving, season, and the risk of highway accidents. Sleep 2001;24(4):401–6.

112. National Transportation Safety Board. Factors that affect fatigue in heavy truck accidents. NTSB/SS-95/01. Washington (DC): National Transportation Safety Board; 1995.

113. National Transportation Safety Board. Grounding of the US tankship Exxon Valdez on Bligh Reef, Prince William Sound near Valdez, Alaska, March 24, 1989. NTSB/MAR-90/04. Maritime Accident Report. Washington (DC): National Transportation Safety Board; 1990.

114. National Transportation Safety Board. Evaluation of US Department of Transportation: efforts in the 1990s to address operation fatigue. NTSB/SR-99/01. Washington (DC): National Transportation Safety Board; 1999.

115. Bjerner B, Holm A, Swensson A. Diurnal variation in mental performance: a study of three-shift workers. Br J Ind Med 1955;12(2):103–10.

116. Brown RC. The day and night performance of teleprinter switchboard operators. J Occup Health Psychol 1949;23:121–6.

117. Wojtczak-Jaroszowa J, Pawlowska-Skyga K. Night and shift work. I. Circadian variations in work. Med Pr 1967;18:1–10.

118. Ong CN, Phoon WO, Iskandar N, et al. Shiftwork and work injuries in an iron and steel mill. Appl Ergon 1987;18(1):51–6.

119. Wojtczak-Jaroszowa J, Jarosz D. Chronohygienic and chronosocial aspects of industrial accidents. Prog Clin Biol Res 1987;227(B):415–26.

120. Andlauer P. The effect of shift working on the workers' health. European Productivity Agency. TU Information Bulletin 1960;29.

121. Gold DR, Rogacz S, Bock N, et al. Rotating shift work, sleep, and accidents related to sleepiness in hospital nurses. Am J Public Health 1992;82(7):1011–4.

122. Smith P. Study of weekly and rapidly rotating shift workers. Ergonomics 1978;21(10):874–9.

123. Mitler MM, Carskadon MA, Czeisler CA, et al. Catastrophes, sleep, and public policy: consensus report. Sleep 1988;11(1):100–9.

124. Smith L, Folkard S, Poole CJ. Increased injuries on night shift. Lancet 1994;344(8930):1137–9.

125. Akerstedt T, Fredlund P, Gillberg M, et al. A prospective study of fatal occupational

accidents: relationship to sleeping difficulties and occupational factors. J Sleep Res 2002;11(1): 69–71.

126. Barger LK, Cade BE, Ayas NT, et al. Extended work shifts and the risk of motor vehicle crashes among interns. N Engl J Med 2005;352(2):125–34.

127. Dawson D, Reid K. Fatigue, alcohol and performance impairment. Nature 1997;388(6639):235.

128. Arnedt JT, Owens J, Crouch M, et al. Neurobehavioral performance of residents after heavy night call vs after alcohol ingestion. JAMA 2005;294(9):1025–33.

129. Leger D. The cost of sleep-related accidents: a report for the National Commission on Sleep Disorders Research. Sleep 1994;17(1):84–93.

130. Knauth P. Speed and direction of shift rotation. J Sleep Res 1995;4(Suppl 2):41–6.

131. van Amelsvoort LG, Jansen NW, Swaen GM. Direction of shift rotation among three-shift workers in relation to psychological health and work-family conflict. Scand J Work Environ Health 2004;30(2):149–56.

132. Wilkinson RT. How fast should the night-shift rotate. Ergonomics 1992;35(12):1425–46.

133. Wedderburn AAI. How fast should the night-shift rotate: a rejoinder. Ergonomics 1992;35(12):1447–51.

134. Folkard S. Is there a best compromise shift system. Ergonomics 1992;35(12):1453–63.

135. Smith L, Folkard S, Tucker P, et al. Work shift duration: a review comparing 8-hour and 12-hour shift systems. Occup Environ Med 1998;55(4):217–29.

136. Tucker P, Smith L, Macdonald I, et al. Distribution of rest days in 12 hour shift systems: impacts on health, well-being, and on shift alertness. Occup Environ Med 1999;56(3):206–14.

137. Dembe AE, Erickson JB, Delbos RG, et al. The impact of overtime and long work hours on occupational injuries and illnesses: new evidence from the United States. Occup Environ Med 2005; 62(9):588–97.

138. Gundel A, Drescher J, Maass H, et al. Sleepiness of civil airline pilots during 2 consecutive night flights of extended duration. Biol Psychol 1995; 40(1-2):131–41.

139. Son M, Kong JO, Koh SB, et al. Effects of long working hours and the night shift on severe sleepiness among workers with 12-hour shift systems for 5 to 7 consecutive days in the automobile factories of Korea. J Sleep Res 2008;17(4):385–94.

140. Scott LD, Hwang WT, Rogers AE, et al. The relationship between nurse work schedules, sleep duration, and drowsy driving. Sleep 2007;30(12):1801–7.

141. American Psychiatric Association. Diagnostic and statistical manual of mental disorders. 4th edition. Washington (DC): American Psychiatric Association; 2000.

142. Sack RL, Auckley D, Auger R, et al. Circadian rhythm sleep disorders. Part I. Basic principles,

shift work and jet lag disorders: an American Academy of Sleep Medicine Review. Sleep 2007; 30(11):1456–79.

143. Tucker P, Smith L, Macdonald I, et al. Effects of direction of rotation in continuous and discontinuous 8 hour shift systems. Occup Environ Med 2000;57(10):678–84.

144. Folkard S, Lombardi DA, Tucker PT. Shiftwork: safety, sleepiness and sleep. Ind Health 2005; 43(1):20–3.

145. Costa G, Sartori S, Akerstedt T. Influence of flexibility and variability of working hours on health and well-being. Chronobiol Int 2006;23(6):1125–37.

146. Tucker P, Folkard S, Macdonald I. Rest breaks and accident risk. Lancet 2003;361(9358):680.

147. Tucker P, Smith L, Macdonald I, et al. The impact of early and late shift changeovers on sleep, health, and well-being in 8- and 12-hour shift systems. J Occup Health Psychol 1998;3(3):265–75.

148. Akerstedt T, Torsvall L, Gillberg M. Shift work and napping. In: Dinges DF, Broughton RJ, editors. Sleep and alertness: chronobiological, behavioral, and medical aspects of napping. New York: Raven Press; 1989. p. 205–20.

149. Purnell MT, Feyer AM, Herbison GP. The impact of a nap opportunity during the night shift on the performance and alertness of 12-h shift workers. J Sleep Res 2002;11(3):219–27.

150. Schweitzer PK, Randazzo AC, Stone K, et al. Laboratory and field studies of naps and caffeine as practical countermeasures for sleep-wake problems associated with night work. Sleep 2006; 29(1):39–50.

151. Dinges DF, Orne MT, Whitehouse WG, et al. Temporal placement of a nap for alertness: contributions of circadian phase and prior wakefulness. Sleep 1987;10(4):313–29.

152. Wertz AT, Ronda JM, Czeisler CA, et al. Effects of sleep inertia on cognition. JAMA 2006;295(2): 163–4.

153. Tietzel AJ, Lack LC. The short-term benefits of brief and long naps following nocturnal sleep restriction. Sleep 2001;24(3):293–300.

154. Wright KP Jr, Badia P, Myers BL, et al. Combination of bright light and caffeine as a countermeasure for impaired alertness and performance during extended sleep deprivation. J Sleep Res 1997; 6(1):26–35.

155. Bonnet MH, Arand DL. The use of prophylactic naps and caffeine to maintain performance during a continuous operation. Ergonomics 1994;37(6):1009–20.

156. Smith MR, Lee C, Crowley SJ, et al. Morning melatonin has limited benefit as a soporific for daytime sleep after night work. Chronobiol Int 2005;22(5): 873–88.

157. Bjorvatn B, Stangenes K, Oyane N, et al. Randomized placebo-controlled field study of the effects of

bright light and melatonin in adaptation to night work. Scand J Work Environ Health 2007;33(3): 204–14.

158. Lowden A, Akerstedt T, Wibom R. Suppression of sleepiness and melatonin by bright light exposure during breaks in night work. J Sleep Res 2004; 13(1):37–43.

159. Santhi N, Aeschbach D, Horowitz TS, et al. The impact of sleep timing and bright light exposure on attentional impairment during night work. J Biol Rhythms 2008;23(4):341–52.

160. Reyner LA, Horne JA. Evaluation "in-car" counter-measures to sleepiness: cold air and radio. Sleep 1998;21(1):46–50.

161. Anund A, Kecklund G, Vadeby A, et al. The alerting effect of hitting a rumble strip: a simulator study with sleepy drivers. Accid Anal Prev 2008;40(6): 1970–6.

162. Batejat DM, Lagarde DP. Naps and modafinil as countermeasures for the effects of sleep deprivation on cognitive performance. Aviat Space Environ Med 1999;70(5):493–8.

Circadian Disruption and Psychiatric Disorders: The Importance of Entrainment

Anna Wirz-Justice, PhD*, Vivien Bromundt, MSc, Christian Cajochen, PhD

KEYWORDS
- Circadian rhythms • Sleep regulation • Actigraphy
- Major depression • Dementia • Psychiatric illness

There is a need for more knowledge of sleep medicine to be integrated into psychiatric training and practice. Although many psychiatrists are aware that most patients have some sort of a sleep problem, these mainly are addressed separately from the primary diagnosis, with appropriate choice of sleep-promoting psychopharmacologic agents or additional treatment with benzodiazepines or newer hypnotics. Consideration of circadian rhythms and their impact on sleep–wake behavior in psychiatric disorders is still rare in psychiatric practice.

This is somewhat surprising, because observations linking rhythmic behavior and psychopathology have a long tradition in clinical psychiatric research, particularly in major depression. These observations have been reviewed comprehensively,[1–3] albeit with rather ambiguous conclusions. The precise nature of the links remains elusive, and it may be too simplistic to expect that the enormous variety of psychiatric disorders have common dysfunctions related to the biological clock. It is not only the problem of clearly defining patient groups within and among diagnoses, but also, different treatments make it difficult to define a specific circadian rhythm abnormality. It may be more the symptoms such as anxiety and depressed mood rather than the diagnosis that are related to sleep disorders. In addition, methodological issues cloud most investigations, because masking effects of behavior and environment on the rhythms measured often have not been controlled for.

Thus, this article will not address evidence for circadian disruption as etiology. Do clock genes play a role in bipolar disorder?[4] What is the evidence for phase–delayed rhythms in winter depression?[5,6] Do different dementias have different rhythm abnormalities?[7] Rather, circadian disruption of rest–activity cycles will be considered as a clinical symptom, which leads to pragmatic use of circadian-based treatments to support re-entrainment.

Hypotheses of biological clock disorder postulate alterations in suprachiasmatic nuclei (SCN) function that may result in a low amplitude or abnormal phase of the observed circadian rhythm. Alterations in SCN function may be caused not only by malfunction of the clock per se, but by means of changes in factors that set the clock. Importantly, the SCN—and all the peripheral clocks in the brain and the rest of the body—require zeitgebers (synchronizing agents) to ensure circadian entrainment (coupling of an endogenous rhythm to an environmental oscillator with the result that both oscillations have the same frequency), internally among themselves and externally with respect to the light-dark cycle. With insufficient zeitgebers, even correctly functioning biological clocks can become

Centre for Chronobiology, Psychiatric Hospital of the University of Basel, Wilhelm Klein Strasse 27, CH-4025 Basel, Switzerland
* Corresponding author.
E-mail address: anna.wirz-justice@unibas.ch (A. Wirz-Justice).

Sleep Med Clin 4 (2009) 273–284
doi:10.1016/j.jsmc.2009.01.008
1556-407X/09/$ – see front matter © 2009 Elsevier Inc. All rights reserved.

desynchronized. This points to the important role for the major zeitgeber light, and the usefulness of melatonin, which feeds back on the SCN. Non-photic zeitgebers such as physical exercise, sleep, or food also contribute to entrainment of peripheral clocks. Social zeitgebers (eg, personal relationships, jobs, social demands) act indirectly on the SCN, because they determine the timing of meals, sleep, physical activity, and out- and indoor light exposure. In addition, the zeitgebers must impact on correct functioning receptors to be effective (eg, retinal photoreceptors for light perception).

A major tenet of chronobiology is that appropriate entrainment or synchronization to the 24-hour day–night/light–dark cycle is important for health. This may be particularly relevant to psychiatric illness.[8] Circadian malentrainment does not necessarily cause the individual psychopathology, but may perpetuate or exacerbate the clinical symptoms. In general, entrainment is not only a prerequisite for good nighttime sleep and daytime alertness, but also for adequate mood state, cognition, and neurobehavioral function.

The chronobiological strategy of attending to entrainment of patients, independent of psychiatric diagnosis, is not entirely new, because it merely reformulates the classical clinical strategy of establishing stable daily structures to support the process of clinical improvement. The primary postulate is that integrity of the circadian rest–activity cycle promotes healthy functioning in all psychiatric disorders.

Here the focus lies on the importance of well-entrained sleep–wake cycles for mental health, with examples from various diagnostic categories. The accent will be on actigraphy, as a well-established, relatively easy and noninvasive objective measure of the circadian rest–activity cycle.

ACTIGRAPHY AS A CLINICAL TOOL

Actigraphs are small, lightweight, wrist-worn solid-state recorders that record movement-induced accelerations (**Fig. 1**). The wrist-worn accelerometer generates activity counts, which are proportional to the intensity, frequency, and duration of motion (the higher the black bars, the more active). The activity counts are summed over a given time interval (eg, 2-minutes) and depicted either as single plots (24-hours) or double plots (48-hours represent day 1 and day 2 next to one another); time of day (x axis) begins at midnight. The subsequent days (y axis) are plotted beneath each another.

In general, two sets of parameters can be derived—one representing sleep measures such as sleep fragmentation and movement time, which correlate reasonably well with electroencephalogram (EEG) data[9]—and one set defining circadian rhythm characteristics, such as interdaily stability (IS), intradaily variability (IV), the timing of the most active and most inactive episodes, and the relative amplitude (RA).[10] IS indicates the degree of resemblance between activity patterns on different days, documenting the consistency across days of the daily circadian signal and the strength of its coupling to stable zeitgebers. A higher value indicates a more stable rhythm. IV indicates the degree of fragmentation of the rhythm (ie, the frequency of transitions between periods of rest and periods of activity during a given day). A lower value indicates a less fragmented rhythm. The sequence of the most active

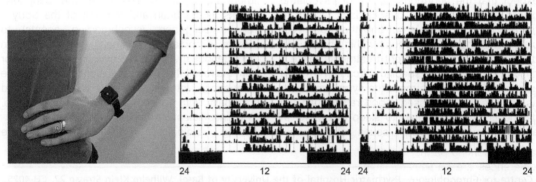

Fig. 1. The circadian rest–activity cycle is documented using an actigraph worn on the wrist of the nondominant hand (inset, Cambridge Neurotechnology Limited, Cambridge, UK, with light meter). Social zeitgebers in a married couple showing weekday work times affecting the onset of daily activity in the employed partner (63-year-old man), *left*, and free choice of wake-up time in the at-home partner (65 year-old woman), *right*. (*Data from* A. Wirz-Justice, unpublished data, 2009.)

10 hours (day) indicates the mean hourly peak of the rhythm, and the sequence of the least active 5 hours (night) indicates the nadir of the rhythm.[10] These two values are used to calculate the third important characteristic, the RA.

Many psychiatric illnesses are accompanied or characterized by changes in the circadian sleep–wake cycle. The advantage of actigraphy is to reveal 24-hour patterns that cannot be obtained otherwise, and which provide objective data for the patient's sleep disturbance. The technique is noninvasive, reliable, and can be interpreted within the paradigm of animal circadian rest–activity cycles, where a large literature can be invoked to interpret the entrainment patterns seen. Importantly, actigraphy can be implemented in everyday life, thus not altering behavior as a laboratory situation might do so, and is accepted by most psychiatric patients, even the most difficult.

CAVEATS IN ACTIGRAPHY

Outcome measures gathered with actigraphs (eg, sleep latency, IS, and IV) often are masked by everyday influences such as physical activity, meals, work schedules, and social demands. To add to the complexity, some of these environmental factors simply mask circadian rhythms without shifting them, but some of these factors (eg, environmental lighting conditions) will acutely affect and phase shift circadian rhythms. Thus, it is sometimes impossible to differentiate between a circadian disruption caused by malfunction of the biological clock or by environmental factors, or both. The circadian clock of a shift worker may work perfectly well, although his or her rest–activity cycle shows severe disruption as indexed by measures like the IS and IV.

To increase the quality in interpreting actigraphy measures, it is recommended to collect as much information as possible about the patient's daily routine by means of diaries. Furthermore, if feasible, one should add a circadian marker such as dim light melatonin onset (determined with the aid of a salivary melatonin diagnostic kit, for example SleepCheck Bühlmann Laboratories, Allschwil, Switzerland) to better discriminate between masking and circadian effects.

Fig. 1 shows rest–activity cycles of a working and nonworking partner in a healthy couple. The differences are particularly seen in the morning wake-up time and the contrast between workdays and weekends. This is an important point for comparing different clinical diagnoses, because the control subjects must live under similar conditions of employment to elucidate whether the differences found are related to the illness and not the sociological circumstances.

Thus, to avoid pitfalls with actigraphy, information of the patient's daily routine (diaries) should be gathered, a circadian marker measured, and if feasible, to compare patient groups only when they live under similar conditions of employment or ward schedules.

PHARMACOLOGIC TREATMENTS, DRUG ABUSE, AND CIRCADIAN REST–ACTIVITY CYCLES

There is mounting evidence that successful pharmacologic treatment in patients suffering psychiatric disorders also improves circadian entrainment, which is important for therapeutic efficacy. The mood stabilizers lithium and sodium-valproate used in bipolar patients have repeatedly been shown to alter circadian period, leading to a long period in humans.[11,12] The antidepressant fluoxetine also affects circadian output by producing a phase advance in the firing of neurons in the SCN.[13] Thus, antidepressants in the selective serotonin reuptake inhibitor class also may exert some of their effects on depression through modulation of the circadian clock. In contrast, circadian rhythm sleep disorders have been reported as a possible adverse effect of fluvoxamine but not fluoxetine.[14] The list of pharmacologic agents with repercussions on circadian clock function certainly will grow in the future.

A pharmacologic example suggests that a patient's response to different neuroleptic medications can impact significantly on the rest–activity pattern (**Fig. 2**). This patient suffering from Alzheimer's disease was prescribed haloperidol for behavioral disturbances after having a reasonably intact rest–activity cycle on risperidone. The disrupted circadian rest–activity cycle suggests an iatrogenic effect related to the drug rather than an effect of the illness per se,[15] because similar negative effects have been found in schizophrenic patients,[16] and even in a neurologic case with Gilles de la Tourette syndrome.[17] More important, the integrity of the circadian rest–activity cycle was related to cognitive function. This patient showed complete arrhythmicity developing with haloperidol concomitant with cognitive decline, that was reversed with clozapine, when cognitive improvement occurred.[15]

Another aspect of how drugs can alter circadian rest–activity cycles comes from patients who have addictive disorders. Even though it is known that these patients develop extreme sleep disturbances during drug withdrawal, there is no literature on possible disturbances of the circadian

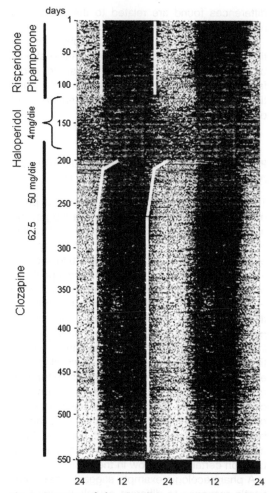

Fig. 2. Patterns of the circadian rest–activity cycle in a long-term recording over 550 days in a patient (54-year-old woman) with early onset Alzheimer's disease change with medications (double plot). The rhythms were entrained when the patient was on risperidone and clozapine. Changing to haloperidol treatment induced apparent total arrhythmicity. Note the rhythm re-emerging with clozapine treatment as a brief free run, and phase advancing with increasing dose (*From* Wirz-Justice A, Savaskan E, Knoblauch V, et al. Haloperidol disrupts, clozapine reinstates the circadian rest–activity cycle in a patient with early onset Alzheimer's disease. Alzheimer Dis Assoc Disord 2000;14:213; with permission.)

rest–activity cycle in drug dependence. An overlap of many psychiatric disorders with anxiety and addictive behavior has been noted.[18] Interestingly, an association between alterations in the human clock gene Per2 and increased alcohol intake in people was identified recently.[19] Given this evidence linking clock genes to reward behavior, a reappraisal of how sleep medicine could apply chronobiological principles to help these patients is warranted.

Again, in a single case study, an opiate-dependent patient whose rehabilitation and stabilization on methadone were successful, the persistent sleep disturbances and irregular sleep and wake times suggest that optimum stability had not been attained (**Fig. 3**). This is certainly an area requiring further study.

PATTERNS OF REST–ACTIVITY CYCLES IN INDIVIDUALS SUFFERING FROM DIFFERENT PSYCHIATRIC DISORDERS

Circadian rhythms are disrupted consistently in a spectrum of psychiatric disorders. In many cases, these disruptions may not be related directly to the circadian clock but to neural circuitries regulating output rhythms, or they may arise from conflicts between the internal biological clocks and environmental and social zeitgebers. Nevertheless, it has been difficult to establish whether circadian system disturbances can contribute to psychiatric disorders or whether they are merely symptomatic of the disease process. Disruption of circadian oscillators, however, clearly modifies disease severity, and in some instances, may play a more primary role in the etiology of the disease. More and more investigations of sleep timing in different psychiatric populations reveal a high incidence of comorbidity. For example, there is good evidence for comorbid delayed sleep phase syndrome in both childhood[20] and adult attention-deficit disorder,[21] and in obsessive–compulsive disorder.[22]

The following section shows individual actigraphs of patients suffering from different psychiatric illnesses to familiarize the reader with interpreting patterns of rest–activity cycles observed in daily routine psychiatry.

Bipolar Manic-Depressive Illness

Most studies looking at circadian rhythm disturbances in psychiatry have focused on depression, because of the clinical phenomenology (ie, diurnal variation of mood, early morning awakening, periodicity of the illness).[1,3] Most evidence for abnormalities in rhythms is available for bipolar manic-depressive patients. Cross-sectional studies reveal a preponderance of evening chronotypes, particularly during the depressed phase.[23,24]

The long-term actigraphy recording of an untreated bipolar patient (**Fig. 4**) illustrates circadian patterns already recognized and analyzed in the very early studies of actigraphy at the National Institute of Mental Health.[25–27] During the manic phase, sleep is short, fragmented, wake-up time extremely phase advanced, and nights

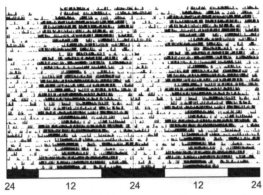

Fig. 3. Double plot of the circadian rest–activity cycle in a socially integrated methadone-substituted patient (28-year-old woman). (*Data from* A. Wirz-Justice, unpublished data, 2009.)

often characterized by spontaneous total or partial sleep deprivation.[27] This circadian rest–activity cycle resembles the extremely disturbed patterns seen in a mouse model of mania, the clock mutant mouse.[4] In contrast, as the patient switches into depression, the sleep phase lengthens, becomes more consolidated, and gradually phase delays. These dramatic alterations in sleep–wake behavior have been noted by the patient for more than 25 years and have occurred every 9 or 10 months independent of season. The patient never has been treated either pharmacologically or behaviorally for her illness. Although during her manic phase she was very compliant and motivated to collect saliva samples for melatonin assessments, during the depressed phase, she refused to collaborate, and it was difficult to convince her to continue wearing the actigraph. Thus, the question cannot be answered as to whether the marked change in her rest–activity cycles was caused by changes in the circadian clock (eg, shortened circadian period during manic phases as opposed to depressed phases). Interestingly, the increase in sleep length preceded the patient's recognition of having depression and lack of motivation by about 2 to 3 weeks.

Actigraphy studies in bipolar patients support the previously observed marked state-related shift in the circadian rest–activity cycle, a phase advance in mania,[28] and a phase advance after successful treatment for depression.[29]

Schizophrenia

Schizophrenia is perhaps the most devastating neuropsychiatric illness. Worldwide, the prevalence rate is approximately 1%. Although the etiology remains unknown, schizophrenia involves the interplay of susceptibility genes and environmental factors. Over 90 years ago, however, Bleuler pointed out: "in schizophrenia, sleep is

habitually disturbed." In times of severe psychotic agitation, schizophrenic patients may experience a profound insomnia or total sleeplessness. Severe insomnia is one of the prodromal symptoms associated with psychotic relapse. Patients also may develop sleep–wake reversals with a preference for sleeping during the day. Thus, the tendency toward a late sleep phase could be psychological (avoidance of interpersonal contact) or related to light-oriented behavior. In a series of careful studies, including measurement of melatonin rhythms at weekly intervals, Wulff and colleagues have shown that the timing of light exposure is reflected in the timing of sleep-wake

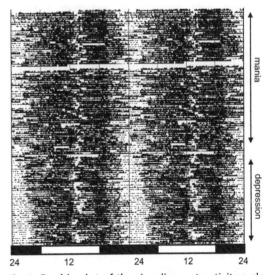

Fig. 4. Double plot of the circadian rest–activity cycle over many months in a bipolar patient (55-year-old woman). Clear changes in duration and timing of rest are seen in the shift from mania (*above*) to the depressive phase (*below*). (*Data from* C. Cajochen, unpublished data, 2009.)

A

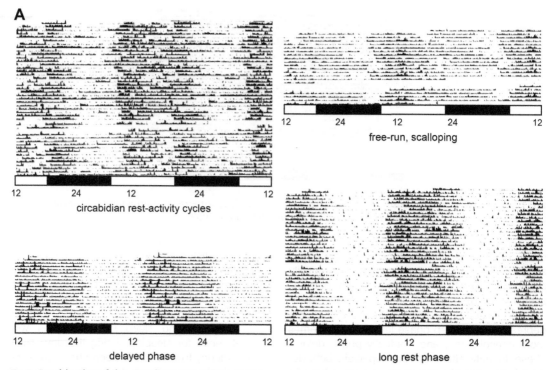

circabidian rest-activity cycles

free-run, scalloping

delayed phase

long rest phase

Fig. 5. Double plot of the circadian rest–activity cycle in seven patients diagnosed with schizophrenia. All patients were hospitalized and treated with monotherapy. (*A*) The four panels represent patients treated with the classical neuroleptics haloperidol or fluphenazine. (*B*) The three panels represent patients treated with the atypical neuro- leptic clozapine. Occasional missing data are left blank. (*From* Wirz-Justice A, Haug HJ, Cajochen C. Disturbed circadian rest–activity cycles in schizophrenia patients: an effect of drugs? Schizophr Bull 2001;27: 499; with permission.)

cycles.[30] By getting up late, the patients lack morning light exposure to establish a phase advance, and drift to later. The most striking example was a single patient whose rest–activity cycle and melatonin rhythms free ran in winter (when, presumably, the opportunity to have suffi- cient light was reduced) but did entrain during summer (K. Wulff, personal communication, 2009). By measuring rest–activity rhythms in unemployed but otherwise healthy controls, they were able to show that patients with schizophrenia are not phase delayed only because of lack of social zeitgebers.[31] Thus, light-oriented behavior may be one important factor in these sleep–wake cycle abnormalities.

Nurses and physicians clearly recognize that some of their schizophrenic patients exhibit abnormal sleep–wake cycles. The first long-term (longer than 1 year) wrist activity recording in one schizophrenic patient revealed virtually continuous activity without prolonged bouts of rest and no day–night differences.[32] Despite this abnormal sleep–wake behavior, the patient's circadian profile of melatonin secretion showed a clear 24- hour rhythm, indicating that his circadian clock

functioned properly. Also, when the patient was studied in the chronobiology laboratory under a 31-hour bed rest protocol with free choice of sleep times, core body temperature exhibited a circadian modulation, albeit with very small amplitude, but his sleep–wake propensity rhythm showed a clear reversal (wake at night, sleep during the day). In the same patient, the authors documented that a change from haloperidol to clozapine treatment improved rhythmicity.[32] In a follow-up study, rest–activity cycles were re- corded in a larger patient cohort.[16] Many patients who had schizophrenia (whether hospitalized or under home conditions) showed unusual rest- activity cycles. Furthermore, a given patient's response to neuroleptic medications impacted significantly on their rest–activity patterns. The circadian rest–activity cycle of patients stabilized for more than a year on monotherapy with a clas- sical neuroleptic (haloperidol, flupenthixol) or with the atypical neuroleptic clozapine was docu- mented by continuous activity monitoring for 3 to 7 weeks. The three patients treated with clozapine had remarkably highly ordered rest–activity cycles (**Fig. 5**B), whereas the four patients on classical

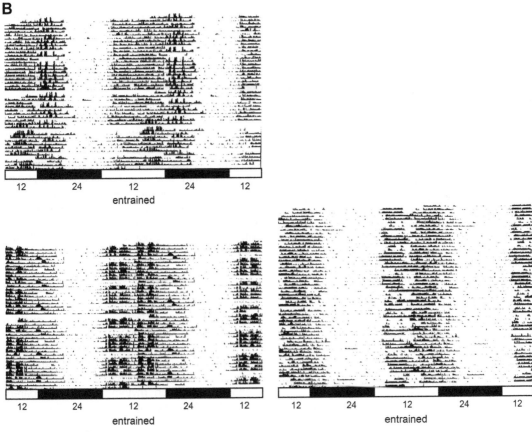

B

12   24   12   24   12
entrained

12   24   12   24   12
entrained

12   24   12   24   12
entrained

Fig. 5. (*continued*)

neuroleptics had minor to major circadian rhythm abnormalities (see **Fig. 5A**).[16] This observation could be conceptualized in terms of the two-process model of sleep regulation. High-dose haloperidol treatment may have lowered the circadian alertness threshold, initiating polyphasic sleep episodes, whereas clozapine increased circadian amplitude (perhaps through its high affinity to dopamine D_4 and serotonin $5HT_7$ receptors in the SCN), thereby improving entrainment.

What are the chronobiological disturbances in schizophrenia? The etiology is probably neither primarily an abnormality of the homeostatic process (although reduced slow-wave sleep or EEG slow-wave activity has been documented) nor an abnormality of the circadian process (although medicated patients in free run show a shorter endogenous periodicity).[2] The combination of diminished social zeitgebers, late sleeping, and light exposure in the evening rather than morning all interacting with medication effects leads to altered internal and external phase relationships. In turn, these altered sleep patterns may reinforce the difficulties with cognitive function and social engagement, and the depressive symptoms associated with schizophrenia.

Ongoing actimetry studies reveal that the higher the relative amplitude of the rest–activity cycle, the better the cognitive function in this patient group.[33] These preliminary data (**Fig. 6**) suggest that efforts to enhance robustness of entrainment may provide a means of improving behavior, that, in turn, allows better rehabilitation, even though not directly treating the underlying illness.

Broadly viewed, these studies provide consistent evidence of circadian dysregulation in schizophrenic patients. Although commonly present, however, it is not clear whether the observed circadian alterations are just an epiphenomenon of the disease (or its treatment) or causally involved, or both.

Borderline Personality Disorder

Many research groups studying delayed sleep phase syndrome have noted the prevalence of accompanying personality disorders, but without finding a reliable strong relationship. The converse

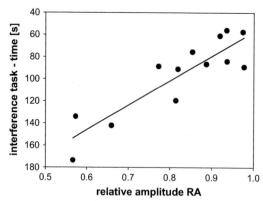

Fig. 6. The Stroop color word interference task is a measure of executive function/reaction inhibition. Reaction time in the Stroop test is faster in patients with schizophrenia whose circadian rest–activity cycles are more stable, as measured by the relative amplitude of the rhythm (N = 13; r = 0.758, P = .003). (*Data from* V. Bromundt, unpublished data, 2009.)

also may be true; in an ongoing study of circadian rest–activity cycles in borderline personality disorder, delayed sleep phase syndrome was rather prominent. Closer investigation, however, revealed a variety of patterns, ranging from relatively normal to extremely disturbed (**Fig. 7**).

Preliminary findings suggest that the use of light therapy has positive effects not only on (actigraphy-defined) sleep characteristics but also on aspects of the borderline symptoms themselves (V. Bromundt and colleagues, unpublished data, 2009).

Alzheimer's Disease

There is a large body of evidence demonstrating a reduction of SCN function with aging that is exacerbated in Alzheimer's disease (AD), and

many studies have used zeitgebers to stimulate and thus better entrain the remaining SCN neurones (see the article by Zee and Vitiello in this issue), notably the recent long-term trial of light with or without concomitant melatonin treatment showing stabilization of cognitive function, mood, and the rest–activity cycle.[34]

At a late stage of life, however, it is not only diminished SCN function that determines the altered sleep-wake cycle in Alzheimer's patients, or specific medication (as in **Fig. 2**). A combination of multimorbidity, combined medications, isolated life style with few social zeitgebers, and little outdoor light exposure can interact to produce the kind of rest–activity cycle seen in **Fig. 8**. Circadian studies of major disease entities are in their infancy, and the complexities of comorbidity and poly-medication have not been addressed.

Korsakoff's Psychosis

Not every dementia is a circadian disturbance. The dramatic disruptions in the rest–activity cycle of patients who have AD (see the article by Zee and Vitiello in this issue) are not the same as in patients who have vascular dementia.[7] In patients who have Korsakoff's psychosis, no evidence of abnormal circadian rhythm phase is apparent; the rest-activity cycle is extremely well-entrained, more so, even, than the matched control subjects (**Fig. 9**). What is characteristic, however, is a marked amplitude diminution—low daytime activity and a long rest phase.[35]

ZEITGEBERS AS THERAPY

The previous examples and indications point toward the use of chronobiological therapies in many of the sleep disorders associated with psychiatric illness. Chronotherapeutics—treatments based on the principles of circadian rhythm

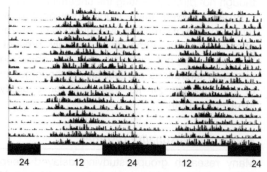

Fig. 7. Double plot of the circadian rest–activity cycle in two patients with borderline personality disorder, ranging from relatively well entrained (*left*) to extremely disrupted (*right*). (*Data from* V. Bromundt, unpublished data, 2009.)

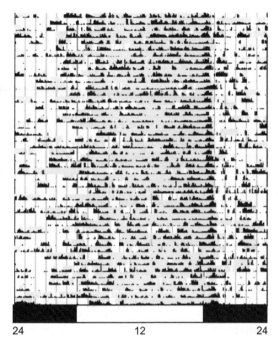

24   12   24

Fig. 8. Single plot of the circadian rest–activity cycle in a patient with probable Alzheimer's Disease (79-year-old woman). Grey background = light exposure. Which of the other illnesses in addition to Alzheimer's disease in this patient (coronary heart disease, occlusive arterial disease, kyphoskoliosis with lumbago, glaucoma) could have contributed to the clearly disturbed sleep? Furthermore, which of the patient's medications (haloperidol, trimipramine, oxazepam, omeprazole, aspirin) and/or their interaction with previously mentioned illnesses impacted the most on the circadian rest–activity cycles? Her main zeitgeber was the 1-hour visit of her son faithfully every evening around 7 PM (*Data from* A. Wirz-Justice, unpublished data, 2009.)

organization and sleep physiology—offer mental health practitioners a set of nonpharmacological, rapid, and effective antidepressant modalities for monotherapy or as adjuvants to conventional medication, particularly in major depression.[36]

Light Therapy

Light therapy can be considered the most successful clinical application of circadian rhythm concepts. The most obvious application in sleep medicine has been to phase shift and re-entrain sleep–wake cycle disorders, whether delayed or advanced sleep phase syndrome, or age-related alterations.[37] Light is the treatment of choice for winter depression.[38,39] There is already good evidence for efficacy in bulimia and preliminary evidence for usefulness in pre- and post-partum depression, both clinical indications where nonpharmaceutical therapies are needed.[40] Particularly promising are the antidepressant effects when used as an adjuvant in nonseasonal major depression.[41,42] Improving the irregular rest–activity cycles often found in patients who have AD[34,43] and demented elderly in general represents another important application of light therapy.[44,45] Light is being recognized not only as a major zeitgeber necessary for daily well-being (with applications in the work place and in architecture) but also as a "drug" that can be prescribed in dose, timing, duration, and spectral composition for specific diagnoses.[41,42]

Dark Therapy

Single case studies of rapidly cycling bipolar patients have shown that extending darkness (or rest, or sleep) immediately stops the recurring pattern, a rather astonishing result in these therapy-resistant patients.[46,47] Further support for the relevance of these findings is that extended darkness (not rest, and not sleep) in manic bipolar patients can control their symptoms within days.[48] A novel approach, which is perhaps easier than shutting up manic patients in dark rooms, is the use of blue-blocking sunglasses.[49] The recent discovery of a blue wavelength-sensitive photopigment in retinal ganglion cells, melanopsin, responsible for the major nonvisual photic input to the SCN, suggests that some of the circadian effects of light can be prevented by filtering out the blue wavelengths.

Melatonin

In circadian physiology, melatonin is important for timing the cascade of events initiating sleep. The nocturnal onset of melatonin secretion opens the gate for sleep propensity, which involves peripheral thermoregulatory mechanisms.[50,51] The warm feet effect of melatonin underlies its soporific action and usefulness in various sleep disorders.[51,52] The few studies administering melatonin to depressed patients have found improvements in sleep, but not in mood.[53,54] Melatonin is a zeitgeber and can enhance entrainment (see the examples of its sleep–entraining properties in blind persons in the article by Uchiyama and Lockley in this issue). Given the development of low-dose and controlled-release formulations, there is an important future for melatonin as a useful long-term sleep/rhythm promoting agent with fewer adverse effects than the hypnotics, and in addition, for the newer melatonin agonists (see the article by Rajaratnam, Cohen, and Rogers elsewhere in this issue).

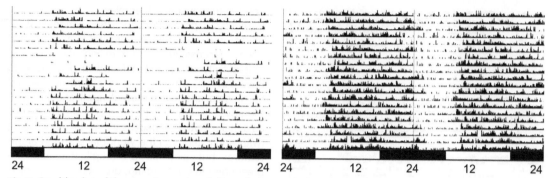

Fig. 9. Double plot of the circadian rest–activity cycle in a patient with Korsakoff's psychosis (61-year-old man, *left*) and an age-matched community-living control subject (*right*). (*Data from* A. Wirz-Justice, unpublished data, 2009.)

CIRCADIAN RHYTHMS AND PSYCHIATRY: WHAT IS IMPORTANT?

The different individual examples hopefully have provided a purview of the enormous variety of sleep–wake cycle disturbances in psychiatric patients. This indicates an important role for actigraphy in defining the circadian rest–activity cycle pattern in many psychiatric disorders. The quality of entrainment may provide information that cannot be obtained otherwise about sleep timing and organization; it also may prove to be an outcome measure of successful treatment. The strategy of attending to entrainment of patients is a restatement, with better understanding of putative mechanisms, of establishing daytime activities as part of the therapeutic strategy. In fact, development of interpersonal and social rhythm therapy for improving occupational functioning in bipolar patients has focused on this aspect.[55]

The rules for good entrainment are adapted from those generally in use in sleep medicine (**Box 1**).[8]

Box 1
Circadian rhythms and psychiatry—what is important?

Stable external and internal phase relationships:

Appropriate entrainment of the sleep–wake cycle to the external light–dark cycle

Enough light during the day, enough darkness during the night

Adequate retinal function

Sufficient social zeitgebers

Reconsider the zeitgeber function of timed activity and meals

---

SUMMARY

Although actigraphy is being used more often now in sleep medicine, its use in psychiatry remains rare. Examples from daily clinical practice illustrate that circadian sleep–wake cycle disturbances are widespread in psychiatric illness. The problems of entrainment that are revealed by actigraphy—irregular, arrhythmic, phase delayed, advanced, or even free-running rest–activity cycles—can arise from different causes. The usefulness of these measurements is not only to better understand underlying etiology but to point the way to treatment possibilities. Many physicians increasingly are using light therapy to treat depression; melatonin is being used for delayed sleep phase or free-running rhythms. Although these treatments are effective for many individuals, they still have limitations. We can generalize, however, that all techniques promoting entrainment can be used as pragmatic adjuvants to the illness-specific medication and psychotherapies. An understanding of how these techniques alleviate psychiatric symptoms and how proper entrainment may result in changes in mood and cognitive behavior will allow the design of less-invasive and more effective treatment modalities for these devastating psychiatric illnesses.

REFERENCES

1. Germain A, Kupfer DJ. Circadian rhythm disturbances in depression. Hum Psychopharmacol 2008;23:571–85.
2. Boivin DB. Influence of sleep-wake and circadian rhythm disturbances in psychiatric disorders. J Psychiatry Neurosci 2000;25:446–58.
3. Wirz-Justice A. Biological rhythms in mood disorders. In: Bloom FE, Kupfer DJ, editors.

Psychopharmacology:the fourth generation of progress. New York: Raven Press; 1995. p. 999–1017.

4. McClung CA. Circadian genes, rhythms, and the biology of mood disorders. Pharmacol Ther 2007; 114:222–32.

5. Avery DH, Dahl K, Savage MV, et al. Circadian temperature and cortisol rhythms during a constant routine are phase-delayed in hypersomnic winter depression. Biol Psychol 1997;41:1109–23.

6. Wirz-Justice A, Kräuchi K, Brunner DP, et al. Circadian rhythms and sleep regulation in seasonal affective disorder. Acta Neuropsychiatrica 1995;7:41–3.

7. Harper DG, Stopa EG, McKee AC, et al. Differential circadian rhythm disturbances in men with Alzheimer disease and frontotemporal degeneration. Arch Gen Psychiatry 2001;58:353–60.

8. Wirz-Justice A. Chronobiology and psychiatry. Sleep Med Rev 2007;11:423–7.

9. Ancoli-Israel S, Cole R, Alessi C, et al. The role of actigraphy in the study of sleep and circadian rhythms. Sleep 2003;28:1017–8.

10. Van Someren EJW, Swaab DF, Colenda CC, et al. Bright light therapy: improved sensitivity to its effects on rest–activity rhythms in Alzheimer patients by application of nonparametric methods. Chronobiol Int 1999;16:505–18.

11. Johnsson A, Engelmann W, Pflug B, et al. Influence of lithium ions on human circadian rhythms. Z Naturforsch [C] 1980;35:503–7.

12. Kripke DF, Mullaney DJ, Atkinson M, et al. Circadian rhythm disorders in manic depressives. Biol Psychiatry 1978;13:335–51.

13. Sprouse JS, Braselton JP, Reynolds LS. Fluoxetine modulates the circadian biological clock via phase advances of suprachiasmatic nucleus neuronal firing. Biol Psychiatry 2006;60:896–9.

14. Hermesh H, Lemberg H, Abadi J, et al. Circadian rhythm sleep disorders as a possible side effect of fluvoxamine. CNS Spectr 2001;6:511–3.

15. Wirz-Justice A, Werth E, Savaskan E, et al. Haloperidol disrupts, clozapine reinstates the circadian rest–activity cycle in a patient with early onset Alzheimer disease. Alzheimer Dis Assoc Disord 2000;14:212–5.

16. Wirz-Justice A, Haug HJ, Cajochen C. Disturbed circadian rest–activity cycles in schizophrenia patients: an effect of drugs? Schizophr Bull 2001; 27:497–502.

17. Ayalon L, Hermesh H, Dagan Y. Case study of circadian rhythm sleep disorder following haloperidol treatment: reversal by risperidone and melatonin. Chronobiol Int 2002;19:947–59.

18. Nestler EJ, Barrot M, DiLeone RJ, et al. Neurobiology of depression. Neuron 2002;34:13–25.

19. Spanagel R, Pendyala G, Abarca C, et al. The clock gene Per 2 influences the glutamatergic system and modulates alcohol consumption. Nat Med 2005;11: 35–42.

20. Van der Heijden KB, Smits MG, Van Someren EJ, et al. Idiopathic chronic sleep-onset insomnia in attention-deficit/hyperactivity disorder: a circadian rhythm sleep disorder. Chronobiol Int 2005;22: 559–70.

21. Rybak YE, McNeely HE, Mackenzie BE, et al. Seasonality and circadian preference in adult attention-deficit/hyperactivity disorder: clinical and neuropsychological correlates. Compr Psychiatry 2007;48:562–71.

22. Mukhopadhyay S, Fineberg NA, Drummond LM, et al. Delayed sleep phase in severe obsessive–compulsive disorder: a systematic case-report survey. CNS Spectr 2008;13:406–13.

23. Mansour HA, Wood J, Chowdari KV, et al. Circadian phase variation in bipolar I disorder. Chronobiol Int 2005;22:571–84.

24. Ahn YM, Chang J, Joo YH, et al. Chronotype distribution in bipolar I disorder and schizophrenia in a Korean sample. Bipolar Disord 2008;10:271–5.

25. Wehr TA, Wirz-Justice A, Goodwin FK, et al. Phase advance of the circadian sleep–wake cycle as an antidepressant. Science 1979;206:710–3.

26. Wehr TA, Wirz-Justice A. Circadian rhythm mechanisms in affective illness and in antidepressant drug action. Pharmacopsychiatria 1982;12:31–9.

27. Wehr TA, Goodwin FK, Wirz-Justice A, et al. 48-hour sleep–wake cycles in manic-depressive illness: naturalistic observations and sleep deprivation experiments. Arch Gen Psychiatry 1982;39:559–65.

28. Salvatore P, Ghidini S, Zita G, et al. Circadian activity rhythm abnormalities in ill and recovered bipolar I disorder patients. Bipolar Disord 2008;10:256–65.

29. Benedetti F, Dallaspezia S, C FM, et al. Phase advance is an actimetric correlate of antidepressant response to sleep deprivation and light therapy in bipolar depression. Chronobiol Int 2007;24:921–37.

30. Wulff K, Joyce E, Middleton B, et al. The suitability of actigraphy, diary data, and urinary melatonin profiles for quantitative assessment of sleep disturbances in schizophrenia: a case report. Chronobiol Int 2006;23:485–95.

31. Wulff K, Joyce EM, Middleton B, et al. Circadian activity and sleep cycle disturbances in schizophrenia patients in comparison to unemployed healthy controls. Int J Neuropsychopharmacol 2008;11(Suppl 1):150.

32. Wirz-Justice A, Cajochen C, Nussbaum P. A schizophrenic patient with an arrhythmic circadian rest–activity cycle. Psychol Res 1997;73:83–90.

33. Bromundt V, Köster M, Stoppe G, et al. Disturbances in sleep–wake rhythms correlate with impairment of cognitive functioning in schizophrenic patients. J Sleep Res 2008;17(Suppl 1):145.

34. Riemersma-van der Lek RF, Swaab DF, Twisk J, et al. Effect of bright light and melatonin on cognitive and noncognitive function in elderly residents of group

care facilities: a randomized controlled trial. JAMA 2008;299:2642–55.

35. Wirz-Justice A, Schröder CM, Fontana Gasio P, et al. The circadian rest–activity cycle in Korsakoff's psychosis. Am J Geriatr Psychiatry 2009, in press.

36. Wirz-Justice A, Benedetti F, Terman M. Chronotherapeutics for affective disorders. A clinician's manual for light and wake therapy. Basel: Karger; 2009.

37. Gooley JJ. Treatment of circadian rhythm sleep disorders with light. Ann Acad Med Singap 2008; 37:669–76.

38. Tuunainen A, Kripke D, Endo T. Light therapy for nonseasonal depression. Cochrane Database Syst Rev 2004;CD004050.

39. Golden RN, Gaynes BN, Ekstrom RD, et al. The efficacy of light therapy in the treatment of mood disorders: a review and meta-analysis of the evidence. Am J Psychiatry 2005;162:656–62.

40. Lam RW. Seasonal affective disorder and beyond. Light treatment for SAD and non-SAD conditions. Washington DC: American Psychiatric Press; 1998.

41. Terman M, Terman JS. Light therapy for seasonal and nonseasonal depression: efficacy, protocol, safety, and side effects. CNS Spectr 2005;10:647–63.

42. Terman M. Evolving applications of light therapy. Sleep Med Rev 2007;11:497–507.

43. Dowling GA, Burr RL, van Someren EJ, et al. Melatonin and bright light treatment for rest–activity disruption in institutionalized patients with Alzheimer's disease. J Am Geriatr Soc 2008;56:239–46.

44. Ancoli-Israel S, Gehrman P, Martin JL, et al. Increased light exposure consolidates sleep and strengthens circadian rhythms in severe Alzheimer's disease patients. Behav Sleep Med 2003;1:22–36.

45. Fontana Gasio P, Kräuchi K, Cajochen C, et al. Dawn–dusk simulation light therapy of disturbed circadian rest–activity cycles in demented elderly. Exp Gerontol 2003;38:207–16.

46. Wehr TA, Turner EH, Shimada JM, et al. Treatment of rapidly cycling bipolar patient by using extended bed rest and darkness to stabilize the timing and duration of sleep. Biol Psychiatry 1998;43:822–8.

47. Wirz-Justice A, Quinto C, Cajochen C, et al. A rapid-cycling bipolar patient treated with long nights, bed rest, and light. Biol Psych 1999;45:1075–7.

48. Barbini B, Benedetti F, Colombo C, et al. Dark therapy for mania: a pilot study. Bipolar Disord 2005;7:98–101.

49. Phelps J. Dark therapy for bipolar disorder using amber lenses for blue light blockade. Med Hypotheses 2008;70:224–9.

50. Kräuchi K, Cajochen C, Werth E, et al. Warm feet promote the rapid onset of sleep. Nature 1999;401: 36–7.

51. Kräuchi K, Cajochen C, Pache M, et al. Thermoregulatory effects of melatonin in relation to sleepiness. Chronobiol Int 2006;23:475–84.

52. Cajochen C, Kräuchi K, Wirz-Justice A. Role of melatonin in the regulation of human circadian rhythms and sleep. J Neuroedocrinol 2003;15:432–7.

53. deVries MW, Peeters FP. Melatonin as a therapeutic agent in the treatment of sleep disturbance in depression. J Nerv Ment Dis 1997;185:201–2.

54. Dolberg OT, Hirschmann S, Grunhaus L. Melatonin for the treatment of sleep disturbances in major depressive disorder. Am J Psychiatry 1998;155:1119–21.

55. Frank E, Soreca I, Swartz HA, et al. The role of interpersonal and social rhythm therapy in improving occupational functioning in patients with bipolar I disorder. Am J Psychiatry 2008; 165:1559–65.

Winter Depression: Integrating Mood, Circadian Rhythms, and the Sleep/Wake and Light/Dark Cycles into a Bio-Psycho-Social-Environmental Model

Alfred J. Lewy, MD, PhD*, Jonathan S. Emens, MD,
Jeannie B. Songer, BA, Neelam Sims, BS,
Amber L. Laurie, BA, Steven C. Fiala, BA,
Allie Buti, BS

KEYWORDS

- Melatonin • Light • Dim light melatonin onset (DLMO)
- Winter depression (SAD) • Phase-angle difference (PAD)
- Bio-psycho-social-environmental model

The diagnosis of winter depression (seasonal affective disorder, or SAD) is based on its annual pattern of recurrence in the fall/winter and spontaneous remission in the spring/summer. At temperate latitudes, about 5% of the population is estimated to have SAD, with another 15% of the population manifesting less severe symptoms (subsyndromal SAD).[1] There is a strong female predominance, at least in patients between the ages of puberty and menopause. In addition to the usual characteristics of depression, particularly what is termed "atypical" or "retarded" major depression (in which the hallmark vegetative changes in sleep and appetite are in the direction of increased sleep and appetite), patients who have SAD crave foods that contain complex carbohydrates (such as pasta, baked goods, and sweets) and gain weight in the winter.[2] Fruits and vegetables are preferred in the spring and summer. Weight loss, if it occurs at all, takes place during the spring and summer, often resulting in a summer wardrobe of smaller sizes. Fatigue, particularly difficulty getting up in the morning, is omnipresent, despite a tendency to lengthen sleep (which is not restorative) by as much as 3 hours in the winter. Although SAD generally is not as severe as other major affective disorders (eg, suicide is less common in SAD than in bipolar and nonseasonal unipolar major depression), patients who have SAD isolate themselves socially to a considerable degree; typically,

This work was supported by Grants No. 5R01 HD042125, 5-R01-AG021826-02, and 5R01EY018312 from the National Institutes of Health. A.J.L. also was supported by a National Alliance for Research on Schizophrenia and Depression Distinguished Investigator Award, and J.S.E. was supported by a National Alliance for Research on Schizophrenia and Depression Junior Investigator Award.
Sleep and Mood Disorders Laboratory, Department of Psychiatry, Oregon Health & Science University, L469, 3181 SW Sam Jackson Park Road, Portland, OR 97239, USA
* Corresponding author.
E-mail address: lewy@ohsu.edu (A.J. Lewy).

they report that they withdraw on weekends and as soon as they get home from work. Many are quite often irritable with family, friends, and co-workers. SAD seems to be more common at the higher latitudes of the temperate zone[3] and affects all ages, sometimes manifesting as school anxiety (during the fall and winter) in young children.[4,5]

SAD seems to run in families and therefore is thought to have a strong genetic component. Symptom severity is measured by a number of mood scales, primarily by one or another version of the Structured Interview Guide for the Hamilton Depression Rating Scale, Seasonal Affective Disorders version (SIGH-SAD), which originally was a composite of the standard 21-item Hamilton Depression Scale (Ham-21) and eight items thought to be highly representative of SAD.[6]

An understanding of the phase-shift hypothesis (PSH) for winter depression or SAD can benefit sleep researchers and clinicians in several ways:

1. The circadian mechanism causing SAD also may be a cause of nonrestorative sleep.
2. The melatonin laboratory test useful in SAD, which depends in part on the mid-point between sleep onset and wake time, may be applicable to nonrestorative sleep.
3. The other part of this laboratory test, the dim-light melatonin onset (DLMO), also indicates the times of the light and melatonin phase-response curves (PRCs) and therefore provides the optimal schedules for using these phase-resetting agents in treating circadian misalignment disorders (such as SAD) as well as advanced sleep phase syndrome (ASPS) and delayed sleep phase syndrome (DSPS).
4. The bio-psycho-social-environmental model suggested by SAD and the PSH now seems relevant to other disorders, including sleep disorders.

It is hoped that this article will stimulate further research in disorders that may have a circadian misalignment component (such as nonrestorative sleep) as well as canonical circadian phase sleep disorders, ASPS, DSPS, and hypernychthermal syndrome.

SAD seems to be caused, at least in part, by a mismatch between the sleep/wake cycle and the circadian rhythms that are tightly coupled to the endogenous circadian pacemaker.[7] Phase-resetting agents (such as exposure to bright light and the administration of low-dose melatonin) are the treatments of choice, provided the patient who has SAD is properly phase typed so that these agents can be administered at the correct time. It is also possible that these agents can phase shift

rhythms too much, causing circadian misalignment in the opposite direction. The prototypical phase-delayed patient with SAD has a DLMO that is delayed with respect to mid-sleep (the mid-point between sleep onset and sleep offset). A smaller subgroup has a DLMO that is phase advanced with respect to mid-sleep (**Fig. 1**). This line of thought builds on 3 decades of research in which endogenous melatonin has been the primary dependent variable and exogenous melatonin the primary independent variable; therefore, by way of introduction, the following review is in order.

HISTORICAL PERSPECTIVES

The second half of the 1970s was seminal for the field of chronobiology. Daniel Kripke,[8,9] Thomas Wehr[10] (working with Frederick Goodwin) and their research teams hypothesized that major affective disorders could be caused by a mismatch between the circadian rhythms associated with core body temperature and those related to the sleep/wake cycle. Specifically, the phase-advance hypothesis stated that the temperature rhythm

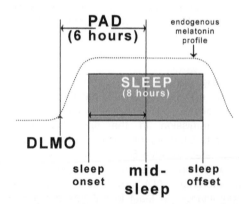

Fig. 1. Schematic diagram of normal phase relationships (rounded to the nearest integer) between sleep phase markers and the 10-pg/mL plasma dim-light melatonin onset (DLMO) derived from historical controls. The present study used the melatonin/mid-sleep interval (phase-angle difference, or PAD) of 6 hours as the hypothesized therapeutic window for optimal circadian alignment. Sleep times were determined actigraphically. Plasma melatonin levels were obtained under dim light every 30 minutes in the evening. The operational definition of the melatonin onset is the interpolated time of continuous rise above the threshold of 10 pg/mL; for example, if the melatonin level was 5 pg/mL at 8 PM and was 15 pg/mL at 8:30 PM the melatonin onset would be 8:15 PM. (*Adapted from* Lewy AJ, Lefler BJ, Emens JS, et al. The circadian basis of winter depression. Proc Nat Acad Sci USA 2006:103:7415; with permission.)

(and its related circadian rhythms) was phase advanced with respect to the sleep/wake cycle. It was difficult to test this hypothesis, because the only available phase-resetting treatment at the time was to shift the timing of the sleep/wake cycle.[10] When sleep was scheduled earlier, theoretically to correct the misalignment, the resulting clinical benefit was only transient. Shifting sleep was the only treatment available because chronobiologists had concluded that, unlike all other animals, humans did not make primary use of light/dark periods for synchronizing their biologic rhythms. Instead, social cues were thought to be more important.[11] In animals, seasonal rhythms were known to be cued to the time of the year via night length as it affected the duration of nighttime melatonin production;[12] the duration of melatonin production in the summer was shortened because of the acute suppressant effect of light on melatonin production in the morning and in the evening. The acute melatonin-suppressant effect of light was not demonstrated in humans until after the phase advance hypothesis was formulated, which in turn depended on the development of a sufficiently accurate and sensitive assay for measuring melatonin in humans.

The gas chromatographic–negative ion mass spectrometric (GCMS) assay for melatonin met the specifications and became the reference standard for laboratory analysis and measurement of melatonin in human plasma.[13] The other assays that were available to researchers in the 1970s lacked adequate specificity and/or sensitivity. Some reported high daytime circulating levels of melatonin and relatively little difference in levels between day and night,[14–17] even though it was known that whole pineal glands contain large amounts of melatonin at night compared with the daytime levels. The GCMS assay was used in some of the most influential studies of human melatonin physiology and directly and indirectly enabled the development of less costly and more convenient radioimmunoassays with sufficient specificity and sensitivity.

The GCMS assay was used to validate the use of circulating levels of melatonin as a measure of pineal output,[18,19] unaffected by so-called "extrapineal contributions"[20] that turned out to be immunoreactive substances that were not melatonin. In 1980, it was reported that human nighttime melatonin could be suppressed by exposure to light, providing the light was sufficiently intense (**Fig. 2**).[21] Previous studies apparently had used room light of ordinary intensity,[22–24] which was not sufficiently intense to suppress melatonin. Chronobiologists immediately understood the implication of this report: that humans might have

biologic rhythms cued to the natural cycle of (brighter) sunlight and darkness that were relatively unperturbed by exposure to ordinary-intensity room light. Furthermore, this finding led directly to the use of bright artificial light to manipulate biologic rhythms experimentally and therapeutically.

Kripke,[8,9] was the first investigator to treat nonseasonal depressives with morning exposure to bright light. In December, 1980 Lewy[25] and co-workers at the National Institute of Mental Health (NIMH) were afforded the opportunity to treat Herbert Kern, the first patient self-identified as having SAD, using 2500 lux exposure between 6 and 9 AM and 4 and 7 PM, based on animal models in which seasonal rhythms respond to the time interval between the twilight transitions (and the duration of nighttime melatonin production). The patient's depression began to remit in a few days, and the response was complete within 2 weeks, a time course that continues to hold for patients who have SAD. The first controlled study of light therapy in SAD was conducted by Rosenthal and co-workers,[2] who used relatively dim yellow light as a placebo.

At Oregon Health & Science University (OHSU), the thinking of the Lewy and Sack research team began to diverge from that of the Kripke and NIMH groups. Kripke,[8,9] chose morning as the best time to schedule light for treating nonseasonal depressives. Although this choice may turn out to be valid, it was based on the idea that there is a critical photosensitive interval for light exposure, consistent with a photoperiodic model. The NIMH group focused on a seasonal/photoperiodic, rather than a circadian, approach (although the two are interrelated), and on a "photon counting" hypothesis in which light at any time of the day (preferably at the most convenient time in the evening) would be therapeutic in patients who had SAD, provided that the exposure was of sufficient intensity and duration. The OHSU team focused instead on the circadian phase-resetting effects of light. Because the OHSU team thought that most seasonal depressives were phase delayed, they hypothesized that for most patients who have SAD morning light would provide a greater antidepressant effect than evening light.[26,27] Specifically, the PSH states that most patients who have SAD become depressed in the winter because later dawn causes their circadian rhythms to drift out of phase with the sleep/wake cycle.[26,27] The PSH was inspired by the work of Kripke and Wehr,[9,10] but in this case the pertinent affective disorder is SAD. Furthermore, although the PSH leaves open the possibility that a patient may be either phase advanced or phase delayed, patients who had SAD were thought to be

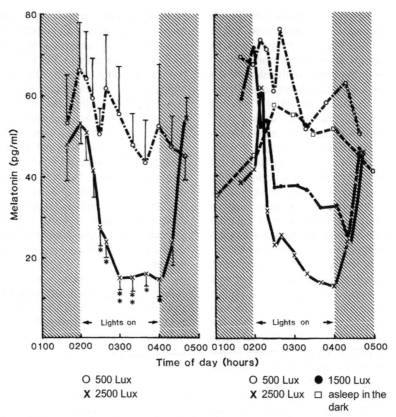

Fig. 2. (*Left*) Effect of light on melatonin secretion. Each point represents the mean concentration of melatonin (± SE) for six subjects. (*Right*) Effect of different light intensities on melatonin secretion. The averaged values for two subjects are shown. O, 500 lux; X, 2500 lux; ●, 1500 lux; and □, asleep in the dark. Melatonin levels were measured by mass spectrometry.[13] These early studies were responsible for an increased awareness of the importance of the light/dark cycle as a zeitgeber (time cue) for human circadian rhythms and for the use of the dim light melatonin onset (DLMO) as a circadian phase marker and of bright light as a circadian phase-resetting agent in the treatment of circadian phase disorders, including winter depression (SAD) and the circadian disorders experienced by totally blind people. (*From* Lewy AJ, Wehr TA, Goodwin FK, Newsome DA, et al. Light suppresses melatonin secretion in humans. Science 1980;210:1268; with permission.)

primarily of the phase delayed type, not of the phase-advanced type as hypothesized by Kripke and Wehr for patients who had nonseasonal depression.

An early refinement of the PSH for SAD was recognizing the possibility that these patients might have a phase-advanced disorder.[25,26] Such patients at first were thought to constitute a very small, indeed negligible, subgroup that could be included in studies without violating the integrity of the experimental design. In the first major publication comparing morning versus evening light treatment, one of eight SAD patients seemed to have a better antidepressant response to evening light.[27] This 1-to-8 proportion was deemed initially to be relatively high, and some researchers began to regard the PSH as the phase-delay hypothesis (for SAD).

Avery[28,29] made an important contribution by emphasizing the importance of hypersomnia in these presumably phase-delayed individuals. Initially, wake time was regarded as a good way to phase type individuals, and patients who had hypersomnia were considered to be phase delayed based on a late wake time, even if there was an early bedtime. Although the use of bright light in the morning was becoming accepted,[27–31] some investigators remained skeptical.[32,33] For example, the NIMH group focused on testing a melatonin/photoperiod hypothesis. At first the results were nonsupportive,[34] but during the last decade this hypothesis became the one preferred for testing at the NIMH.[35] Other investigators dismissed the importance of the timing of the light exposure, based on their studies that showed no difference between morning and evening light;[33] still other investigators thought those studies were confounded by the profound placebo response accompanying exposure to bright light, a response documented by Eastman.[36]

Consensus on the preferential benefit of morning versus evening light was finally was achieved in 1998, when large studies were published by three independent groups.[37–39] This consensus, however, did not necessarily validate the PSH, because it could be argued that morning is a time of increased light sensitivity. It became clear that another type of test of the PSH was needed. Fortunately, a second PRC to melatonin was obtained that replicated and extended the findings in the first melatonin PRC study in humans,[40] providing a way to use low-dose daytime melatonin to cause phase shifts (**Fig. 3**) and to test the antidepressant effects of phase shifts in response to melatonin in a protocol in which a placebo control group is possible.

The history of testing the phase-resetting effects of melatonin in humans has already been reviewed.[41] Many investigators think that the demonstration in a mammalian (rodent) species under free-running conditions was the inspirational landmark study by the Armstrong team,[42] although credit also should be given to Underwood[43] for his work in lizards and to the numerous studies in birds.[44,45] Sack and colleagues[46] initially chose to investigate blind people, to follow up on the Armstrong study as closely as possible. Before and while the studies were being conducted in blind people, the Arendt and colleagues[47] and Claustrat[48] teams were testing the circadian phase-shifting effects of melatonin in sighted people.

Sack and colleagues[71] showed that 6 of 7 free-running blind subjects could be entrained to a nightly dose of 10 mg melatonin. Lewy and colleagues[49] later showed that the seventh blind free-running subject could be entrained to 0.5 mg of melatonin. Based on their PRC to melatonin,[50,51] they surmised that when melatonin is administered on the advance zone of the melatonin PRC, there will always be a phase advance; however, its magnitude may be reduced if there is too much spillover on the delay zone of the melatonin PRC. In addition to avoiding spillover,[49] another heuristically useful pharmacokinetic principle for optimizing melatonin pharmacodynamics is to ensure that there is overlap between the exogenous melatonin pulse and either the onset or the offset of the endogenous melatonin profile so as to optimize the magnitude of the desired phase advance or phase delay, respectively.[41]

The dose–response curve for the phase-shifting effects of melatonin indicates a log-linear relationship for doses in the physiologic range.[52] An added benefit of using low doses of melatonin is that they are less likely to result acutely in sleepiness, which would be undesirable when melatonin is given during the day or early evening (although this possibility has not been examined systematically). This side effect seems to occur in about

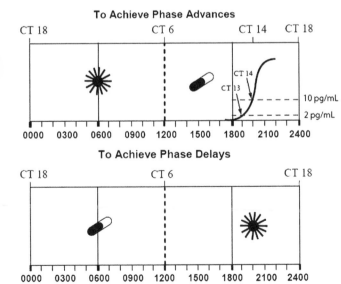

Fig. 3. The optimal times to schedule bright light exposure and low-dose melatonin administration to cause circadian phase shifts are based on their respective phase–response curves (PRCs), which are about 12 hours out of phase with each other. The 10 pg/mL plasma (3 pg/mL saliva) melatonin onset–marking circadian time (CT) 14 hours can be used to indicate when advance and delay responses occur, to maximize phase shifts. The crossover times are 8 hours before (CT 6 hours), and 4 hours after (CT 18 hours) the melatonin onset. Also indicated are clock times typical for individuals who awaken at 6 AM (0600). Optimally, exogenous melatonin should overlap with either the onset or the offset of the endogenous melatonin profile. High doses (> approximately 5 mg) may be less effective than lower doses because of spillover onto the wrong zone of the melatonin PRC. The crossover times for the light PRC are based on the one published by Czeisler and colleagues[78] in the Johnson Atlas of PRCs.[79] The optimal times for scheduling light are based on earlier work,[27] and the melatonin crossover and optimal scheduling times are based on the melatonin PRC.[40,50] ☀, melatonin; ✐, bright light. (*Adapted from* Lewy AJ. Melatonin and human chronobiology. Cold Spring Harb Symp Quant Biol 2007;72:626; with permission.)

a third of the population, and there is no way to predict who will be sensitive to it, although the higher the dose, the greater the proportion of individuals who are affected, and the greater the magnitude of the soporific effect.

TESTING THE PHASE-SHIFT HYPOTHESIS WITH LOW-DOSE MELATONIN ADMINISTRATION

The use of low-dose daytime melatonin to cause phase shifts in blind and sighted people based on the melatonin PRC[50,51] makes possible a critical test of the PSH. Patients who had SAD were given three or four doses of melatonin (0.75–0.3 mg) every 2 hours, beginning at wake time or in the afternoon to cause phase delays or phase advances, respectively.[7] After the data were collected, they initially were analyzed under the assumption that nearly all subjects would be phase delayed and that the inclusion of any phase-advanced subjects would be discounted. Therefore, for the group as a whole, afternoon/evening melatonin should be more antidepressant than morning melatonin. This comparison did not reach statistical significance. Hence, subjects were phase typed retrospectively according to the number of hours between their DLMO and mid-sleep, or their phase-angle difference (PAD). A PAD of 6 hours is the average in historical healthy controls; therefore subjects who had a PAD greater than 6 hours were designated as phase advanced (the DLMO is relatively advanced with respect to mid-sleep), and patients who had a PAD of 6 hours or less were designated as phase delayed (the DLMO is relatively delayed with respect to mid-sleep) (see **Fig. 1**). Surprisingly, one third of the subjects were phase advanced at baseline before they entered the treatment phase of the study. Remarkably, for both phase-advanced and phase-delayed subjects, the more the baseline PAD deviated from 6 hours, the greater was the depression rating. That is, in the phase-advanced group, the more phase advanced the DLMO was relative to mid-sleep, the greater were the depression ratings; in the phase-delayed group, the more phase delayed the DLMO was relative to mid-sleep, the greater were the depression ratings.

SLEEP DISORDERS AND CIRCADIAN MISALIGNMENT

Previously, phase typing usually was possible only in cases of extremely misaligned sleep (eg, people who had ASPS or DSPS). A PAD of 6 hours offers a way to phase type individuals who have conventional sleep times. Furthermore, both DLMOs and sleep times are required for PAD phase typing.

Although sleep times are appropriate for diagnosing ASPS and DSPS and for determining the correct scheduling of phase-resetting treatments, they do not take into consideration the possibility that internal circadian misalignment may require a different treatment schedule.

In fact, there are at least three ways in which circadian misalignment can cause sleep and alertness difficulties. First, circadian misalignment can lead to ASPS and DSPS, because sleep propensity occurs at an unconventional time. Second, circadian misalignment might affect PSG measures of sleep quality, even if sleep times are conventional. Third, other measures of nonrestorative sleep and daytime alertness might be affected by circadian misalignment, even if sleep times and PSG measures are not.

THE PHASE-SHIFT HYPOTHESIS AND SEASONAL AFFECTIVE DISORDER: MORE RECENT FINDINGS

Treatment response was evaluated after subjects in the SAD study who happened to be assigned randomly to the correct treatment were subgrouped retrospectively to the incorrect treatment or to placebo.[7] The correct treatment was afternoon/evening melatonin for subjects who were prototypically phase delayed before treatment (at baseline) and morning melatonin for subjects who were phase advanced before treatment. The incorrect treatment was morning melatonin for subjects who were phase delayed before treatment and afternoon/evening melatonin for subjects who were phase advanced before treatment. One third of the subjects were assigned to each treatment regimen.

The placebo response was about 13%, perhaps because the photoperiod was increased over the course of the 4-week study.[7] This percentage was expectedly low, certainly in comparison with studies in which subjects are exposed to light, which has a strong placebo effect. Another reason for the low placebo response was the instructions given to patients and raters: the investigators did not expect to see large changes in patients' mood in either direction. These instructions were compatible with the study design, which was not to optimize the efficacy of melatonin treatment but rather to test the antidepressant mechanism of action for light treatment. Thus, all that was needed was a statistically significant difference between treatment groups. In fact, the investigators found about a 20% separation in depression ratings between treatment groups, and the most conservative effect size was 0.61. Both findings are impressive when compared with studies of treatment with fixed-dose antidepressant drugs.

Thus, in addition to establishing the PSH for SAD, this study established therapeutic efficacy for appropriately timed low-dose daytime melatonin treatment.

This study was the first in which symptom severity in a psychiatric disorder was shown to correlate before and in the course of treatment in the same subjects. In fact, the circadian misalignment component was shown to be causal, in that the change in scores indicating treatment efficacy depended on the degree to which circadian misalignment was corrected. Among the 10 phase-delayed (correctly treated) subjects who received afternoon/evening melatonin and the 12 phase-advanced (correctly treated) subjects who received morning melatonin, only one subject (who shifted the most away from PAD 6) actually worsened on the wrong treatment; no subjects worsened on the correct treatment. After adjustments were made for the 13% placebo response, however, 5 of 21 subjects worsened, and 4 of these subjects shifted away from a PAD of 6 hours (**Fig. 4**).

When the depression ratings of the prototypical phase-delayed group taking the treatment of choice (afternoon/evening melatonin) were plotted against PAD, the parabolic minimum occurred at a PAD of 6 hours. At the vertex, the depression score was 13, which is not far from the normal range. According to this parabola, in these 11 subjects, 65% of the variance in these inherently noisy depression ratings was explained by the degree of circadian misalignment. Thus, it is possible that this component accounts for most (or perhaps all) of the basis for SAD. Because the PAD average and range is the same in healthy controls and in patients who have SAD, at least one other biologic or psychologic variable must render the patients who have SAD vulnerable to becoming depressed in the winter when they experience circadian misalignment. By way of

analogy, not everyone experiences jet lag when they travel across time zones.

The significance of an optimum PAD of 6 hours seems to hold for SAD, in that it was found in the baseline scores when the extant data from an earlier light treatment study[38] of 49 patients[53,54] were tested a priori. Furthermore, the r-square of the parabola was statistically significant. Moreover, two thirds of the subjects were phase delayed. Therefore, a PAD of 6 hours seems to be heuristically useful, at least for SAD. Perhaps some data sets, particularly for disorders other than SAD, are best fit by a linear regression and not a parabola. But first a review of proposed revisions is in order, along with other criticisms of the PSH.

PROPOSED REVISIONS TO THE PHASE-SHIFT HYPOTHESIS FOR SEASONAL AFFECTIVE DISORDER

Some investigators have had difficulties with the fact that treatment with evening bright light did not worsen depression in more subjects. In the first study of morning versus evening light, for example, after a baseline week, subjects were assigned randomly to a week of either morning light or evening light and then were crossed over to the other treatment. During the fourth and final week of the study, subjects received bright light exposure at both times (6–8 AM and 8–10 PM). The second bright light pulse is scheduled much later in this study than in the original case report (4–7 PM), so it is more likely to cause a phase delay. Some investigators noted that subjects who received evening light first did not worsen on average. Nor were these investigators impressed by the fact that subjects who received morning light first worsened when switched to evening light,[55] because mean ratings in the latter condition were not different from mean ratings at baseline. The explanation of an accompanying placebo component to light

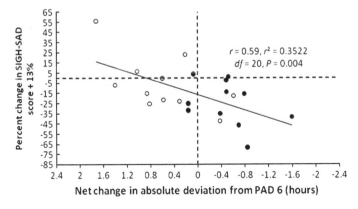

Fig. 4. Percent change in SIGH-SAD score as a function of net change in absolute deviation toward and away from a PAD of 6 hours in phase-advanced and phase-delayed subjects treated with evening melatonin. Thirteen percent has been added to the change in SIGH-SAD score to remove the average placebo response. Pretreatment versus posttreatment shifts with respect to a PAD of 6 hours account for 35% of the variance. O, phase-advanced subjects; ●, phase-delayed subjects. (*Adapted from* Lewy AJ, Lefler BJ, Emens JS, et al. The circadian basis of winter depression. Proc Nat Acad Sci USA 2006:103:7417; with permission.)

Net change in absolute deviation from PAD 6 (hours)

$r = 0.59, r^2 = 0.3522$
$df = 20, P = 0.004$

treatment that would counteract evening light's depressogenic effects (as would be predicted by the PSH) was not persuasive. In the authors' opinion, the placebo component is the same for equal durations of morning and evening light, particularly in the early studies before it became known that morning light was superior (that is, before 1998). In agreement with Eastman,[36] the authors think the placebo component to light varies among studies, in contrast to what some investigators have implied.[56]

Although some investigators thought the lack of a placebo control in the first major (crossover) study of morning versus evening light was problematic, other investigators (the present authors included) thought that the lack of a placebo control in parallel studies that showed no difference between morning and evening light was problematic, rendering interpretation of the results extremely difficult. Furthermore, a parallel-design study is vulnerable to the following confound: raters, and perhaps even subjects, expect the initial phase of the study to precede treatment that is increasingly effective as the study progresses. In one of these studies, for example, treatments were given to separate groups in parallel, following an initial baseline week.[33] Lack of a placebo control in this study would not have been problematic had one treatment proved to work better than another, because raters were unaware of whether the treatment week was testing morning or evening light exposure, as in the crossover studies. Because there was no difference in depression ratings comparing the two treatments, raters and patients could have been influenced by their knowledge of which weeks were baseline and which were light treatments. Furthermore, without a placebo comparison, it is not possible to tell whether the results should be interpreted as meaning that the two treatments were equally effective or that they were equally ineffective.

Nevertheless, for several years proponents of parallel-design studies[57] were concerned about an order effect in crossover studies. These concerns arose because some of the earlier crossover studies showed a greater benefit of morning versus evening light in the second treatment period than in the first treatment period. Critics of the PSH favored the importance of the first treatment period (which showed less difference between morning and evening light), positing that the second treatment period was confounded by an order effect. Subsequently, however, the antidepressant superiority of morning light was shown to be statistically significant in parallel-design studies, as well as in the first treatment period in crossover studies, thus rendering this criticism

moot. In fact, the three 1998 studies effectively created consensus that morning light is more antidepressant than evening light, at least for most patients who have SAD.[37–39]

Based on what was thought to be an order effect (but later was not replicated),[58] the first revision to the PSH was posited by the Terman[59] research group, to wit, that bright light is antidepressant in SAD except when it causes phase delays. In other words, evening light has increased efficacy when it is scheduled as a first treatment because it causes smaller phase delays than when it is scheduled as a second treatment (in the latter situation, the light PRC has been advanced by morning light given in the first treatment period, thus exposing more of the delay zone to stimulation by evening light). In any event, in their 2001 study the Terman group retracted this revision in favor of a second revision.[58] The present authors' group, incidentally, attributed any reduction, statistically significant or not, in the superiority of morning light in the first treatment period to the placebo component of light.[38] As a first treatment, any light treatment is expected to be somewhat antidepressant. As a second treatment, however, evening light suffers in comparison with the subject's prior benefit with morning light.

Before moving on to the discussion of the revision of the PSH, a brief review of the use of the DLMO may be helpful. The DLMO was assessed in many of the earliest studies of the PSH.[27,60,61] Compared with the average in normal, healthy controls, the average time of the DLMO was slightly delayed in patients who had SAD. In some studies, however, this finding was not statistically significant, a matter of concern to some critics of the PSH, even though the PSH posited that the DLMO reflects an ipsative (intra-individual, probably state-dependent) and not necessarily normative difference; that is, most patients who had SAD became depressed in the fall/winter at least in part because of a phase delay compared with a time in the spring/summer when they were euthymic.[25] Therefore, in the authors' opinion, a DLMO in patients who have SAD that is not delayed compared with controls does not invalidate the PSH. It would not be surprising if the DLMOs of most controls were delayed in the winter as well. In fact, it would not be surprising if the DLMOs of most controls were also delayed in the winter compared with the summer. There are very few studies of circadian phase across the seasons. In a study that compared patients who had SAD with controls, the dim light melatonin offset (DLMOff) and melatonin synthesis offset (SynOff), but not the DLMO, advanced in the summer in the patients compared with controls.[35]

Clearly, more studies across the seasons are needed.

In addition to dichotomous comparisons of the mean DLMOs between patients who had SAD and controls, correlational analyses were undertaken also, even in the earliest studies. The first such correlation showed a statistically significant correlation between depression ratings and the DLMO clock time of the group means for each treatment condition (ie, first baseline, 2 hours of morning light, 0.5 hour of morning light, and second baseline).[55] Of note, to keep the raters blind in this parallel study, half of the subjects began with a light treatment week followed by a baseline week. Nevertheless, even though raters could not know which weeks were treatment weeks, the subjects knew. The second such correlation comparing morning and evening light following a baseline week in a crossover study also was statistically significant.[30]

The more meaningful correlational analysis using a separate data point for each individual was first provided by Terman,[59] utilizing the data from the authors' first two major studies of morning versus evening light.[27,30] A similar analysis in a larger number of their own subjects published in 2001 helped refocus attention on the importance of correlational, rather than dichotomous, analyses, even though the Termans and colleagues[58] were not able to show antidepressant superiority of morning versus evening light. In this study, the second revision of the PSH was posited: the Termans and colleagues proposed that improvement in patients who had SAD depends on the magnitude of the phase advance produced by morning light. In other words, patients who advance their DLMO by 3 hours will do better than those who advance by 2 hours, and patients who advance their DLMOs by 1 hour will not do as well as either of the other two groups. The PAD between the DLMO and sleep is not thought to be important, and wake time often has to be scheduled earlier to accommodate an early clock time of morning light exposure to provide a sufficient phase advance. According to the original PSH, however, an advance in either bedtime or wake time should be minimized, because this advance would work against increasing PAD to 6 hours.

This revision differs from the PSH in three ways. First, it does not take into account a phase-advanced subgroup of patients who have SAD who require a corrective phase delay, which is part of the original PSH. Second, the PSH is based on the PAD between the DLMO (and its related rhythms) and the sleep/wake cycle (and its related rhythms), whereas this revision is concerned only with the clock time of the DLMO. Third, the PSH envisions a "sweet spot" for the time of the DLMO relative to sleep (allowing for the possibility of overshifting past the sweet spot), whereas this revision explicitly states that the greater the phase advance, the greater the antidepressant response (in plots of clinical response versus phase, overshifting past the sweet spot with very large phase shifts would be described by a parabolic fit of the data, not by a linear regression).

The differences between the original PSH and this revision have several important clinical implications. The revision recommends only morning light—for all patients. The original PSH recommends evening light for the phase-advanced type and provides a way to identify them (a baseline DLMO that is more than 6 hours before midsleep), whereas work-ups based on this revision do not include a way to phase type. Nor does this revision allow for the possibility that a patient could become overly phase shifted. According to this revision, patients who have the earliest DLMOs should receive morning light at the earliest times. Evening light would probably be the treatment of choice for these patients, because according to the PSH they likely would be phase typed as phase advanced based on a DLMO/mid-sleep interval greater than 6 hours. For patients who would qualify for morning light according to both the PSH and this revision, according to the PSH sleep times should not be shifted in the same direction as the DLMO, whereas the proponents of this revision, to accommodate relatively early morning light exposures, would have patients awaken earlier than usual to achieve the maximal possible phase advance in the clock time of the DLMO.

Although sleep times are the way to phase type patients who have ASPS and DSPS to determine the correct times to administer phase-resetting agents, phase typing of patients who have SAD should be based on whether the PAD is greater or less than 6 hours. Sleep times alone are not a reliable way to do phase typing. In fact, if patients who have SAD have delayed sleep, they may be even more likely to have a DLMO that is relatively advanced with respect to sleep. The Terman group continues to recommend sleep times and morningness/eveningness ratings (that to some extent correlate with sleep time) to specify how early a patient should be awakened to accommodate relatively early light exposures, although recently some exceptions recommending evening light exposure have been considered.[62]

Morningness/eveningness ratings are influenced by sleep times. As predicted by the PSH and as recently shown,[63] the typical patient who has SAD has circadian rhythms that are delayed (perhaps the result of a long intrinsic circadian period) but is required to sleep at an earlier time than desired in the winter. Interestingly, all three individuals who had long intrinsic circadian periods who were morning types were retrospectively determined to have SAD.[64] These three individuals would be expected to have a DLMO that is phase delayed with respect to mid-sleep, because persons who have longer intrinsic circadian periods should have a delayed phase-angle of entrainment. In any event, morningness/eveningness ratings (which correlate with both DLMO clock times and sleep times) may be of questionable benefit in predicting whether a patient who has SAD will benefit preferentially from morning rather than evening light.

As mentioned earlier, the sweet spot of a PAD of 6 hours now has been found in two different groups of patients who had SAD. It may turn out, however, that other patients should be phase typed on a more individual basis. So far, this seems to be the case with patients who have unipolar nonseasonal depression, in that their data are best fit linearly and not parabolically.[65] Because it has only been 7 years since the Terman linear correlational study was published[58] and only 2 years since the authors' parabolic correlation,[7] the jury is out as to how many patients who have SAD are of the phase-advanced type and how likely is overshifting of the phase-delayed types.

It may turn out that the Terman revision of the PSH for SAD may be more applicable to other groups of patients, at least with respect to a linear versus a parabolic plot of the data. Even with linear analyses, however, the authors recommend that future studies plot data differently than done by the Terman group.[58] Although their posttreatment change scores in depression ratings were based on the change from the initial baseline condition for all subjects, these scores apparently were plotted against change in DLMO clock time from the initial baseline condition only for those subjects who received morning light first. For those subjects who received evening light first, this condition (that is evening light), instead of the baseline condition, apparently was used in the change scores for DLMO clock times, even though the baseline condition was used in the change scores for depression ratings in the same individuals. Therefore, if this discussion is correct, the change scores are not consistent, and for half of the subjects the change scores for the DLMO clock times are not based on the same initial condition and time point as the change scores for the depression ratings.

It also may be that the DLMO clock time has greater statistical significance than the PAD when plotted against depression ratings, particularly in linear plots. Nevertheless, the authors continue to think that the PAD is to be preferred over the DLMO clock time for several reasons (even though the authors and others have found DLMO clock times to lead to significant analyses when sleep times are held constant, rendering the difference between DLMO circadian and clock times moot, at least for changes during the course of the study). The same cannot be said for initial phase typing, however. The PAD also takes into account different preferred sleep times in individuals in whom sleep may have nothing to do with their disorder. The PAD also takes into account various influences on sleep times that may or may not have to do with their disorder or clinical state and are more likely to be causal of sleep and psychiatric symptoms, whereas changes in the DLMO clock time easily could result from changes in sleep times vis-à-vis the perceived light/dark cycle.

In any event, the recommendations the authors made 2 decades ago[66] seem to be current, with one modification (**Box 1**), first suggested for SAD by the Terman group.[31] The first SAD studies used light of 2000 to 2500 lux.[2,27,67] The Terman group suggested using 10,000 lux in the treatment of SAD.[31] There probably is intensity/duration reciprocity, so that an exposure of 10,000 lux can have a shorter duration than originally recommended for 2000 lux, at least for maintenance after induction of the treatment response (which can take up to 2 weeks to be complete).

Research continues to uphold the original treatment recommendations for SAD,[66] which considered the possibility that patients could be overly phase shifted with too much light. Most (at least two thirds) of patients who have SAD are phase delayed (that is, have a DLMO that is delayed with respect to the sleep/wake cycle). Therefore, bright light should be tried first in the morning, even in patients with early sleep times. In fact, these patients probably have a DLMO that is delayed with respect to the sleep/wake cycle; that is, they probably have a sleep/wake cycle that is advanced with respect to the DLMO. In fact, modal patients are prevented from indulging their inclination to sleep later in the winter because of work or family obligations. Years ago, the authors found preliminary evidence for the therapeutic efficacy of delaying sleep in SAD,[68] which is another way of accomplishing the goal of having the wake time coincide with bright light exposure (even on a cloudy, winter day, sunlight exposure an hour or more after dawn is at least 10,000 lux). These recommendations will be refined as

---

Box 1
Treatment guidelines for patients who have seasonal affective disorder

- If patients do not have early morning awakening, schedule 1 to 2 hours of exposure to 2500 to **10,000** lux immediately upon awakening.
- If patients begin treatment on the weekend, they may not have to arise earlier to accommodate the morning light exposure; early rising may retard the response for a few days.
- The response begins 2 to 4 days after beginning light therapy and usually is complete within 2 weeks.
- These patients should minimize any advance in their sleep time and should avoid bright light in the evening.
- Patients who do not respond to treatment may need a longer duration of exposure to morning light.
- If patients respond only transiently or begin to complain of early morning awakening or severe fatigue in the evening, they may be becoming overly phase advanced because of too much morning light. The duration of morning light should be reduced, but exposure still should begin immediately upon awakening. Alternately, some late evening light exposure could be added.
- Some patients may respond to an immediate "energizing" effect (possibly a placebo effect) of exposure to bright light, which, if not administrated too late in the evening, might be helpful.
- Once a response has been achieved, the duration and frequency of light exposures can be reduced. Always begin light exposure immediately upon awakening or a little later if a patient becomes overly phase advanced.
- If there is still no response, a trial of bright light in the evening (7–9 PM) may be necessary. These patients should minimize any delay in their sleep time and should avoid bright light in the morning.
- Appropriate precautions should be taken to avoid any possibility of eye discomfort or injury (eg, an eye history and examination if indicated, instructions never to stare at the sun, use of safe artificial light sources, and recommendation of follow-up visits).

Adapted from Lewy AJ. Treating chronobiologic sleep and mood disorders with bright light. Psychiatr Ann 1987;17:664–9; with permission.

---

salivary DLMOs become commercially available. Samples can be collected at home. In almost all cases, the DLMO occurs before sleep onset, so collections can be completed before bedtime. Another very important feature that will make this test much more convenient is the use of orange goggles[69,70] that will obviate the need for dim light, or at least light that is so dim that reading is uncomfortable, which is the standard recommendation.

THE PHASE-SHIFT HYPOTHESIS AS APPLIED TO OTHER DISORDERS THAT MAY HAVE A CIRCADIAN MISALIGNMENT COMPONENT

As in the study of blind people (see the article by Uchiyama and Lockley in this issue), SAD is a useful model for studying the effects of light deprivation on the circadian system of humans. Totally blind people who completely lack light perception provide an unfortunate but useful experiment of nature which is the only way to study human circadian rhythms in the absence of the confounding effects of light.[49,71–75] Of course, light deprivation in the winter compared with the summer is not comparable to the experience of a totally blind person. SAD, however, is an excellent model for a circadian rhythm affective disorder and perhaps for a certain type of circadian rhythm

sleep disorder, that is, nonrestorative sleep caused by internal circadian misalignment.

People who have circadian misalignment, even when they have little difficulty going to sleep and waking up at conventional times, may have nonrestorative sleep, which seems to be part of the dysphoric mood constellation of symptoms in patients who have SAD and in those who have unipolar nonseasonal depression.[65] In an item analysis of the SIGH-SAD baseline ratings of the subjects in the melatonin administration study,[7] three items accounted for the results found for the 29 items, even though the former 21 items had a range that was one tenth of the latter 3 items.[54] These three items were depression severity, psychic anxiety severity, and severity of agitation observed by the interviewer. These three items might constitute the nub of an endotype that corresponds to the circadian misalignment component for SAD. Of note, these three items resulted in a statistically significant parabolic correlation with the PAD in the baseline data from the authors' latest light treatment SAD study.[39] Perhaps a subgroup of people have nonrestorative sleep when their circadian rhythms become misaligned, even in the absence of any other symptoms. It would not be surprising, therefore, if the salivary DLMO were incorporated into the standard PSG test routinely done in clinical sleep laboratories, particularly if there is a low level of suspicion that the PSG will reveal any abnormalities. The PSG, following a few days of documenting sleep and wake times, will allow calculation of the PAD. The sleep laboratory PAD could be followed up with additional assessments to provide even more information about the relationship between the patient's sleep and psychiatric symptoms and circadian misalignment.

SUMMARY

Clearly, the DLMO/mid-sleep PAD needs to be assessed in a variety of sleep and psychiatric disorders. Thus far, the authors have found that symptom severity (as measured by the Connor's Parent Rating Cognitive Problems/Inattention Subscale and the Attention Deficit Hyperactivity Disorder Index Subscale in attention deficit hyperactivity disorder,[76] the Ham-21 depression scores in nonseasonal depression,[66] and the Profile of Mood States Brief Form ratings in healthy medical students) correlates with the PAD, in that the more the DLMO is phase delayed with respect to mid-sleep, the greater is the symptom severity.[77] Correlations, either linear or parabolic, with symptom severity should lead to the safe and effective use of bright light and/or melatonin, at least as add-on treatments, assuming that the circadian misalignment is causal, as it is in SAD, even if it accounts for a small component of the disorder. Patients probably will have to be phase typed on an individual basis, in which a PAD of 6 hours may or may not be as useful as it is in SAD. An alternative way to phase type on an individual basis would be to determine whether there is a positive or negative slope, even if not statistically significant, on at least three or four data points in which symptom severity is plotted against the PAD: individuals who tend to be more symptomatic when more delayed could be phase typed as delayed, and vice versa. Low-dose melatonin (or bright light) could then be scheduled at the correct time (to cause an increase or a decrease in the PAD, respectively) to validate phase type and treatment parameters and to determine causality between PAD and symptom severity. Also, mid-sleep may not be the best marker for sleep phase when calculating the PAD, although it does take into account inter- and intra-individual differences in sleep duration. For continued monitoring of therapeutic efficacy, the DLMO and the PAD probably will be important, in addition to the clinical assessment of improvement or relapse. The DLMO also is the best way to identify the phase of the light and melatonin PRCs and thus will help optimize the scheduling of treatment times more precisely. In conclusion, such work may lead to an extension of a heuristically useful model in medicine and psychiatry. The roles of light, melatonin, and biologic rhythms in a bio-psycho-social-environmental model have yet to be understood and appreciated fully.

REFERENCES

1. Rosen LN, Rosenthal NE. Seasonal variations in mood and behavior in the general population: a factor-analytic approach. Psychiatry Res 1991;38:271–83.
2. Rosenthal NE, Sack DA, Gillin JC, et al. Seasonal affective disorder: a description of the syndrome and preliminary findings with light therapy. Arch Gen Psychiatry 1984;41:72–80.
3. Kasper S, Wehr TA, Bartko JJ, et al. Epidemiological findings of seasonal changes in mood and behavior. Arch Gen Psychiatry 1989;46:823–33.
4. Rosenthal NE, Carpenter CJ, James SP, et al. Seasonal affective disorder in children and adolescents. Am J Psychiatry 1986;143(3):356–8.
5. Swedo SE, Pleeter JD, Richter DM, et al. Rates of seasonal affective disorder in children and adolescents. Am J Psychiatry 1995;152:1016–9.
6. Williams JBW, Link MJ, Rosenthal NE, et al. Structured interview guide for the Hamilton Depression Scale—Seasonal Affective Disorder version (SIGH-SAD). New York: New York State Psychiatric Institute; 1988.
7. Lewy AJ, Lefler BJ, Emens JS, et al. The circadian basis of winter depression. Proc Natl Acad Sci U S A 2006;103:7414–9.
8. Kripke DF, Mullaney DJ, Atkinson M, et al. Circadian rhythm disorders in manic-depressives. Biol Psychiatry 1978;13(3):335–51.
9. Kripke DF. Phase-advance theories for affective illness. In: Wehr TA, Goodwin FK, editors. Circadian rhythms in psychiatry. Pacific Grove (CA): Boxwood Press; 1983. p. 41–69.
10. Wehr TA, Wirz-Justice A, Goodwin FK, et al. Phase advance of the circadian sleep-wake cycle as an antidepressant. Science 1979;206(9):710–3.
11. Wever R. The circadian system of man: results of experiments under temporal isolation. New York: Springer-Verlag; 1979.
12. Goldman BD, Darrow JM. The pineal gland and mammalian photoperiodism. Neuroendocrinology 1983;37:386–96.
13. Lewy AJ, Markey SP. Analysis of melatonin in human plasma by gas chromatography negative chemical ionization mass spectrometry. Science 1978;201:741–3.
14. Arendt J, Paunier L, Sizonenko PC. Melatonin radioimmunoassay. J Clin Endocrinol Metab 1975;40:347–50.
15. Wetterberg L, Arendt J, Paunier L, et al. Human serum melatonin changes during the menstrual cycle. J Clin Endocrinol Metab 1976;42:185–8.

16. Arendt J, Wetterberg L, Heyden T, et al. Radioimmunoassay of melatonin: human serum and cerebrospinal fluid. Horm Res 1977;8(2):65–75.

17. Smith JA, Padwick D, Mee TJX, et al. Synchronous nyctohemeral rhythms in human blood melatonin and in human post-mortem pineal enzyme. Clin Endocrinol 1977;6(3):219–25.

18. Lewy AJ, Tetsuo M, Markey SP, et al. Pinealectomy abolishes plasma melatonin in the rat. J Clin Endocrinol Metab 1980;50(1):204–5.

19. Neuwelt EA, Lewy AJ. Disappearance of plasma melatonin after removal of a neoplastic pineal gland. N Engl J Med 1983;308:1132–5.

20. Ozaki Y, Lynch HJ. Presence of melatonin in plasma and urine of pinealectomized rats. Endocrinology 1976;99:641–4.

21. Lewy AJ, Wehr TA, Goodwin FK, et al. Light suppresses melatonin secretion in humans. Science 1980;210:1267–9.

22. Arendt J. Melatonin assays in body fluids. J Neural Transm Suppl 1978;13:265–78.

23. Wetterberg L. Melatonin in humans: physiological and clinical studies [review]. J Neural Transm Suppl 1978;13:289–94.

24. Akerstedt T, Fröberg JE, Friberg Y, et al. Melatonin excretion, body temperature, and subjective arousal during 64 hours of sleep deprivation. Psychoneuroendocrinology 1979;4:219–25.

25. Lewy AJ, Kern HA, Rosenthal NE, et al. Bright artificial light treatment of a manic-depressive patient with a seasonal mood cycle. Am J Psychiatry 1982;139(11):1496–8.

26. Lewy AJ, Sack RL, Singer CM, et al. The phase shift hypothesis for bright light's therapeutic mechanism of action: theoretical considerations and experimental evidence. Psychopharmacol Bull 1987;23(3):349–53.

27. Lewy AJ, Sack RL, Miller S, et al. Antidepressant and circadian phase-shifting effects of light. Science 1987;235:352–4.

28. Avery DH, Khan A, Dager SR, et al. Bright light treatment of winter depression: morning versus evening light. Acta Psychiatr Scand 1990;82:335–8.

29. Avery D, Khan A, Dager S, et al. Morning or evening bright light treatment of winter depression? The significance of hypersomnia. Biol Psychiatry 1991;29:117–26.

30. Sack RL, Lewy AJ, White DM, et al. Morning versus evening light treatment for winter depression: evidence that the therapeutic effects of light are mediated by circadian phase shifts. Arch Gen Psychiatry 1990;47:343–51.

31. Terman M, Terman JS, Quitkin FM, et al. Light therapy for seasonal affective disorder: a review of efficacy. Neuropsychopharmacology 1989;2(1):1–22.

32. Thalén BE, Kjellman BF, Mørkrid L, et al. Light treatment in seasonal and nonseasonal depression. Acta Psychiatr Scand 1995;91:352–60.

33. Wirz-Justice A, Graw P, Kraeuchi K, et al. Light therapy in seasonal affective disorder is independent of time of day or circadian phase. Arch Gen Psychiatry 1993;50:929–37.

34. Wehr TA, Jacobsen FM, Sack DA, et al. Phototherapy of seasonal affective disorder: time of day and suppression of melatonin are not critical for antidepressant effects. Arch Gen Psychiatry 1986;43:870–5.

35. Wehr TA, Duncan WC, Sher L, et al. A circadian signal of change of season in patients with seasonal affective disorder. Arch Gen Psychiatry 2001;58:1108–14.

36. Eastman CI. Is bright-light therapy a placebo?. In: Partonen T, Magnusson A, editors. Seasonal affective disorder practice and research. New York: Oxford University Press; 2001. p. 103–12.

37. Eastman CI, Young MA, Fogg LF, et al. Bright light treatment of winter depression: a placebo-controlled trial. Arch Gen Psychiatry 1998;55(10):883–9.

38. Lewy AJ, Bauer VK, Cutler NL, et al. Morning versus evening light treatment of patients with winter depression. Arch Gen Psychiatry 1998;55:890–6.

39. Terman M, Terman JS, Ross DC. A controlled trial of timed bright light and negative air ionization for treatment of winter depression. Arch Gen Psychiatry 1998;55:875–82.

40. Lewy AJ, Bauer VK, Ahmed S, et al. The human phase response curve (PRC) to melatonin is about 12 hours out of phase with the PRC to light. Chronobiol Int 1998;15(1):71–83.

41. Lewy AJ, Sack RL. Exogenous melatonin's phase shifting effects on the endogenous melatonin profile in sighted humans: a brief review and critique of the literature. J Biol Rhythms 1997;12:595–603.

42. Redman J, Armstrong S, Ng KT. Free-running activity rhythms in the rat: entrainment by melatonin. Science 1983;219:1089–91.

43. Underwood H. Circadian rhythms in lizards: phase response curve for melatonin. J Pineal Res 1986;3:187–96.

44. Gwinner E, Benzinger I. Synchronization of a circadian rhythm in pinealectomized European starlings by injections of melatonin. J Comp Physiol 1978;127:209–13.

45. Cassone VM, Menaker M. Is the avian circadian system a neuroendocrine loop? J Exp Zool 1984;232:539–49.

46. Sack RL, Lewy AJ, Hoban TM. Free-running melatonin rhythms in blind people: phase shifts with melatonin and triazolam administration. In: Rensing L, an der Heiden U, Mackey MC, editors. Temporal disorder in human oscillatory systems. Heidelberg (Germany): Springer-Verlag; 1987. p. 219–24.

47. Arendt J, Bojkowski C, Folkard S, et al. Some effects of melatonin and the control of its secretion in man. In: Evered D, Clark S, editors. Photoperiodism, melatonin and the pineal. London: Ciba Foundation Symposium 1985. p. 266–83.

48. Mallo C, Zaidan R, Faure A, et al. Effects of a four-day nocturnal melatonin treatment on the 24 h plasma melatonin, cortisol and prolactin profiles in humans. Acta Endocrinol (Copenh) 1988;119(4):474–80.

49. Lewy AJ, Emens JS, Sack RL, et al. Low, but not high, doses of melatonin entrained a free-running blind person with a long circadian period. Chronobiol Int 2002;19(3):649–58.

50. Lewy AJ, Ahmed S, Jackson JML, et al. Melatonin shifts circadian rhythms according to a phase-response curve. Chronobiol Int 1992;9(5):380–92.

51. Lewy AJ, Sack RL, Latham JM. Exogenous melatonin administration shifts circadian rhythms according to a phase response curve [abstract 021]. The Fifth Colloquium of the European Pineal Study Group. Guildford, England; 1990.

52. Lewy AJ, Emens JS, Lefler BJ, et al. Melatonin entrains free-running blind people according to a physiological dose-response curve. Chronobiol Int 2005;22(6):1093–106.

53. Lewy A, Woods K, Kinzie J, et al. DLMO/Mid-sleep interval of six hours phase types SAD patients and parabolically correlates with symptom severity. Sleep 2007;30(Abstract Supplement):A63–4.

54. Lewy A, Rough J, Songer J, et al. The phase shift hypothesis for the circadian component of winter depression. Dialogues Clin Neurosci 2007;9:291–300.

55. Lewy AJ, Sack RL, Singer CM, et al. Winter depression and the phase shift hypothesis for bright light's therapeutic effects: history, theory and experimental evidence. J Biol Rhythms 1988;3(2):121–34.

56. Lam RW, Levitt AJ, Levitan RD, et al. The Can-SAD study: a randomized controlled trial of the effectiveness of light therapy and fluoxetine in patients with winter seasonal affective disorder. Am J Psychiatry 2006;163(5):805–12.

57. Rafferty B, Terman M, Terman JS, et al. Does morning light therapy prevent evening light effect? Society for Light Treatment and Biological Rhythms Abstracts 1990;2:18.

58. Terman JS, Terman M, Lo E-S, et al. Circadian time of morning light administration and therapeutic response in winter depression. Arch Gen Psychiatry 2001;58(1):69–75.

59. Terman M. Overview: light treatment and future directions of research. In: Wetterberg L, editor. Light and biological rhythms in man, vol. 63. New York: Pergamon Press; 1993. p. 421–36.

60. Terman M, Quitkin FM, Terman JS, et al. The timing of phototherapy: effects on clinical response and the melatonin cycle. Psychopharmacol Bull 1987; 23(3):354–7.

61. Dahl K, Avery DH, Lewy AJ, et al. Dim light melatonin onset and circadian temperature during a constant routine in hypersomnic winter depression. Acta Psychiatr Scand 1993;88:60–6.

62. Terman M, Terman JS. Light therapy for seasonal and nonseasonal depression: efficacy, protocol, safety, and side effects. CNS Spectr 2005;10(8):647–63.

63. Lewy AJ. Melatonin and human chronobiology. Cold Spring Harb Symp Quant Biol 2007;72:626–36.

64. Brown SA, Kunz D, Dumas A, et al. Molecular insights into human daily behavior. Proc Natl Acad Sci U S A 2008;105(5):1602–7.

65. Emens J, Rough J, Arntz D, et al. Circadian misalignment correlates with symptom severity in non-seasonal depression. Sleep 2008;31:A314 [Abstract Supplement].

66. Lewy AJ. Treating chronobiologic sleep and mood disorders with bright light. Psychiatr Ann 1987;17: 664–9.

67. Lewy AJ, Kern HA, Rosenthal NE, et al. Bright artificial light treatment of a manic-depressive patient with a seasonal mood cycle. Am J Psychiatry 1982;139(11):1496–8.

68. Lewy AJ, Sack RL, Singer CM. Bright light, melatonin, and winter depression: the phase-shift hypothesis. In: Shafii MA, Shafii SL, editors. Biological rhythms, mood disorders, light therapy, and the pineal gland. Washington DC: American Psychiatric Press; 1990. p. 143–73.

69. Kayumov L, Casper RF, Hawa RJ, et al. Blocking low-wavelength light prevents nocturnal melatonin supression with no adverse effect on performance during simulated shift work. Journal of Clinical Endocrinology and Metabolism 2005;90:2755–61.

70. Sasseville A, Paquet N, Sevigny J, et al. Blue blocker glasses impede the capacity of bright light to suppress melatonin production. J Pineal Res 2006; 41:73–8.

71. Sack RL, Brandes RW, Kendall AR, et al. Entrainment of free-running circadian rhythms by melatonin in blind people. N Engl J Med 2000;343:1070–7.

72. Lewy AJ, Bauer VK, Hasler BP, et al. Capturing the circadian rhythms of free-running blind people with 0.5 mg melatonin. Brain Res 2001;918:96–100.

73. Lewy AJ, Hasler BP, Emens JS, et al. Pretreatment circadian period in free-running blind people may predict the phase angle of entrainment to melatonin. Neurosci Lett 2001;313:158–60.

74. Lewy AJ, Emens JS, Sack RL, et al. Zeitgeber hierarchy in humans: resetting the circadian phase positions of blind people using melatonin. Chronobiol Int 2003;20(5):837–52.

75. Lewy AJ, Emens JS, Bernert RA, et al. Eventual entrainment of the human circadian pacemaker by melatonin is independent of the circadian phase of treatment initiation: clinical implications. J Biol Rhythms 2004;19(1):68–75.

76. Keepers GA, Evans C, Colling E, et al. Circadian rhythm disturbances in adolescents with ADHD. Presented at the 159th Annual Meeting of the

American Psychiatric Association, Toronto May 24, 2006.

77. Emens J, Lewy AJ, Rough J, et al. Sub-clinical dysphoria correlates with phase-delayed circadian misalignment in healthy subjects. Presented at the 47th Annual Meting of the American College of Neuropsychopharmacology, Scottsdale, Arizona, December 5, 2008.

78. Czeisler CA, Kronauer RE, Allan JS, et al. Bright light induction of strong (type O) resetting of the human circadian pacemaker. Science 1989;244: 1328–33.

79. Johnson CH. An atlas of phase response curves for circadian and circatidal rhythms. Nashville (TN): Department of Biology, Vanderbilt University; 1990.

A Glossary of Circadian Rhythm Terminology for the Researcher and Clinician

Kenneth P. Wright, Jr., PhD[a],*, Tina M. Burke, MS[a],
Teofilo Lee-Chiong, MD[b]

This glossary is not meant to be all inclusive, but it includes many terms used in chronobiology, sleep, and circadian medicine.

acrophase: peak of a rhythm or time series; often the peak of a fitted curve, rather than absolute peak of a physiological or behavioral rhythm

actigraphy: accelerometer usually worn on the nondominant wrist to record activity levels in humans

actogram: graph of activity levels across one or more days (in nonhumans, activity may represent running wheel activity; laser beam crossings, eg, breaking of a beam by movement across a room or between rooms; or measures of activity with an accelerometer)

advanced sleep phase disorder (ASPS/ASPD): circadian rhythm sleep disorder resulting in wakefulness and sleep times that are much earlier relative to the desired/imposed times

amplitude: magnitude between the mesor to the peak of a rhythm

ASPS/ASPD: *see* advanced sleep phase disorder

biological clock: self-sustained oscillator that generates circadian rhythms under constant conditions

biological day: term used in diurnal species to represent the internal circadian time when wakefulness and associated functions are promoted

biological night: term used in diurnal species to represent the internal circadian time when sleep and associated functions are promoted

CBT: core body temperature

chronobiology: field of biology that studies the biological timing of life processes

chronotherapy: treatment timed according to internal biological time to maximize treatment outcome and minimize side effects

circadian degrees: nomenclature used to divide the circadian cycle into circadian hours with 15 degrees representing 1 circadian hour (360 degrees = 24 hours or one complete circadian cycle; zero degrees is often used to denote the timing of the core body tempeature minimum in humans)

circadian period (τ): cycle length; the time it takes to cycle from circadian phase on one day to the same circadian phase on the following day, also called tau and intrinsic circadian period

circadian phase (φ): time within the circadian cycle at which a particular event occurs (eg, minimum, maximum, onset)

This work was supported by NIH HL081761.
[a] Department of Integrative Physiology, Sleep and Chronobiology Laboratory, University of Colorado, 1725 Pleasant Street, Clare Small 114, Boulder, CO 80309, USA
[b] Division of Sleep Medicine, National Jewish Health University of Colorado Denver School of Medicine, 1400 Jackson Street, Room J221, Denver, CO 60206, USA
* Corresponding author.
E-mail address: Kenneth.Wright@Colorado.EDU (K.P. Wright).

Sleep Med Clin 4 (2009) 301–304
doi:10.1016/j.jsmc.2009.03.002

circadian rhythm: physiological or behavioral oscillation with a periodicity near 24 hours; a self-sustained physiological or behavioral oscillation with a periodicity near 24 hours that is clock-driven (clock-driven implies that the rhythm is driven by the circadian timekeeping system and not caused by external factors; a circadian rhythm will persist in constant conditions)

circadian time (CT): nomenclature used to divide the circadian cycle into circadian hours relative to the light–dark cycle (CT0= subjective dawn and CT12 = subjective dark) in a 12-hour light/12-hour dark light–dark cycle

circannual: physiological or behavioral oscillation with a periodicity near one year

clock-controlled genes: genes whose rhythmic expression are regulated by the internal circadian time-keeping system

clock genes: genes within biological tissue whose expression osscilates with a circadian rhythm (clock genes mechanistically underlie circadian oscillations within cells and tissue)

constant dark/darkness: experimental procedure used in nonhuman research designed to estimate circadian period and phase-shifting agents under environmenal conditions of continuous darkness exposure

constant light: experimental procedure used in nonhuman research designed to estimate circadian period and phase-shifting agents under environmenal conditions of continuous light exposure

constant routine: experimental protocol used in human circadian research to examine circadian variation in physiological or behavioral processes (the constant routine procedure controls, eg, constant dim light, ambient temperature, posture, wakefulness–sleep state [constant wakefulness], or equally distributes factors that infleunce the measure of interest across the circadian cycle, eg, meal intake)

CRSD: circadian rhythm sleep disorder

CT: *see* circadian time

delayed sleep phase disorder (DSPS/DSPD): circadian rhythm sleep disorder resulting in wakefulness and sleep times that are much later relative to the desired/imposed times

dim light melatonin offset (DLMOff): a marker of endogenous circadian phase defined at the time when melatonin levels decline to daytime levels (as with the DLMO, thresholds of 10 pg/ml in plasma [~3 pg/ml in saliva] are most common measures of DLMOff, and relative measures have also been used)

dim light melatonin onset (DLMO): a marker of endogenous circadian phase defined as the time when melatonin levels are consistently above daytime levels; dim light refers to the requirement to assess melatonin levels in low-light levels since room light or brigher can mask or acutely suppress melatonin levels (a threshold of 10 pg/ml in plasma [~3 pg/ml in saliva] is the most common measure of DLMO; other DLMO measures take into account large individual differences in melatonin amplitude and use a relative measure for DLMO, eg, 25% of the fitted peak to trough amplitude referred to as $DLMO_{25\%}$; on average, DLMO occurs ~2 hours prior to habitual bedtime in healthy subjects sleeping at night)

diurnal: day-related, eg, diurnal vs. nocturnal activity pattern

diurnal rhythm: term used to describe an observed daily rhythm with an unknown mechanism (a diurnal rhythm may be driven by eviromental factors, eg, light–dark; sleep–wake state, eg, the evening increase in growth hormone is sleep dependent; or may be circadian-driven, eg, glucose use in the SCN); *see* constant routine and forced desynchrony for examples of experimental procedures that can be used to distinguish between environmental, sleep–wakefulness, and circadian rhythms

double plot: graph of daily parameters in which records from subsequent days are plotted next to and beneath another (the double plot improves illustration of changes in physiology and behavior that span over more than one day)

DSPS/DSPD: *see* delayed sleep phase disorder

entrainment: term used to describe the process by which environmental time cues, such as the light–dark cycle, produce stable timing of an internal circadian oscillator (entrainment occurs when the circadian system is aligned with the light–dark cycle so that the daily phase-shift [$\Delta\varphi$] is equal to the difference between the imposed cycle length, eg, T = 24 hours, and the intrinsic period of the circadian system [τ], T = τ - $\Delta\varphi$)

forced desynchrony: experimental protocol used mostly in human research to estimate circadian period as well as the independent contribution of circadian phase and sleep–wakefulness state on physiology and behavior (wakefulness and sleep in a forced desynchrony protocol are scheduled at day lengths [T-cycles] that are far from the circadian period of the internal clock and environmental conditions, eg, dim light, that are insufficient to entrain the circadian clock to the imposed day length; the forced period of the sleep–wakefulness cycle is chosen to be far from the circadian period of the internal clock, and the T-cycle is also not a harmonic of the clock period; common T-cycles for forced desynchrony protocols include 20, 28, and 42.85 hours)

free-running protocol: experimental protocol used to estimate circadian period in nonhumans and humans (nonhumans are studied under constant conditions of DD or LL; human subjects are permitted to self-select sleep and wakefulness times and exposure to associated light–dark cycles)

infradian: physiological or behavioral oscillation with a periodicity of longer than one day

irregular sleep wake disorder (ISWD/irregular sleep wake type): CRSD characterized by sleep times that occur in multiple, fragmented, and short episodes over the 24-hour day, suggesting a primary disruption of the circadian clock or its output rhythms

ISWD: *see* irregular sleep wake disorder

jet lag: temporary impairment of sleep and wakefulness, as well as other biological functions, associated with rapid eastward or westward travel across multiple time zones

LD cycle: light–dark cycle

lux: international system unit of illumination used to indicate the intensity of light as a function of the spectral characteristics of human visual photoreceptors (one lux is equal to the light exposure received when gazing at a standard candle that is one meter away from the eye; room light is typically around 200 lux, sunrise and sunset as well as commercially available light exposure devices are approximately 10,000 lux; a midday bright blue sky is approximately 100,000 lux)

masking: acute alteration in the timing and/or shape of a rhythm without persistent alteration of the circadian clock

melanopsin: photopigment in the vertebrate eye present in a subset of retinal ganglion cells that project directly to the SCN via the RHT; photoreceptor that contributes to circadian vision, however, rods and cones also have input into the SCN

melatonin: hormone produced predominantly by the pineal gland (melatonin synthesis and secretion is controlled by the SCN, and, therefore, melatonin is often used to indicate internal biological time)

mesor: value midway between the peak and trough of a fitted rhythm or time series

nadir: minimum/trough of a rhythm or time series; often the minimum of a fitted curve, rather than absolute minimum, of a physiological or behavioral rhythm

non-24–hour (non-24–hour type/free running disorder): CRSD that occurs when the internal circadian clock fails to maintain entrainment to the 24 hour day

non-photic: non-light (eg, non-light input into the circadian timekeeping system)

observed rhythm: physiological or behavioral oscillation influenced by extrinsic resetting stimuli acting on the circadian clock during the time of observation

pacemaker: cells that drive the period of other cells

PER: protein encoded by the per gene

per gene: period clock gene involved in the molecular feedback loops determining the circadian period

period: *see* circadian period

phase advance: shift in the timing of the circadian clock in that circadian phase is earlier on the subsequent day (eg, an eastward shift) denoted by a plus sign

phase angle (ψ): time within the circadian cycle relative to other events (biological or environmental) at which a circadian phase occurs (eg, the average timing of the DLMO with habitual sleep onset is ~2h)

phase delay: shift in timing of the circadian clock in that circadian phase is later on the subsequent day (eg, a westward shift) denoted by a negative sign

phase response curve: graph illustrating how the biological timing of light exposure determines the direction and magnitude of circadian phase resetting (phase advances are denoted by a plus sign, and phase delays are denoted by a negative sign)

phase shift: resetting of internal biological time

phase tolerance: apparent ability of some humans to be less impaired by wakefulness during the biological night and sleep during the biological day

photic: light (eg, light input into the circadian timekeeping system)

PRC: phase response curve

process C: term used in mathematical and theoretical models to represent the circadian system

process S: term used in mathematical and theoretical models to represent the sleep homeostatic system

retinal hypothalamic tract (RHT): monosynaptic pathway from retinal ganglion cells to the SCN

RHT: *see* retinal hypothalamic tract

SCN : *see* suprachiasmatic nucleus

shift work disorder: clinically meaningful impairment in wakefulness and/or sleep associated with required work schedules outside of the normal daytime hours (eg, night and early morning shifts)

sleep-dependent: change in physiology that is dependent upon sleep and not circadian timing

suprachiasmatic nucleus (SCN): intrinsic oscillator located in the hypothalamus that coordinates circadian rhythms in brain and peripheral tissues

tau: *see* circadian period

T-cycle: period of a time giver (eg, day length)

ultradian: physiological or behavioral oscillation with a periodicity of less than one day

watt: international system unit of power used to indicate the intensity of light in absolute energy units per meter squared

zeitgebers: inputs to circadian clocks that alter the timing of rhythmic biological ossilations

Index

Note: Page numbers of article titles are in **boldface** type.

A

Accidents, at work, effect of shift work disorder on, 263–264

Acetylcholine, in circadian rhythms, 100–105

Acrophase, definition of, 301

Actigraphy, as clinical tool for circadian disruption in psychiatric disorders, 274–275
  caveats in, 275
  definition of, 301

Actogram, definition of, 301
  in irregular sleep wake rhythm disorder, 213–214

Advance-related sleep complaints, **219–227**

Advanced sleep phase disorder, **219–227**
  definition, 310
  definition of, 301
  diagnosis and assessment, 220–222
  epidemiology, 219–220
  potential mechanisms, 222–223
    familial, 222–223
  treatments, 223–225
    behavioral, 225
    chronotherapy, 225
    hypnotics, 225
    light and darkness exposure, 224
    longitudinal care, 225
    oral melatonin, 224–225
    phototherapy, 223–224
    stimulants, 225

Agomelatine, 186–187

Alzheimer's disease, circadian rhythm and severity of, 151–152
  irregular sleep wake rhythm disorder in, 213
  patterns of rest-activity cycles in, 280

Anatomy, of circadian system, 129–132, 166
  integration of circadian regulation, 130–132
  suprachiasmatic nucleus, 129

Angiotensin-converting enzyme inhibitors, in chronotherapy for cardiovascular disorders, 147

Animal models, physiologic and health consequences of circadian disruption, **127–142**
  anatomic organization, 129–132
  behavioral phase shift and reversal, 132
  circadian regulation and energy metabolism, 136–137
  circadian synchronization, 127–128
  clock genes, 132–135

effects of shift work desynchronization, 128
perspective and summary, 138
regulation of sleep-wake homeostasis, 135–136
research approaches, 128–129

Aspirin, in chronotherapy for cardiovascular disorders, 147

Asthma, circadian rhythm and severity of, 147–150
  chronotherapy for, 149–150
  day-night rhythm and, 147–148
  versus behavioral influences on pulmonary function and severity of, 148–149

B

Behavioral phase shift, in animal models of circadian desynchronization, 132

Behavioral strategies, for delayed sleep phase disorder, 235–236

Behavioral treatment, for advanced sleep phase disorder, 225

Beta-adrenoreceptor antagonists, in chronotherapy for cardiovascular disorders, 146–147

Bio-psycho-social-environmental model, of seasonal affective disorder, **285–299**

Biological clock, definition of, 301

Biological timekeeping. *See* Circadian rhythms.

Bipolar manic-depressive illness, patterns of rest-activity cycles in, 276–277

Blind patients, non-24 hour sleep-wake syndrome in, **195–211**

Borderline personality disorder, patterns of rest-activity cycles in, 279–280

Bright-light therapy, morning, for delayed sleep phase disorder, 232–234
  to minimize or avoid jet lag, 247–234

C

Caffeine, as countermeasure for shift work sleep disorder, 265

Calcium channel blockers, in chronotherapy for cardiovascular disorders, 146

Cancer, circadian rhythm and severity of, 150

Cardiovascular disease, influence of circadian system on severity of, 143–147

Sleep Med Clin 4 (2009) 305–311
doi:10.1016/S1556-407X(09)00063-0